CORRECTIONAL PSYCHIATRY

CRITICAL ISSUES IN AMERICAN PSYCHIATRY AND THE LAW

was edited for

THE AMERICAN ACADEMY OF PSYCHIATRY AND THE LAW (TRI-STATE CHAPTER)

Volume 1 Edited by Richard Rosner, M.D.

Volume 2 Edited by Richard Rosner, M.D.

Volume 3 GERIATRIC PSYCHIATRY AND THE LAW
Edited by Richard Rosner, M.D., and Harold I. Schwartz, M.D.

Volume 4 JUVENILE PSYCHIATRY AND THE LAW
Edited by Richard Rosner, M.D., and Harold I. Schwartz, M.D.

Volume 5 CRIMINAL COURT CONSULTATION
Edited by Richard Rosner, M.D., and Ronnie B. Harmon, M.A.

Volume 6 CORRECTIONAL PSYCHIATRY
Edited by Richard Rosner, M.D., and Ronnie B. Harmon, M.A.

A Continuation Order Plan is available for this series. A continuation order will bring delivery of each new volume immediately upon publication. Volumes are billed only upon actual shipment. For further information please contact the publisher.

CORRECTIONAL PSYCHIATRY

Edited by

RICHARD ROSNER, M.D.

Clinical Professor, Department of Psychiatry,
New York University School of Medicine
Diplomate, American Board of Forensic Psychiatry
and Medical Director, Forensic Psychiatry Clinic for the New York Criminal
and Supreme Courts (First Judicial Department)
Department of Mental Health, Mental Retardation,
and Alcoholism Services of the City of New York
New York, New York

and

RONNIE B. HARMON, M.A.

Administrative Director, Forensic Psychiatry Clinic for the
New York Criminal and Supreme Courts (First Judicial Department)
Department of Mental Health, Mental Retardation,
and Alcoholism Services of the City of New York
New York, New York

PLENUM PRESS • NEW YORK AND LONDON

Library of Congress Catalog Card Number 88-657025
ISBN 0-306-43070-3

A Division of Plenum Publishing Corporation
233 Spring Street, New York, N.Y. 10013

Printed in the United States of America

To our parents,

Henry J. and Rose L. Rosner

and

Chester and Zelda Harmon

Contributors

Jane A. Barker • Mental Health Services, Victim Services Agency, New York, New York
Michael H. Bell • Department of Psychiatry and Mental Health Services, University of Medicine and Dentistry of New Jersey, Newark, New Jersey
Harvey Bluestone • Department of Psychiatry, Albert Einstein College of Medicine, Yeshiva University, Bronx, New York; Department of Psychiatry, Bronx-Lebanon Hospital Center, Bronx, New York
Christina B. Casals-Ariet • Department of Psychiatry, Albert Einstein College of Medicine, Bronx, New York
Thomas A. Coughlin III • New York State Department of Correctional Services, Albany, New York
Judith F. Cox • Bureau of Forensic Services, N.Y. State Office of Mental Hygiene, Albany, New York
Bruce L. Danto • Patton State Hospital, Patton, California
Nancy N. Dubler • Department of Social Medicine, Montefiore Medical Center, Bronx, New York
Thomas A. Johnson • Criminal Justice Division, California State University, Sacramento, California
Jay E. Kantor • Department of Philosophy, New York University, College of Arts and Sciences, New York, New York
Michael Kaye • Forensic Center, Mendota Mental Health Institute, Madison, Wisconsin
Sara L. Kellermann • New York City Department of Mental Health, Mental Retardation and Alcoholism Services, New York, New York
Gerald Landsberg • New York City Department of Mental Health, Mental Retardation and Alcoholism Services, New York, New York
Gary J. Maier • Forensic Center, Mendota Mental Health Institute, Madison, Wisconsin; Department of Psychiatry, University of Wisconsin-Madison, Madison, Wisconsin

Dennis W. McCarty • State Law Enforcement Accreditation Program, N.Y. State Division of Criminal Justice, Albany, New York

Robert D. Miller • Forensic Center, Mendota Mental Health Institute, Madison, Wisconsin; Department of Psychiatry and School of Law, University of Wisconsin-Madison, Madison, Wisconsin; Department of Psychiatry, Medical College of Wisconsin, Milwaukee, Wisconsin

Barbara Morrow • Forensic Center, Mendota Mental Health Institute, Madison, Wisconsin

William S. Packard • Mental Health Unit, Suffolk County Correctional Facility, Riverhead, New York

M. Peter Paravati • Medical Review Board, New York State Commission of Correction, Albany, New York

Jacques M. Quen • Department of Psychiatry, Cornell University School of Medicine, New York, New York

Susan O. Reed • Department of Public Affairs, Criminal Justice Program, University of Wisconsin-Oshkosh, Oshkosh, Wisconsin

Marjorie A. Rock • New York City Department of Mental Health, Mental Retardation and Alcoholism Services, New York, New York

Sheldon Travin • Department of Psychiatry, Bronx-Lebanon Hospital Center, Bronx, New York; Department of Psychiatry, Albert Einstein College of Medicine, Bronx, New York

Robert Weinstock • Department of Psychiatry, University of California, Los Angeles, California

Margaret D. Wishart • Montefiore Medical Center, Bronx, New York; Rikers Island Health Services, East Elmhurst, New York

Foreword

Ralph Slovenko, commenting on the spate of malpractice lawsuits, has said, "Malpractice actions may be unjust and harrassing, yet they can also be a powerful outside force for critical and responsible self-examination and surveillance." However one may argue with that position or complain that we have come to a point where the disadvantages to society far exceed the purported benefits, it cannot be gainsaid that successful lawsuits against local, state, and federal corrections departments have not only ushered in an era of critical and responsible self-examination and surveillance, but have opened new vistas for the establishment and modernization of health and mental health services in jails and prisons in the United States. Recent experience in many states has shown that corrections administrators are, on their own initiative, albeit frequently in response to court orders, taking steps to bring their medical programs into conformity with standards promulgated by one or another nongovernmental national organization; for example, the American Medical Association, the American Public Health Association, the National Commission on Correctional Health Care, and the American Correctional Association. The time is ripe for psychiatric organizations to develop a consensus as to how best to allocate manpower and provide first-class mental health services for corrections.

Our credibility would be much enhanced if we were to come to rationality in our approach to the insanity defense. Why is clarification and resolution of this matter important? Simply put, although the vast majority of criminal offenders do not invoke the insanity plea, the consequences of the cases in which the plea is raised, whether successful or unsuccessful, have a devastating impact on society's willingness to provide funds for mental health services in corrections. There is no doubt that the insanity defense fosters the illusion that all convicted inmates are "sane" and treatment services are warranted only for supposedly nonblameworthy and deserving "insane" acquittees.

This volume provides us with a wide array of topics covering areas of interest to the mental health professional working in corrections. Although a touch of pessimism and skepticism will, from time to time, be noted, based on the authors' experiences under past and even current conditions, the reader will be heartened that problems have been clearly delineated and that there is reason to hope that solutions can be worked out—as they must—by legislators, administrators, and mental health professionals. Contrary to the pronouncements of the doomsayers, deterrence, retribution, and confinement are not irreconcilable with treatment and rehabilitation. What is needed is that people of good will address the problems, so well spelled out in this book, with Weinstock's Law as a starting point: "The difficult is not the impossible."

Abraham L. Halpern, M.D.
Department of Psychiatry
United Hospital Medical Center
Port Chester, New York

Introduction

Correctional Psychiatry is an outgrowth of a project that began at the February 1984 meeting of the American Academy of Forensic Sciences, which created a Joint Committee of the Psychiatry and General Sections on Mental Health Services to Correctional Facilities. The initial fruit of that project was a collection of papers, *Mental Health Services to Correctional Facilities Report,* that appeared in the *Journal of Forensic Sciences,* Volume 32, Number 1, January 1987. Revisions of some of the papers in that collection appear in this book. The scope of the present volume is broader and the issues are considered in greater depth and detail here than was possible in the earlier work.

There is a fundamental difference between the ends of clinical psychiatry, which are therapeutic, and the ends of the correctional system, which include specific deterrence, general deterrence, incapacitation, retribution, and reformation. Only the last of those correction system goals has traditionally been regarded as related to the therapeutic goal of clinical psychiatry. Thus, for many psychiatric clinicians, working in the field of correctional psychiatry has been viewed as compromising their professional commitment. There are serious ethical concerns regarding whether or not a physician can ever participate in nontherapeutic activities. There are some individuals who maintain that the Hippocratic oath and its equivalents (e.g., the oath of Maimonides, the ethical prescriptions of the American Medical Association, or of the American Psychiatric Association, or of the American Academy of Psychiatry and the Law) place an indelible mark on the soul, so that one is forever and in all instances bound to adhere to them. Such persons would suggest that a doctor is always obliged to function in a therapeutic role. For such people, the very concept of forensic psychiatry is an oxymoron. It is a thesis of this book that such a viewpoint is erroneous.

The therapeutic work of clinical psychiatry can and should be pursued within the correctional system. A mentally disordered inmate of a correctional system is as worthy of the therapeutic concern of psychiatrists as is a mentally disordered person anywhere else. To abandon correctional inmates to inadequate mental health services, on the grounds that a correctional setting is intrinsically antitherapeutic, is inconsistent with the physician's ethical commitment to provide services to those in need. It is tantamount to refusing to provide the Armed Forces with mental health services in wartime, on the grounds that military service is antitherapeutic.

Much of the difficulty in functioning as a psychiatrist in a correctional setting derives from a confusion between clinical psychiatry, which is directed to therapeutic ends, and forensic psychiatry, which is directed to legal ends. The correctional system may reasonably expect the doctor to act in a therapeutic capacity as one part of his work and to function in a nontherapeutic capacity as another part of his work. For example, the psychiatrist may treat an inmate with antidepressant medications (functioning in a therapeutic role) and may also provide input into a review of whether or not an inmate should be granted parole status (functioning in a forensic role).

In general, it would be preferable if correctional systems hired different doctors to do different categories of work. Failing that option, it falls upon the individual physician to keep clear in his or her own mind that he or she is working in two separate roles within one job. The concept of one person having more than one role should not be incomprehensible. One can be a physician, a spouse, an employer of some persons, an employee of other persons, a child of parents, and a parent of children; a different set of rights and responsibilities is applicable in each distinct role. Analogously, a different set of rights and responsibilities is applicable in the clinical psychiatric role than in the forensic psychiatric role.

The forensic psychiatrist does not have a doctor–patient relationship with the person being examined. The person being examined must be informed about this fact, often repeatedly, so as to insure as best as possible that the forensic psychiatrist is not inadvertently misconstrued as being a clinical psychiatrist. When one and the same doctor is obliged, by the nature of the job, to function sometimes as a forensic psychiatrist and sometimes as a clinical psychiatrist, the doctor must make sure that each role is clear to the person being examined.

Whereas the clinical psychiatrist has the therapeutic interests of his patient as the focus of concern, the forensic psychiatrist has the interests of the legal system as the focus of concern. The forensic specialist may be reporting to an attorney (defense or prosecution), a judge, a probation officer, a parole officer, or an administrator. To the extent that a clinical psychiatrist is devoted to health, a forensic psychiatrist is devoted to justice. Because the ends of health are not always identical with the ends of justice, the forensic psychiatrist may be called on to apply his knowledge and skills in endeavors contrary to the interests of the specific person being examined.

The actual practice of forensic psychiatry can be understood as being based on a four-step analysis of psychiatric-legal problems:

1. What is the psychiatric-legal issue?
2. What are the legal criteria that determine the issue?
3. What are the relevant clinical data?
4. What is the reasoning process by means of which the expert opinion has been formed?

Using this method, one psychiatric-legal issue might be the competence of an inmate in a correctional facility to refuse psychiatric treatment. The criteria would be set forth in the applicable mental health laws of the local, state, or federal government. The relevant clinical data are those related to evidence that the inmate has a diagnosable mental disorder of the required severity to qualify as a legally recognized "mental illness," and those related to evidence that the inmate meets the criteria for incompetence to refuse treatment as set forth in law. The reasoning process is the explication in specific language, so as to make the matters comprehensible to the court, of how the clinical data, when applied to the legal criteria, resolve the issue.

In some instances, it may be difficult initially to identify the legal issue to be addressed. A doctor working in the correctional system may feel that his job is purely clinical, rather than forensic; he is there is examine and treat patients who just happen to be in a jail or prison. That viewpoint, however ignores the fact that the doctor is there because of a legal requirement; namely, the government's obligation to care for those individuals whose deprivation of liberty prevents them from caring for themselves. If the same person whom the doctor is asked to treat in a correctional setting were free in the community, the government would not have the same affirmative obligation to evaluate his need for health services and provide such services as are indicated. In this unique clinical context, the provision of therapeutic services may be regarded as a forensic work product in the manner that the provision of a psychiatric-legal opinion is a forensic work product in a consultative context.

The forensic administrator has a somewhat different problem. Increasingly, jail and prison systems are coming under legislative, administrative, and judicial scrutiny, and the provision of medical and mental health services has become a politically important issue.

The range of psychiatric-legal issues has been expanding with the growth of regulation of correctional systems in the form of statutes, case law, and administrative directives. The system is no longer a world unto itself. Rather, concepts that have been spawned in other settings are now relevant to the correctional system. The right to treatment, the right to refuse treatment, and due process protections (notice of hearings, confrontation of one's accusers, representation by counsel), for example, have been recognized as relevant to correctional settings. In order to function effectively, it has become necessary for correctional administrators to become knowledgeable in these basic principles of mental health law.

Practical problems for the administrator include the legal and public relations consequences of suicidal, homicidal, and assaultive behaviors in prison, the determination of whether a given prisoner is competent to be executed, and the management of offenders with disruptive personality disorders.

The administrator of a jail or prison must be prepared to work with mental health professionals in the design and implementation of a plan for the delivery of mental health services. Such a plan must frequently be written under the watchful eye of judges or legislators who have mandated its structure and goals. Whether a mental health service system should be run by the correctional agency itself, by a public mental health agency, or by a private service provider is a choice that has administrative and fiscal consequences that cannot be ignored. Whether the mental health services in the correctional setting are adequate and conform to legal requirements may be evaluated by funding sources, by outside accrediting agencies, by inmates' attorneys, and by news media. The correctional mental health system is being subjected to more intrusive inspection than ever before, even as many argue that it is in need of yet greater scrutiny.

Although the reader might benefit from an acquaintance with the contents of the prior volumes in this series, nonetheless, this volume was designed to be freestanding. *Correctional Psychiatry* does not pretend to be a comprehensive review of all facets of the field, nor does it pretend that the chapters in this volume represent professional consensus. Rather, we have addressed selected issues that we believe are among the most important that merit consideration and we have asked each author to present a particular viewpoint vigorously and cogently. Each of the essays is designed to be read as an independent unit, with the result that there is some overlap in the contents of the various chapters. It is our belief that such intentional redundancy is an appropriate educational tool, designed to reenforce those matters that are fundamental to the field. Our goal in this volume, as in all other volumes of *Critical Issues in*

American Psychiatry and the Law, is to stimulate constructive encounters between the ideas of the authors and the mind of the reader.

RICHARD ROSNER
RONNIE B. HARMON

Contents

SECTION IV. SERVICE DELIVERY SYSTEMS

I

Perspectives: Past and Present

1

Insane Criminals and the Criminally Insane

A Persistent Problem for Psychiatry, Law, and Society

JACQUES M. QUEN

INTRODUCTION

This chapter will review the categories of the insane criminal and the criminally insane, the import of that distinction, and the substantial difficulties that efforts to distinguish between these two groups have posed for psychiatry, law, and society.

The insane criminal is an individual who has become insane after committing a crime, or whose insanity is not sufficiently integral to the offense to hold him nonresponsible. Most often these are people who have become insane after sentencing and imprisonment.

The second category, the criminally insane, refers to those mentally ill whom society recognizes as afflicted with an insanity that imposes criminal behavior. These are people who commit an act that may be criminal but which the law and society (as represented by the jury) decide is not a crime because it was imposed by a disease and, therefore, did not fit the definition of the crime. The criminally insane are those who are tried and acquitted because of their insanity (not guilty by reason of insanity or NGRI), or whose insanity is recognized by the prosecuting attorney and the judge. These officials use their discretionary powers and do not bring these individuals to criminal trial but arrive

JACQUES M. QUEN • Department of Psychiatry, Cornell University School of Medicine, New York, NY 10021.

at a disposition through civil law channels. These people are not criminals, nor have they committed a crime. They have, however, committed an antisocial act that threatens the community and, thus, invoked its police powers.*

PROBLEM

The immediate problem for society, in the distinction between the insane criminal and the criminally insane, lies in determining the role of the insanity in the specific offense and, thus, deciding the proper societal response, as well as the culpability or nonculpability of the offender. The law holds as nonculpable, those who do not have "an understanding will" regarding the offense in question. Consequently, children, idiots, and the insane (among others) must be evaluated for that understanding will to determine their culpability or nonculpability in individual offenses.† It is this principle that includes all those who may have been coerced, physically, verbally, or otherwise, to act in a criminal way.

The insane criminal is the criminal, convicted of a crime, who has subsequently become insane. There are various purposes and definitions of the criminal law that must be considered when deciding whether or not they should be applied to a particular incident and response by the government. These purposes, at various times, have been described as punitive, rehabilitative, protective (of society), and deterrent (i.e., the punishment meted out and publicized will serve as a deterrent for those who might consider committing a similar crime).

The criminally insane individual has *not* committed the alleged crime, as defined by law, and has been judged to have been, at the time of the offense, lacking the state of mind necessary to meet the definition of the crime charged. Such a person is entitled to the *parens patriae* (parental) protections of the state for all who are not competent to look after themselves.‡ Having committed no crime, the criminal law is, or

*"[T]he exercise of the sovereign right of a government to promote order, safety, health, morals and general welfare [is] within constitutional limits and [is] an essential attribute of government" (Black's *Law Dictionary,* p 1041). Today many would maintain that this is a governmental obligation rather than a right.

†Exception is made for children under the age of seven, for whom the Anglo-American common law provides blanket immunity from the consequences of their actions.

‡"A concept of standing utilized to protect those quasi-sovereign interests such as health, comfort and welfare of the people." *Parens patriae* originates from the English common law where the King had a royal prerogative to act as guardian to persons with legal disabilities, such as infants, idiots, and lunatics. In the United States, the *parens patriae* function belongs with the states." Today, many would consider this an obligation of the state, rather than a "prerogative" (Black's *Law Dictionary*, p 1003).

should be, irrelevant to that individual's case and disposition. The parental functions of the state include the care of and treatment for the incompetent individual and his disabling disorder. However, equally significant is the fact of the antisocial act that, simultaneously, invokes the police power of the state.

Legal scholars, for purposes of presentation and discussion, will often speak of these two powers, or roles, as if they operated in mutually exclusive isolation. In the case of the criminally insane, these powers function simultaneously and have concurrent roles to play. However, political purposes and rhetoric are often served by implying such a mutual exclusivity.

The superficial similarities between the insane criminal and the criminally insane frequently result in public misperceptions and misunderstandings. The treatment and improvement or cure of the illness will return the individual, presumably, to the status quo ante: for the insane criminal, to the status of an imprisoned convict, and for the criminally insane, to a noncriminal member of the community. It is here that the distinctions between these two groups are substantially important and speak to the values, standards, and understanding of the community. The confusion that currently exists regarding the meaning of these two terms is, perhaps, most clearly demonstrated by the publication and widespread acceptance of a major research study titled *Careers of the Criminally Insane,* which dealt exclusively with *insane criminals;* not the criminally insane.[1]

One way in which the law determines the criminal culpability of an individual is by means of a criminal trial and the insanity defense. This defense usually acknowledges that an act, in the generally accepted meaning of the word, not in the legal sense, was committed by an individual, not as an expression of will but because of a mental disability.† Although few people question this principle in regard to a five- or six-year-old child, the media and the public are frequently led to an emotional challenge of this same principle when applied to unknown adults. It is not unusual to find that an unknown individual who commits bizarre or apparently senseless violence is referred to as "crazy," "mad,"

**Act* the legal definition of the word occupies almost a full column in Black's *Law Dictionary.* Among other statements, it says, "denotes external mainfestations of an actor's will . . . expression of will or purpose . . . In its most general sense, this noun signifies something done voluntarily by a person: . . . an effect produced in the external world by an exercise of the power of a person objectively, prompted by intention, and proximately caused by a motion of the will. In a more technical sense, it means something done voluntarily by a person, and of such a nature that legal consequences attach to it" (p 24). The definition of *criminal act* includes "external manifestation of one's will which is prerequisite to criminal responsibility" (p 24).

or "insane," but when that person is apprehended, he is attacked by the media who suppose that he will offer an insanity defense. One example of this was seen in the case of the "Son of Sam" killings that were committed by David Berkowitz, who, eventually, chose not to use an insanity defense.

It is not within the scope of this chapter to consider the evolution and jurisprudential philosophy underlying the necessity for an "insanity defense," or some equivalent yardstick for "blameworthiness," to be included in a legal system, but the reader may refer to an earlier publication.[2]

COLONIAL TREATMENT OF THE INSANE

Despite the generally accepted belief that the insane usually were treated in casually, if not viciously, cruel and uncaring ways by the American colonists, careful review of the evidence reveals that this is, at best, only a partial truth. Historians have generally ignored the importance, for the colonial and early American communities, of the distinctions between "kinfolk/neighbor" insane and the "stranger/foreign" insane. The bulk of the evidence supports the interpretation that the colonists, Puritan and otherwise, treated their "kinfolk/neighbor" insane with consideration and sympathy, frequently making significant sacrifices for their care.[3,4,5] They were not at all niggardly in their willingness to help each other in time of need.

What has been overlooked in the historical studies of this period, epitomized, perhaps, by the work of Albert Deutsch,[6] was that life was harsh for everybody in that period. The treatment of their "kinfolk/neighbor" insane did not represent a punitive rejection, nor did it embody a lack of awareness of the natural illness or disability of their mentally ill kinfolk and neighbors. The colonists knew that, unless they were prepared to help each other, there would be no survival for any of them.

Deutsch noted and then appeared to lose sight of the fact that:

> The settlements were . . . populated for the most part by an impecunious people who lived on the ragged edge of existence, engaged in constant struggle to wrench a bare living from the soil.[6 (p 39)]

It was that situation which fostered mutual reliance and reciprocal support for each other within the community. When a neighbor needed help, whether to build a barn or a house, or to take care of a sick family member, to fight a fire, or to cope with some other catastrophe, the members of the community responded with the support that they knew they themselves would want and should be able to expect in like circumstances. That such community caring and involvement in the plight of kin and neighbors was not restricted to any discrete time in history is documented by Roth and Kroll in their discussion of the community response to the insane in medieval times.[7]

In a history of the Eastern State Hospital in Williamsburg, Virginia, one historian said of a local 1760s newspaper:

> Unlike the popular American press a half century later, the *Gazette* refrained from describing the insane murderers as beasts or inhuman creatures upon whom society must revenge itself. It reported dramatic cases in a calm, factual manner. For example: A planter who "we hear, has for some Time been disordered in his Mind . . . this Day [after killing his overseer] delivered himself up to Justice, and is now in the publick Jail." A report of a "Melancholy Accident" relates that a wife "long disordered in her senses" struck her husband in the head with an axe and killed him. Another edition of the *Gazette* calls this "a most shocking murder" and describes how the wife broke her husband's skull to pieces by repeated strokes but seemed "quite insensible of the horridness of the crime she [had] committed."[5 (p 9)]

What appears to have happened is that, as the population increased and the number of stranger/foreign people increased, the lack of concern for the impecunious or sick stranger, who might drain the community's carefully husbanded resources, increased to a near-xenophobic mistrust. A stranger who called for help was a threat. As the communities grew larger, the capacity of its members to expand (numerically) the category of kinfolk/neighbor reached a (biologically?) determined limit on the size of the kinfolk/neighbor group. It is striking to observe that, in times of national or widely publicized crises, the response suggests that all Americans (or other nations for that matter) care deeply for each other, but in communities beyond a critical size, there seems to be almost no sense of a special connection, relatedness, or obligation to help the unknown or barely known neighbor.

EARLY HOSPITALS, ASYLUMS, AND THE ASYLUM MOVEMENT

As early as 1752, the people of Pennsylvania, with a statement written by Benjamin Franklin, petitioned their legislature to charter a private hospital financed by donations that would, among other goals, offer protection and treatment to the insane:

> That some of [the insane] going at large are a Terror to their Neighbours, who are daily apprehensive of the Violences they may commit; and others are continually wasting their Substance, to the great detriment of themselves and Families, ill disposed persons wickedly taking Advantage of their unhappy Condition, and drawing them into unreasonable Bargains, &c.[8]

The statement makes clear that there was, simultaneously, concern for the insane as victims of social predators as well as concern for the substantial violent damage they might do, to person or property or both.

In 1766, Governor Fauquier of the Province of Virginia called upon the House of Burgesses to establish a hospital for the insane. In 1773, the first public hospital devoted solely to the treatment of the insane in the British colonies opened in Williamsburg.[5(pp 6–8)] Thus began the insane asylum movement in America, and with it, the development of psychiatry.

ASSOCIATION OF MEDICAL SUPERINTENDENTS OF AMERICAN INSTITUTIONS FOR THE INSANE

Despite a slow beginning, the asylum movement gained increased momentum with the opening of the Friends' Asylum in 1817, the McLean Hospital in 1818, the New York Hospital's Bloomingdale in 1822, and the Hartford Retreat in 1824. The Retreat owed its existence directly to the Connecticut Medical Society's lobbying and fund-raising efforts. It was they who first proposed the blending of the best of moral treatment (i.e., psychological treatment) with the best of medicinal treatment.[9] It was from that time through the first half of the twentieth century that institutional care of the insane was universally recognized as requiring medical supervision.[10]

In 1844, thirteen asylum superintendents met in Philadelphia to form the Association of Medical Superintendents of American Institutions for the Insane (AMSAII), in order to educate and assist each other with their common problems. That was the beginning of the oldest medical specialty organization in America, the American Psychiatric Association. Almost all the institutions represented by the founders were supported, at least in part, by public donations or state money or both. It is important to remember that psychiatry is a medical specialty born out of service to the community at large, made possible by public, municipal, or state funding, or some combination of these, rather than the usual fee for service to individuals. It was community support that made psychiatry an economically feasible and viable medical service to the American insane.

The asylum movement in the middle third of the 19th century owed its growth to the inspiration, the efforts, and the remarkably dedicated perseverance of one individual above all others, Dorothea L. Dix.[11] She can be credited with being responsible for the establishment of most of the state psychiatric hospitals in America at that time, as well as the founding of some in Europe. She did this as a private citizen, without any formal group or organization. In 1845, she published a booklet, *Remarks on Prison and Prison Discipline in the United States,* another interest of hers which played a crucial role in arousing her determination to help the insane.[12]

ASYLUMS AND PRISONS

Shortly before the founding of the AMSAII, the year 1844 saw the first issue of the *American Journal of Insanity (AJI),* which is the oldest medical specialty journal in America. In 1922, it became the *American Journal of Psychiatry,* to conform to the organization's new name. Amariah Brigham, one of the "original thirteen" founders of the American Psychiatric Association and the first Superintendent of the New York State Lunatic Hospital in Utica, was also the first editor of that journal.[13] The following year, the Philadelphia Prison Society, founded in 1787 by Benjamin Rush, published the first issue of *The Pennsylvania Journal of Prison Discipline and Philanthropy.* One third to one half of its pages were devoted to the condition of the insane.

In a brief review, Brigham attacked that journal as well as the annual reports of the Boston Prison Discipline Society, for the space and prominence they gave to insane asylum statistics and conditions.[14] The linking of the insane and their asylums with the criminal and his prisons was considered to be a disservice to the insane. There was a restrained but strong response in the next issue of the *Prison Journal*[15] and an editorial reply of some length in a later issue of the *AJI.*[16] Although Brigham protested this misleading and damaging association between depraved criminals and the insane, he overlooked the fact that, at the first meeting of the AMSAII, one of the several committees formed was on the insane prisoner, and he was one of its three members.[17] Tension persisted between these human betterment groups, although they clearly had overlapping and parallel interests. This is underscored by the prominence of Dorthea L. Dix and Samuel Gridley Howe in the asylum movement, while they were active in prison reform.

These two movements, developing concurrently, appear to have been fueled by congruent social concerns and moral obligations to look after one's less fortunate fellow humans. Those early psychiatrists were facing the same problem that later physicians, treating tuberculosis and cancer faced; that is, the role played by social stigma in the public's reluctance to seek treatment early, when the best results appeared to be most attainable. But with the shame of insanity coupled to that of criminality, the difficulty of their mission must have seemed, to the early American psychiatrists, frustratingly compounded. For the founders of the AMSAII, it was perceived as vitally important to remove the association between insanity and depravity (criminality) in the public mind. It appears likely that this concern did not originate with them.

Although many writers, including Albert Deutsch, have pointed to the occasional confinement of the 18th-century colonial and 19th-century American insane in jail cells, as proof of an attitude of "punishment, repression, and indifference" toward the mentally diseased, careful examination of historical records refutes this misunderstanding of the actual situation.* Despite the abuses, concern for the sensibilities of the insane and their families was reflected in state statutes and municipal laws and court decisions.

In 1827, long before the founding of the AMSAII, the New York State Legislature passed a statute stating "that no lunatic or mad person, nor any person disordered in his or her senses, shall be confined in the same room with any person charged with or convicted of any criminal offense." The statute went on to define the offense as a misdemeanor, subject to a maximum fine of $250 and/or a year in jail.[18] In the early 19th century, $250 was a remarkably large sum of money, and, even more than now, one year was a long time out of one's life, especially for the middle-class civil servants at risk (i.e., overseers of the poor, constables, and keepers of gaols). Fourteen years later, in 1841, the annual salary of the Medicial Superintendent of the Maine Insane Asylum was about $800.

ISAAC RAY

The second volume of the *American Journal of Insanity* contained an extensive article by Isaac Ray, another founder of the AMSAII, a past superintendent of the Maine Insane Hospital (Augusta), "superintendent-elect" of the projected Butler Hospital, and the founder of American forensic psychiatry as a separate discipline, with its own perspective and its own body of knowledge and skills. As part of his preparation to superintend the yet-to-be-built Butler Hospital, Ray traveled to Great Britain and Europe, studying the facilities for the treatment of the insane, architectural and medical. His article described his observations and thoughts about the major hospitals for the insane in Great Britain, France, and Germany.[19]

Ray included a three-page section on "Criminal Lunatics." He de-

*Quen JM: Albert the Noorman: Colonial American attitudes toward their neighbor insane. Read at the annual meeting of the American Association for the History of Medicine, Philadelphia, PA, May 1, 1987.

fined the term as including "those insane persons who have committed criminal acts while insane, as well as those who have become so while suffering imprisonment for their crimes."[19 (p 383)] It was only later that the importance of distinguishing between those two recognized subgroups became apparent. He noted that their proper disposition was a cause of "no little embarrassment to many of our Superintendents." He may have been referring to the case of Abner Rogers, the insane convict who killed his warden and was acquitted on the ground of insanity.

Rogers, on acquittal, was transferred from prison to the Worcester State Hospital, which was under the superintendency of the man who was to become the first president of the AMSAII, Samuel B. Woodward. During the course of his first few months there, Rogers complained of the presence of corpses, odors, and people poisoning his food. One day, he made similar complaints in the chapel during a religious service. He asked to be taken out of the room. His attendants asked him to wait until the services were over. He suddenly got up and jumped through the second-floor window. He landed on the ground, 14 feet below, and died. Woodward apparently was criticized for everything from allowing an obviously sane convict to make an escape attempt to providing inadequate security for an agitated insane patient.

The problems raised by the experience with Rogers persisted. Ray clarified, in his *AJI* article, that part of the problem was that conditions necessary for the treatment of insane prisoners required security precautions that were inimical to the treatment program of the American psychiatrists. American asylum treatment included strolls in relaxing, peaceful, attractive surroundings, outside work in gardens, farming, freedom from stress, and a respectful, nonpunitive attitude on the part of staff. It also involved avoidance of staff behavior that would reinforce delusions that the individual was the prisoner of a malevolent group. The treatment of insane convicts would require a constant maximum security, a condition that created problems for the indicated treatment of the nonprisoner insane.

Ray went on to say that:

> In the disposal of this class of subjects, security is a prime consideration. Our insane hospitals are made strong enough to retain their inmates with the occasional exception of one of unusual perseverance and ingenuity. To make them so strong and adopt such a system of watching as to render the escape of such persons, impossible, would be to make them real prisons instead of hospitals for weak and disordered minds; in other words, to make them incompatible with the promotion of their rightful purposes which require that they should be as little like a prison, as is possible. [He observed that, if an asylum could be made that secure, that] it would be very doubtful, after all, whether we had done anything more than to convert a good hospital into a poor prison.[19 (pp 384–385)]

EDWARD JARVIS, INSANE TRANSGRESSORS, AND INSANE CONVICTS

A clear distinction was needed between "criminal lunatics" who were insane criminals and those noncriminals whose insanity drove them to criminal acts. In the first case, the insanity was relatively independent of the criminality, whereas in the latter case, the insanity was the direct or proximate cause of it. In the first case, cure would simply restore a criminal to his former dangerous depravity; in the second case, it would restore a respectable member to the community.

In an article published in the *AJI* in 1857, Edward Jarvis, a Massachusetts physician who was a statistician as well as the superintendent of a private asylum in his home, attempted to deal with the problem of the insane criminal and the criminally insane in a comprehensive and definitive way.[20] He suggested that the designations *insane transgressor* and *insane convict* be used to distinguish between these two groups.

Jarvis maintained that although both groups were entitled to appropriate and effective treatment to restore them to their senses, the two categories clearly required different treatment circumstances. The criminal, who, characteristically, had been convicted and subsequently became insane while imprisoned, required an asylum designed to prevent the escape with which "criminals were continually preoccupied," whereas the innocent individual, whose insanity imposed behavior that was criminal, was entitled to treatment in the usual civil hospital, unless the insanity made him far too violent or dangerous.

With remarkable sensitivity, Jarvis went on to say:

> But the insane criminal has nowhere any home; no age or nation has provided a place for him. He is everywhere unwelcome and objectionable. The prisons thrust him out; the hospitals are unwilling to receive him; the law will not let him stay at his house, and the public will not permit him to go abroad. And yet, humanity and justice, the sense of common danger, and a tender regard for a deeply degraded brother-man, all agree that something should be done for him—that some plan must be devised, different from, and better than any that has yet been tried, by which he may be properly cared for, by which his malady may be healed, and his criminal propensity overcome.[20] (p 196)

Jarvis contended that it would be best to provide treatment for the insane criminal *outside* the walls of a penitentiary, since it was quite likely that the criminal, too, needed to be removed from the environment in which he got ill. However, it certainly would require far more security than could be found in the usual civil asylum. Jarvis recognized that it would be too expensive for any one state to provide such an asylum. Consequently, he suggested that multistate districts be formed, one for the Northeast, including the New England states and New York, perhaps New Jersey and Pennsylvania as well. Another one for Delaware south to Florida, and so on. The states in each district would share the costs of building and maintaining such a prison-hospital for their insane convicts.

In the first half of the 19th century, insane prisoners were kept in their cells or were transferred to the state asylums. As Jarvis had observed, the asylums and their superintendents were unwilling to receive the insane convicts. The impropriety of mixing depraved insane criminals with the "innocent insane" was apparently unquestioned among those who were responsible for the asylum programs. This attitude persisted through the first half of the 20th century. Convict patients did impose new and complicated problems on the superintendents and the ward staff, as Isaac Ray had observed. Perhaps equally as important as a determinant of policy, this forced association of the noncriminal insane with the insane criminals might strengthen the lay public's rejection of the insane and their need for asylums. It would make families even more reluctant to send a relative to an asylum for timely effective treatment. It was feared that asylums could and would be destroyed by the withdrawal of public support.

That this was not peculiar to the American psychiatric establishment was quite clear. Jarvis reported that the Association of Superintendents of British Institutions for the Insane had unanimously petitioned their Parliament to relieve them of the burden of caring for the insane convicts and "to establish a central criminal lunatic asylum for all this class of patients." In 1844, the British government formed the British Commissioners in Lunacy, to insure adequate standards of care in the asylums. Jarvis noted that in eight of their first ten annual reports to the Parliament, they had urged this same measure.

Ireland, around 1847, established the Central Asylum at Dundrum, for the safe custody of insane persons charged with offenses. It was reported as having been "eminently successful, and as having realized the object for which it was originally experimentally intended." Its census was 126.[20]

In 1848, a statute was passed in New York (chapter 294), authorizing the prison inspector to investigate any allegedly insane prisoner, and, if satisfied that he was insane, to transfer him to the New York Lunatic Asylum at Utica, where a special ward was to be maintained for prisoners. At the expiration of the sentence, if the prisoner was still insane, the Superintendent of the Asylum could discharge him to the Superintendent of the Poor of the ex-convict's home county.

Ten years later, in 1858, the legislature recognized the inadequacy of the Utica asylum for the task and authorized the building of a state asylum at Auburn. Officially titled the State Lunatic Asylum for Insane Convicts, this facility had 64 single rooms for 64 prisoners[21] and operated in an overcrowded condition almost from the day of its opening in February, 1859. By 1869, subsequent statutes had added the "insane transgressor" as well as the insane convicts to their patient population. By 1874, its role had been expanded further to include the insane charged with arson, murder and attempted murder, and any misdemeanant determined to be insane. By 1884, its mission included civil insane patients who were considered to be too violent for the civil asylum.[21 (p 242)]

In 1855, the Connecticut State Medical Society, critical of the practice of sending insane convicts to the Hartford Retreat and the alternative of keeping them in prison cells, petitioned the state government to explore other solutions. The commission, created in response to this request, suggested the construction of a separate state hospital building on the grounds of the State Prison at Wethersfield. Although the building was completed, it was never used for its intended purpose but became a storehouse instead.[22]

In 1886, the New York State Legislature authorized the building of the Matteawan State Hospital in Fishkill. It was opened in 1892. Within seven years, the need for a larger capacity was apparent. The legislature voted for a new facility to be built outside the walls of the State Penitentiary at Dannemora, for male prisoners who were declared insane while in prison. By 1916, Matteawan, now restricted to female insane convicts and those insane charged with crimes but mentally incompetent to be tried, was again badly overcrowded.[21 (pp 241–245)]

Meanwhile, the Pennsylvania State Hospital Superintendent was having the same kind of difficulties that had plagued the Superintendent of the Utica Asylum. A law had been passed, in 1852, authorizing the transfer of insane prisoners to the State Hospital. In 1874, a modification of that law was before the Pennsylvania Legislature. This time the psychiatrists mounted a major attack against it, with T. S. Kirkbride, John H. Worthington, Isaac Ray, and other Pennsylvania psychiatrists, who petitioned for the establishment of a hospital either separate from the prisons or "in connection with the grounds of one or more of the State penitentiaries, and under the same government as those institutions." They concluded with the statement that all experienced psychiatrists would

> most earnestly protest against the inauguration of any system looking to a provision for insane criminals in any one of the existing State Hospitals, or upon any part of the grounds of these institutions as impolitic, unnecessary, and detrimental to the best interests of the insane.

They lost that battle, but won the war when Pennsylvania opened the Farview State Hospital for insane convicts on December 16, 1912.[21] (pp 500–503)

Ultimately, the distinction between the insane transgressor and the insane criminal is a societal one. It is an issue decided, not by physicians, but by society acting through its jury in the criminal law system. If the jury says that an individual is a criminal, he is: if they say he is to be held nonresponsible for his acts, that he is NGRI, then he is criminally insane. In his role as an expert witness, the psychiatrist has the obligation to assist the jury in arriving at their decision. A forensic psychiatrist can explore and bring to his testimony the multiple facts and interpretations involved in evaluating the extent and significance of the role of psychopathology in influencing or controlling behavior. The jury's decision determines whether that individual goes to jail as a convict (and is thereafter designated an ex-felon for legal purposes) or whether he goes to a hospital as a private citizen for treatment and care.

Few professionals would argue that an individual on high doses of cortisone may become irrational in behavior and yet should not be held liable for his actions at that time. The irrational and possibly dangerous behavior will stop when the effect of the steroid stops. Few would hold that person responsible for his actions when in that toxic state. Yet individuals with behavior imposed by functional mental illness are frequently prejudged and condemned, by the news media and the public, as criminals trying to escape their just deserts. It is particularly disturbing to find mental health professionals eager to arrive at a determination of "criminally insane" or "insane criminal" solely on the basis of abbreviated and frequently distorted news media reports. Nor is it helpful to anyone when psychiatrists subordinate their professional knowledge and skills to the hidden agenda of their political philosophy (right or left) and their *a priori* conviction that criminal offenders are all, *ipso facto,* mentally ill or that those who plead mental illness are all "faking."

The distinction between the criminally insane and the insane criminal is as important now as it was in Edward Jarvis' day. That distinction determines so much about the quality of the treatment that individual receives, that it calls for the exercise of maximum professional skill, caution, and care. The history of the societal responses to the task of distinguishing between insane criminals and the criminally insane does not reflect credit on psychiatry, law, or society. Perhaps medical schools and their departments of psychiatry can initiate a needed change by improving the quality of education of physicians and psychiatrists so that they can appreciate the difference between the insane criminal and the criminally insane, along with the importance of that difference.

REFERENCES

1. Steadman HJ, Cocozza JJ: *Careers of the Criminally Insane: Excessive Social Control of Deviance.* Lexington, Mass, Lexington Books, 1974.
2. Quen JM: Psychiatry and the law: Historical relevance to today, in Freedman LZ (ed): *By Reason of Insanity: Essays on Psychiatry and the Law.* Wilmington, Del, Scholarly Resources, 1983, pp 153–166.
3. Blackmon DME: The care of the mentally ill in America, 1604–1812, in the thirteen original colonies. *Fourth Nursing Research Conference,* 1968, pp 65–113.
4. Jiminez MA: *Changing Faces of Madness: Insanity in Massachusetts, 1700–1850,* dissertation. Brandeis University, Waltham, Mass, 1981.
5. Dain N: *Disordered Minds: The First Century of Eastern State Hospital in Williamsburg, Virginia: 1766–1868.* Williamsburg, Va, Colonial Williamsburg Foundation, 1971, p 9.
6. Deutsch A: *The Mentally Ill in America.* Garden City, NY, Doubleday Doran & Co Inc, 1937, p 39.
7 Roth M, Kroll J: *The Reality of Mental Illness.* London, Cambridge University Press, 1986, p 100.
8. [Franklin B]: *Some Account of the Pennsylvania Hospital; From its First Rise, to the Beginning of the Fifth Month, Called May, 1754.* Philadelphia, B. Franklin & D. Hall, 1754. Facsimile edition. Baltimore, Johns Hopkins Press, 1954, p 4.
9. Dain N: *Concepts of Insanity in the United States: 1789–1865.* New Brunswick, NJ, Rutgers University Press, 1964, p 22.
10. Grob GN: *Mental Institutions in America: Social Policy to 1875.* New York, Free Press, 1973.
11. Browne WJ: A psychiatric study of the life and work of Dorothea Dix. *Am J Psychiatry* 1969; 126:83–89.
12. Dix DL: *Remarks on Prison and Prison Discipline in the United States.* Boston, Monroe and Francis, 1845.
13. Carlson ET: Amariah Brigham, I: Life and works. *Am J Psychiatry* 1956; 112:831–836.
14. Brigham A (reviewer): book review. *Am J Insanity* 1844; 1:381–382.
15. "Journal of Prison Discipline" and lunatic asylums, editorial (unsigned). *Pennsylvania Journal of Prison Discipline and Philanthropy* 1846; 2:49–57.
16. [Brigham A]: "Journal of Prison Discipline" and lunatic asylums, editorial. *Am J Insanity* 1845; 2:175–183.
17. Report of Superintendents' meeting. *Am J Insanity* 1844; 1:251–258, 256.
18. 1827 N.Y. Laws (50th Session) chap. 294: An Act respecting Lunatics (Apr 16, 1827) pp 318–319.
19. Ray I: Observations on the principal hospitals for the insane in Great Britain, France, and Germany. *Am J Insanity* 1846; 2:289–390, 383–386, 383.
20. Jarvis ER: Criminal insane: Insane transgressors and insane convicts. *Am J Insanity* 1857; 13:195–231.
21. Hurd HM, Drewry, WF, Dewey, R, (eds): *The Institutional Care of the Insane in the United States and Canada,* 4 vols. Baltimore, Md, Johns Hopkins Press, 1916, vol 3, pp 241–242.
22. *Ibid.* vol. 2, p 73.

2

A National Perspective on Mental Health Services to Corrections

SHELDON TRAVIN

This chapter will describe some of the emerging trends and major issues related to providing mental health services to corrections. *Corrections* has been defined as that part of the criminal justice system comprised of "all agencies of social control which attempt to rehabilitate and neutralize deviant behavior of adult criminals and juvenile delinquents for the protection of society."[1(p 444)] Although the category of corrections includes such institutions as jails, prisons, and maximum-security hospitals as well as community-based programs, probation, and parole departments, this chapter will focus on the history and current relationship of mental health services to correctional institutions—jails and prisons—for adult males, because the major challenges these institutions pose to mental health workers are both representative and indicative of the issues involved in every attempt to provide mental health services within the corrections system.

The provision of psychiatric services to mentally disordered offenders has become an issue of increasing concern to mental health and correctional professionals. It is important to realize, however, that the term *mentally disordered offenders* (MDO) is used by the criminal justice system to designate individuals who are mentally ill and deviant, that is,

SHELDON TRAVIN • Department of Psychiatry, Bronx-Lebanon Hospital Center, Bronx, NY 10456, and Department of Psychiatry, Albert Einstein College of Medicine, Bronx, NY 10461.

those who have been formally judged, by the judicial system, both guilty of a crime and emotionally disturbed. The MDO category, therefore, does not include inmates who, though mentally ill, have never been formally categorized as mentally disturbed by the courts and have not been transferred from corrections to a hospital.[2] This chapter, therefore, will concentrate on adult criminals who require psychiatric services in correctional institutions, but who have not been formally identified as MDOs, although, as Halleck[2] points out, their psychiatric problems may be as severe as those of MDOs. Such inmates, Halleck notes, "are managed quite differently" than the MDOs within the correctional system; indeed, many of them may go either unnoticed, or untreated, or both, during their incarceration. Because they manifest both disturbed and disruptive behavior, they are certainly among the most undesired clients, which may contribute to a situation in which they frequently receive inadequate care in the mental health and in the correctional systems.[3]

Although estimates vary on the extent of mental illness among convicted offenders, the problem has been recognized as significant, and there is general agreement that the need for mental health services is considerable. Because of the recent emphasis on deinstitutionalization and the stricter criteria being used for admissions to mental hospitals, the number of mentally ill people who get channeled into the criminal justice system has increased.[4] Clearly, these individuals require psychiatric treatment. But the sheer size of our prison population provides perhaps a better idea of the need that exists within the correctional system for mental health services: it is estimated that 2% of all males aged twelve years and over are under some kind of correctional supervision,[5] and estimates of the total population of jails is around 256,615 people in 1985,[6] with an additional population in federal and state prisons of some 546,659 inmates in 1986.[7] Given these figures, the approximately 20,000 inmates, who are formally recognized as mentally disordered offenders per year (inmates, that is, who are institutionalized after being found not guilty by reason of insanity, incompetent to stand trial, or mentally disordered sex offenders, or who have been transferred from prison to a psychiatric hospital)[8] represent only a small proportion of all those individuals under correctional supervision who could benefit from mental health services.

In fact, the inmates themselves provided a major impetus to the improvement of mental health services to corrections through their involvement in the recent prisoners' rights movement, an impetus that was furthered by the courts' willingness to rule on the constitutionality of the prisoners' complaints, in particular, on such legal issues as the prisoners' rights to treatment, the requirement of procedural due process before the transfer of an inmate to a mental hospital, and the necessity of having adequate classification systems in correctional institutions. More recently, however, the federal courts seem to be returning to the traditional "hands-off" doctrine on prisoners' rights issues.[9]

Additional trends across the country that will affect the delivery of mental health services to inmates in the coming years include the discontinuation of many "sexually dangerous" offenders programs and the consequent committing of these offenders into corrections, the increasing implementation of determinate sentencing associated with the phasing out of parole board decisions (which were based on perceptions of the prisoner having been "rehabilitated") for releasing prisoners and the increasing pressure on the corrections system to privatize, that is, to allow private centers to administer certain correctional programs and even entire institutions. These developments have made more clear, and more urgent, the need to implement and maintain adequate standards of health care in corrections. A variety of national professional organizations have responded to this situation; they have promulgated standards of care and treatment and committed themselves to the thrust for correctional facilities to meet these standards and get accredited.

MENTAL ILLNESS IN JAILS AND PRISONS

Planning for mental health services in jails and prisons must take into account the true prevalence rates of mental illness among prisoners in these institutions. Regrettably, published data in this area have varied greatly. Certainly some of the differences evident in the published data are a result of the diverse definitions of mental disorders currently in use, and of the different methods employed in locating cases.[10] The reliability of the published data is further jeopardized by the fact that, although the prisoners who are mentally ill as well as being management problems may be recognized, some of the quietly psychotic prisoners may not be recognized as people suffering from mental illness.

In their monograph, *Developing Jail Mental Health Services: Practice and Principles,* Steadman *et al.*[11] report on the results of six studies that investigated true prevalence rates of mental illness among inmates in particular jail settings. These studies indicated that the true prevalence rates of psychoses in local jails ranges from 1% to 7%, and the prevalence rates of nonpsychotic forms of mental disorders to range as high as 20%.[12] These authors also cite Monahan and Steadman[13] who concluded, after studying the matter, that the true prevalence rate of psychosis among prisoners was not greater than that among class-matched populations in the community. But Steadman and his colleagues believe that, because of the deficiencies of mental health services in jail, this amount of mental illness among the inmates is quite significant. Moreover, as Roth[12] points out, a number of factors may cause the jail experience to be as stressful or even more stressful than prison, including the facts that many of the jail inmates have alcohol or drug problems, that there is an increasing tendency to jail the chronically mentally ill on minor charges, and that there is uncertainty among the jail inmates about their legal predicament.

In the *Sourcebook on the Mentally Disordered Prisoner,* McCarthy[14] reports on the results of a survey that elicited data on mentally ill and mentally retarded offenders in the state and the federal prison systems. The *Sourcebook* was intended to provide pertinent information in this area to the nation's correctional administrators. The survey instrument was a 31-question protocol mailed to the central administrative office of the Department of Corrections in each state, to the Federal Bureau of Prisons, and to the Washington (DC) Department of Corrections. No operational definition of either the term *mentally ill* or the term *mentally retarded* was provided. Some of the major findings of this survey were that, out of a combined total of approximately 400,000 inmates, 2,400 inmates or 6.0% were classified as mentally ill, 9,800 inmates or 2.5% were classified as mentally retarded, and 250 inmates were classified as both mentally ill and mentally retarded. Because most mentally ill inmates are not officially identified as such (that is, they are not officially identified and treated as MDOs), the *Sourcebook* recommends that vigorous efforts be made now to screen and identify them in order to initiate treatment. This screening and identifying process should consist of a review of records, observation by corrections staff, testing interviewing, and referral to mental health professionals for further evaluation as indicated.

In regard to the transfer of mentally ill patients to other agencies, some very interesting data were obtained. According to the responding corrections departments, only 1,019 inmates out of a total of 24,052 inmates classified as mentally ill were transferred out. The reported data revealed that 93.6% of the mentally ill were receiving psychiatric care within their own corrections institutions, but of this 93.6%, more than three-fourths were receiving outpatient psychiatric services and less than one fourth were receiving inpatient psychiatric services.

TRENDS OF REFORMS IN CORRECTIONS

The history of mental health services in the corrections system is inextricable from the history of prison reforms. A brief sketch of this history provides an essential context for any attempt to understand and improve mental health services in the corrections system.

In the introduction to his *Correctional Treatment,* Bartollas[15] places the development of correctional reforms in their historical context so as to reveal each stage of reform as an attempt to implement a new philosophy of treatment. Using Hirsch's comprehensive definition of the phrase "correctional treatment" as "any measure taken to change an offender's character, habits, or behavior patterns so as to dismiss his (or her) criminal propensities,"[16(p 11)] Bartollas explains that early American colonists believed in severe punishment, such as the stocks or gallows, partly because, given their belief in Calvin's stern doctrine of "the natural depravity of the human race," they could not believe that incarceration would be able to rehabilitate a criminal. Opened in 1790, the Walnut Street Jail was the first true correctional institution in the United States. The system of discipline it employed assumed that solitary confinement would enable the prisoner to reflect on, and repent, his crimes. This became known as the "Pennsylvania System," and incorporated many of Dr. Benjamin Rush's ideas about the purpose of punishment.[17] Similarly, Rothman[18] describes the "Penitentiary" stage as a product of the Jacksonian era's view of the origins of crime as attributable to the environment rather than the individual—a view which was prevalent in the early 19th century. The design of the penitentiary and the rigid arrangement of the daily routine were intended to eliminate the unfavorable influences that led the individual to commit a crime. Silence and penitence would then be able to change behavior. From 1870 to 1900, the Reformatory model was established; its goal was to reform offenders through helping them to develop their own self-respect and to determine their own destiny. This model led to the development of such programs as education, training, the "mark" system for good conduct, and the indeterminate sentencing process. It was also during this era that parole began to be implemented. The Progressive era, between 1900 and 1920, was characterized by the onset of the individualized approach to the treatment of offenders. During this period, reformers began to use the medical model to treat offenders, to establish alternatives to incarceration such as community-based programs, and to expand on indeterminate sentencing, parole, and probation. The progressive reforms dominated reformist thinking until the middle 1960s. Rothman[19] believes that the basic premises at the time were not seriously challenged. These premises were that we were able to understand the etiology of deviant behavior, that alternatives to incarceration could coexist easily with institutions, and that a program that combined custodial and rehabilitative services could be accomplished without much difficulty. But by the end of the 1960s, the medical model, whose major goal had been to transform the prison setting into a treatment center, had lost credibility. The reintegration model, which gained considerable encouragement from such commissions as the 1967 President's Commission on Law Enforcement and Administration of Justice,[20] emphasized keeping offenders in the community and helping them reintegrate there. Both the probation officer and the parole officer were therefore to be transformed from caseworkers to community resource managers. With a sizable infusion of federal funds, many community-based programs were established throughout the country. But during the late 1970s, as the public attitude toward criminal offenders hardened, the popularity of the reintegration model began to wane.

In 1974, the entire idea of rehabilitating offenders came under severe attack with the startling pronouncement by Robert Martinson, who was then a professor of sociology at New York's City College, that "with few and isolated exceptions, the rehabilitative efforts that have been reported so far have had no appreciable effect on recidivism."[21(p 25)] This conclusion was based on the results of a survey of the effectiveness of correctional treatment programs around the country from 1945 to 1967.[22] Dr. Ted Palmer,[23] of the California Youth Authority, took issue with Martinson's assertion; he pointed out that some of the programs in the study Martinson cited as failures did indeed work for some offenders. Others argued that Martinson's study was conducted before 1967, when programs were neither adequately organized nor funded.[24]

Today, Bartollas[15] believes that there are four competing ideologies regarding correctional treatment, each associated with a philosophical position: (1) one school of liberals essentially reaffirms the ideology of rehabilitation and wants to continue the system of indeterminate sentencing with parole boards requiring participation in rehabilitation programs; (2) the justice model liberals reject indeterminate sentencing and parole boards but accept voluntary rehabilitative programs; (3) the proponents of the conservative perspective have little use for rehabilitation and believe in determinate sentencing, increased incapacitation, and the use of the death penalty; and (4) the radical advocates believe only in radical change in society itself. Which model will emerge as the dominant model in the corrections system in the United States remains to be seen, but it is clear that the model employed determines, to some extent, the role of mental health services in the corrections system.

LEGAL TRENDS IN CORRECTIONAL PSYCHIATRY

A basic question related to prisoners' rights is put forth in the words of Bronstein,[25] the Executive Director of the National Prison Project of the American Civil Liberties Foundation: "Does the Constitution follow a person into prison?" And just as the answer to that question necessarily shapes the corrections system, so too does it help determine the role of mental health services within this system. Bronstein's answer today is a qualified "yes, to some extent." But he underscores the fact that in 1871, a Virginia judge wrote quite explicitly that "prisoners have no more rights than slaves,"[26] and that up until quite recently "conditions inside prisons were off-limits to judicial scrutiny." In his view, two events significantly helped in changing this "hands-off" policy: "the Attica Rebellion and the Supreme Court's 1961 decision in *Monroe v Pape*[27] which resurrected the Civil Rights Act of 1871." In fact, several legal decisions have proved important to efforts to provide mental health services to prisoners.

Among the leading cases related to psychiatric treatment of prisoners, several cases stand out, for different reasons, as landmark decisions. In *Newman v Alabama,*[28] the federal district court held that failure to provide inmates with the basic elements of medical care, including the treatment of mental illness, would be depriving the prisoner of his or her constitutional right to protection against cruel and unusual punishment guaranteed under the Eighth Amendment. *Estelle v Gamble*[29] was the 1976 Supreme Court case that established the "deliberate indifference to serious medical needs" standard for violation of the Eighth Amendment prohibition of cruel and unusual punishment. The decision in *Bowring v Godwin,* a critical case decided by the Fourth Circuit Court of Appeals in 1977, stated that "we see no underlying distinction between the right to medical care for physical ills and its psychological or psychiatric counterpart."[30(p 47)] Finally, in *Vitek v Jones,*[31] the Supreme Court decided in 1980 that before a prisoner could be transferred to a mental hospital, the prisoner must be allowed the chance to contest the transfer at an administrative hearing. The Supreme Court's decision in this case took into account the change in the prisoner's status and the potential stigma involved in being transferred to a psychiatric hospital, as well as the possibility that the prisoner would be subject to involuntary behavior modification programs, and determined that such a transfer, without a hearing, would compromise a violation of a liberty interest stemming from the Due Process Clause of the Fourteenth Amendment.

In the *Sourcebook of the Mentally Disordered Prisoner,* Cohen[32] cited the leading cases relating to the prison inmate's legal identity, the right to treatment (which includes such areas as classification, records, substance abuse programs, rehabilitation, and suicide), the transfer of inmates to treatment, and the treatment relationship. After reviewing these cases, Cohen discussed factors that emerge in his review as significant to the courts' decisions. For example, if the prison is grossly deficient, a federal judge is more likely to require extensive programs and objectives than if one particular claim for rehabilitation is made, or if the prison in question seems even minimally acceptable. Because rehabilitation and treatment are often dealt with in cases in an overlapping fashion, the differences between the two may be more formal than real.

Although there is no clear constitutional right to rehabilitation as there is to treatment, rehabilitation programs can get into judicial orders and consent decrees if the prison problems are enormous. Such was the case, for example, in *Pugh v Locke,*[33] a case that addressed the continuance of the existing Alabama prison system on the basis that the grossly inadequate conditions of the prison deprived prisoners of their fundamental constitutional rights. Given the critical role the courts have played in establishing prisoners' rights to treatment, it is important to note Cohen's assertion that the Supreme Court now appears to be deciding cases against the inmate position. The Supreme Court's 1979 decision in *Bell v Wolfish,*[34] cited by Carrabba[9] as evidence of the Court's return to the traditional "hands-off" doctrine, stated that the Fourth Amendment right against unreasonable search does not apply to routine strip and body cavity searches of prison inmates. This trend in the Courts' decisions on issues of prisoners' rights suggests, in particular, that the Supreme Court is not likely to expand on the basic legal outline on care and services that has already been established for the mentally ill offender.

Despite the conservative mood of the Supreme Court, there is an enormous amount of litigation in the lower courts. The National Prison Project of the American Civil Liberties Foundation, formed in 1972, has been monitoring the court decrees and pending litigation dealing with overcrowding and/or total conditions of confinement in the nation's prison system, and, more recently, has attempted to do the same with jail litigation across the nation. Parlour and Sperbeck[10] report that, in 1985, a total of 16,741 state prisoners filed civil rights petitions in the United States. Steadman *et al.*[11] observe that, although the role of the courts is not clear in facilitating reforms in jail mental health programs, many more suits are likely to be filed in the future.

As Metzner and Dubovsky[35] explain, the litigation of constitutional inadequacies of psychiatric services in prisons necessarily consists of three different stages: the alleged inadequacies must be proved, the state must be ordered to develop an adequate prison psychiatric service, and the state's compliance must then be evaluated. In their national survey of the existence of standards, compliance with standards, and prevalence of class action suits which involved providing adequate mental health services in prisons, 37 state correctional departments responded by completing the questionnaires. The data obtained in this study showed that 20 states had at least one facility in their correctional system included in a class action suit that alleged failure to provide adequate mental health services; and although 28 states had standards for health services, these standards conformed to those developed by national professional organizations in only 6 of these 28 states. In fact, only 17 states indicated that they were in compliance with their own standards. Not surprisingly, lack of financial resources was the main reason given for not complying with standards.

STANDARDS FOR MENTAL HEALTH CARE SERVICES IN CORRECTIONAL INSTITUTIONS

The efforts to develop national correctional standards grew out of the recognition that standards were needed to assure that at least minimum care would be provided in these institutions.[36] A brief history of the early development of correctional standards can be traced from the publication of the first guidelines for corrections in 1870, through the publication of minimum standards by the Federal Bureau of Prisons in the 1930s; the recommendations by the Wickersham Commission Standards of good correctional practice in 1931; the publication of the first standards for jails by Austin MacCormick, the Commissioner of Correction for New York City in the early 1940s; and the development of standards by the American Prison Association (now the American Correctional Association) in 1946, which were revised to form the basis for accreditation by the Commission on Accreditation for Corrections starting in 1974. In order to develop standards of health care, critical data about the provision of medical services in the nation's correctional institutions were required. Anno and Hornung[37] summarize the findings of the first survey of medical facilities in jails, which was conducted by the Law Enforcement Assistance Administration (LEAA) in 1970, as suggesting that only about half of the jails in this country had any such facility. The American Medical Association's survey of the nation's jails, which was conducted in mid-1972, found that, in almost two thirds of the jails, the only medical facility available within the jail itself was first aid. Petrich[38] reports that this AMA study also revealed that only 13% of the jails reported having psychiatric services for mentally ill inmates.

Anno *et al.*[39] also report on the American Medical Association's pilot study, in 1975, to improve the quality of health care in 30 jails in 6 states; they note that, after two years of operation, this project was evaluated as successful both in regard to the process component of meeting the standards of health care that were established by the AMA, and in regard to the impact component of improvement in the early identification of inmates' health problems. In 1978, the AMA study was expanded from the 30 original sites and the 18 jails, which were added in the second year, to 94 more facilities in the third year. As reported by Anno *et al.*,[39] the results of the study indicated that the AMA program substantially improved both the availability and adequacy of health care services in jails. The major factor in the success of the program, and in these jails achieving accreditation in such a short period of time, seems to have been the fact that this project had been undertaken by organized medicine. In the words of Anno *et al.*: "the key determinant of success appeared to be the extent of cooperation and support received from the medical community."[39(p 24)]

Although there were formerly few standards in corrections available from national organizations, Singer[40] points out that the situation has changed dramatically. In fact, because there are now a variety of standards in use, the courts could have difficulty selecting the one most relevant. Actually, this difficulty is reduced because the national standards agree to a considerable extent, though each standard may stress a particular area. Currently, national standards to corrections in general, such as those established by the National Advisory Commission on Criminal Justice Standards and Goals (1973), are available, as are recommendations or guidelines for jail administrators, such as the National Sheriff's Association Manual on Jail Administration (1970). A third category of national standards relates directly to medical care; this category includes standards promulgated by the American Public Health Association (1976) and the American Medical Association (1979). In addition to the national standards endorsed by these last two medical organizations, McCarthy[41] also selects the national standards of the U.S. Department of Justice (1980), of the American Association of Correctional Psychologists (1980), and of the American Correctional Association (1981) as having special relevance to the delivery of mental health services in adult prisons.

The National Commission on Correctional Health Care (NCCHC) has developed a voluntary accreditation program specifically related to the medical and health care services, including mental health services, in jails, prisons, and juvenile confinement facilities. The correctional health care program originated in the American Medical Association's pilot study of jails in the early 1970s. In 1982, the AMA correctional health care program began to expand to include a number of other national professional organizations, resulting in the establishment of the NCCHC. At present, the Board of Directors of the NCCHC is composed of representatives of a total of 29 of the most prestigious professional organizations involved with the courts, including the American Medical Association, the American Nurses' Association, the American Psychiatric Association, the American Psychological Association, and the American

Academy of Psychiatry and the Law. The most recently revised standards for jails and prisons were published by the NCCHC in January, 1987, and the standards in use for juvenile confinement facilities were published in August, 1984. The effectiveness of these standards can be judged, at least in part, by the fact that, since 1983, there has been a 71% increase in the number of accredited facilities; there are now over 200 such institutions.[42]

Despite the recent emphasis on standards for mental health services in jails, Steadman *et al.*[11] question the usefulness of standards that identify desirable goals but do not offer specific guidelines on how to establish and, equally important, to finance better services. Such standards, they feel, "focus on content to the virtual exclusion of the form that is needed to implement that content."[11(p 32)] On the basis of their study of 43 jails in 42 communities across the nation, Steadman and his colleagues delineated five principles or basic guidelines that they believe local communities should consider during the planning and implementation of mental health programs in jails:

> The mentally disturbed jail inmate must be viewed as a community issue. The jail is and should remain primarily a correctional facility. Serious mental health needs among inmates require limited but high quality professional services in every jail. Correctional administrators should concentrate their efforts on developing mental health service in the areas of identification, crisis intervention, and case management at release. There is no one best way to organize a jail mental health program.[11(pp 115–129)]

Useful though these guidelines are, they do not address the issues mental health workers necessarily confront in their work with inmates. If these standards are to be met, these issues must be examined.

PSYCHIATRIC TREATMENT OF MENTALLY ILL PRISONERS

Psychiatrists who work with mentally ill prisoners have had continual difficulties in clearly defining their role in correctional settings. Indeed, as James and Gregory[43] point out, psychiatry in general has been ambivalent about treating mentally ill offenders. Halleck[44] notes that, during the decade between 1930 and 1940, the rise of considerable psychiatric interest in treating the criminal coincided with the increasing use of psychoanalytic theory to explain criminal behavior. But the next decade saw a waning of interest in the criminal. This development coincided with psychiatrists' moving away from institutions and into private offices to treat motivated patients with individual psychotherapy. At the same time, prison populations were expanding, exacerbating the problems faced by already inadequate psychiatric services. James and Gregory attribute this reluctance on the part of psychiatrists to get involved with treating mentally ill offenders with a number of factors, including the generally poor results of working with sociopaths and the negative attitudes directed toward psychiatrists by correctional administrators and caretakers. Writing in 1951, Powelson and Bendix[45] had described the tremendous tension between the psychiatric and the custodial orientations:

> Custodial employees enter the prison with the clear objective of punishing convicted offenders and protecting society. Perhaps members of the other professions (doctors. . .) enter the prison for equally clear reasons, for instance, to promote the rehabilitation and the health of prisoners. Yet, they cannot, in fact, pursue these goals.[45(p 77)]

Additional issues cited by James and Gregory[43] as contributing to the reluctance of psychiatrists to treat mentally ill prisoners include psychiatrists' uncertainties about how and where inmates should be treated. James and Gregory demonstrate the extent of psychiatric ambivalence in this area by citing Rubin's questioning the need to have psychiatrists work in prisons "when most of the inmates need not, and should not be there"[46(p 218)]; Shervington's questioning whether rehabilitation can, in fact, "ever take place within the walls of a prison"[5(p 49)]; and Tyce's emphatic assertion that "no effective psychiatric intervention exists or can exist in our present correctional system."[47(pp 19–20)] Clearly, psychiatrists' ambivalence about treating mentally ill inmates is based on questions about the ethics, as well as questions about the efficacy, of this work.

In Smith's[48] opinion, such questions can and must be resolved by delineating the proper role and function of the psychiatrist as that of a physician "whose task is to diagnose and heal illness and to ease human suffering."[48(p 717)] Smith believes that psychiatrists should assume the leadership role in providing mental health services to inmates, but also feels that many functions in the mental health service program can be designated to other professionals. Smith points out that because the psychiatrist's primary loyalty should be to the patient, he or she should "decline primary responsibility for administrative decision-making concerning such matters as custody, discipline, institutional placement, and release."[48(p 719)] Halleck, who shares this opinion, feels that the "possibility of ameliorating the suffering of the mentally ill prisoner is a worthy enough goal without worrying about rehabilitation."[49(p 603)] Similarly, Goldstein elaborates on two premises she considers basic to prison psychiatry: "there is a great need for basic psychiatric care within the system," and "it is ethical to work in these institutions."[50(p 753)] In a recent chapter on "Correctional Psychiatry", Roth[51] begins with the declaration that psychiatric practices in prisons must always strive to adhere to standards equivalent to those practiced on the outside.[52] According to Roth, although an effective psychiatric program must be familiar with the special circumstances in prisons, "it must be inmate-oriented in its goals, and it consciously must avoid preoccupation with whether inmates recidivate."[51(p 429)] He suggests that psychiatry should be "more modest in its aims" in prisons and jails, and that, since it is "unlikely that 'rehabilitation' will ever constitute the primary function of these institutions . . . it is in the area of direct services to the mentally ill inmate and in crisis intervention that the psychiatrist's future role in corrections most clearly lies."[51(p 434)]

Thus, it is generally agreed that crisis intervention techniques consisting of crisis evaluations, disposition, and treatment are especially appropriate for the jail setting.[53] As was mentioned earlier, the stresses to inmates in jail may even exceed those stresses to inmates in prisons. Danto's *Jail House Blues*,[54] a study of suicidal behavior among prisoners, points out that suicides in prisons are reported at a rate of 10.5 per 100,000 persons, a figure lower than the overall average of 16 per 100,000 persons in the United States. However, suicides in jails are reported at the rate of 57.5 per 100,000 persons, a figure considerably higher than the overall rate of suicide in the country. Jail suicides occur most commonly in the pretrial period, between 16 days and 12 weeks of confinement; suicides in prisons usually occur after 4 months. Because crisis intervention in jail is initiated, for the most part, to stabilize a severely mentally disturbed jail inmate, often with psychotropic medication and without an attempt to make any long-term personality changes in the prisoner, the goals of jailers and mental health workers tend to converge in such crisis interventions, resulting in minimal conflict between the two systems.[55] Jails are characterized more as "short-term people processing" rather than as "people-changing" organizations; the staff do not have the time to engage in long-term therapy.[56]

Even in situations in which jailers and mental health workers share a common goal, however, there are a number of special ethical considerations with which a mental health professional working in a correctional institution should be familiar, including issues of confidentiality, dual agency, and the treatment of condemned inmates on "death row," as well as specific clinical concerns, such as "prison psychosis,"[52] habitually violent inmates,[57] self-mutilators,[58] neuroleptic medication for most-violent inmates,[59] and the use of indigenous correctional personnel to supplement the efforts of the professional staff.[60]

In regard to the question of psychiatric involvement in the parole release decision, Roth[51] emphasizes that the psychiatrist who participates in this administrative decision should not be the one doing the treatment. He cites the Standards of the American Public Health Association (1976),[61] which clearly makes this prescription. In their study of the significance of an inmate's psychiatric history in parole release decisions, Adams and Flint[62] found that assaultive offense behavior weighed heavily in parole boards' decisions. In light of this finding, they believe it would be important to conduct research to determine the impact of the psychiatrist's report on the decisions made by the parole board about inmates who have received psychiatric services while in prison. One strategy for working with the parole board is reported by Prandoni *et al.*;[63] they describe an interagency team approach that includes the participation of one psychiatrist from a forensic psychiatric bureau, and uses mental health referral criteria to improve the effectiveness of preparole mental health evaluations.

LOCUS OF TREATMENT CONCERNS

The question of models in the provision of health services to mentally ill prisoners still remains under discussion. Indeed, Cormier's[52] account of Baer's[64] description in 1897 of four methods of dealing with mentally ill prisoners sounds almost contemporary: (1) transfer them to mental bospitals; (2) segregate them in special annexes of mental hospitals; (3) place them in special institutions, that is, asylums; or (4) treat them in the medical services of prisons. Cormier believes that the description of the last model proves Baer was ahead of his time. Cormier himself argues that:

> Psychiatric services in correctional services should not be separated from a major penal institution and should operate as they do in the free community offering facilities for full hospitalization, day and night hospital, and outpatient clinic.[52(p 181)]

After discussing the advantages and disadvantages of different approaches to providing mental health care in corrections, Dougherty[65] describes the model used in South Carolina where the responsibility lies directly with the Department of Corrections. This model consists of three levels of care situated within or on the grounds of different correctional institutions throughout the state. Arboleda-Florez and Chato[66] describe another model in which the Forensic Services of the Calgary General Hospital provide inpatient psychiatric services for the prison population.

It seems possible that the 1980 Supreme Court decision in *Vitek v Jones*[31] added momentum to the movement to provide mental health services within the correctional institutions themselves.[67] In *Vitek,* as was pointed out earlier, the court ruled that before a prisoner could be transferred from a prison to a mental hospital, an administrative hearing was required in which the prisoner could contest the transfer. In effect, the court's decision that such a hearing was necessary to protect inmates' rights (guaranteed by the Due Process Clause of the Fourteenth Amendment) made such transfers more complicated and more costly, factors that make mental health services within the correctional institutions seem more feasible than they otherwise would appear. Yet another perspective is offered by Maier and Miller's[68] discussion of the positive and negative aspects of five different models of mental health delivery to convicted mentally disordered offenders. They contend that basically neither the correctional system nor the mental health system wants jurisdiction over these kinds of patients. After discussing these five models—(1) a centralized psychiatric prison, (2) small psychiatric units attached to major prisons, (3) regional forensic psychiatric centers, (4) regional security units at psychiatric hospitals, and (5) a centralized psychiatric security hospital—the authors express their preference for small psychiatric units attached to major prisons with dual management, because this model places less of an emphasis on excessive security, which is a crucial factor in establishing a greater level of trust, better communication among staff members, good morale, and increased possibilities of developing specialized services.

The national trend of abolishing abnormal offender laws and programs poses yet another challenge to mental health workers, because it will result most likely in increased numbers of sex offenders under the supervision of the correctional system. In recent years, abnormal offender programs have been virtually limited to the "sexually dangerous."[69] Michigan was the first state to enact a "sex psychopath" statute in 1937, and thus began the national movement toward diverting mentally disordered sex offenders from the criminal justice system into the mental health system.[70] Steadman *et al.*[8] found that 1,203 persons in the United States were admitted to mental health facilities (most of them under the administration of the Department of Mental Health) as mentally disordered sex offenders in 1978. This number represented 6% of the total number of mentally disordered offenders that were committed to mental health facilities that year. The average length of confinement of mentally disordered sex offenders in mental health facilities was a little over two years. Since California repealed its mentally disordered sex offenders' statute, effective January 1, 1982, sex offenders have been sentenced under the general penal regulations. The number of states that still have some form of mentally disordered sex offenders' statute has contracted to approximately 20 plus the District of Columbia.

Thus, any attempt to improve mental health services within the correctional system will have to address the particular problems presented by a population that includes mentally disordered sex offenders.

THE PRIVATIZATION OF CORRECTIONAL PROGRAMS

Yet another trend that may have a significant effect on mental health services to corrections is *privatization*. The idea of allowing private vendors to operate within correctional facilities has generated considerable debate and gained considerable support. Faced with problems that include severe overcrowding, insufficient funding for programs, and inadequate physical plants, the corrections system has increasingly turned to the public sector for help. Debate has centered on the advantages and disadvantages of this privatization. Travis *et al.*[71] identify the major reasons for the emergence of this trend toward privatization as the promise it holds out of cost-effectiveness, and the somewhat connected belief that privatization enables institutions to "cut the red tape." But Travis and his colleagues also describe three major areas in which problems arise when correctional institutions turn to the public sector for help: (1) legal issues (in particular, questions surrounding liability for the agencies' actions); (2) cost issues (some critics argue that, in the long run, these services will prove more rather than less costly); and (3) issues of accountability for overseeing the contract. Sensibly, Travis *et al.* conclude their discussion with the suggestion that private sector involvement should be viewed as a complementary rather than as an alternative method of providing services, and should be employed only where it is appropriate rather than unilaterally.

In a survey of the extent of private contracts in 54 correctional agencies across the country, Levison[72] found that most of the contracting is done by juvenile agencies, with California having the highest number of private contracts for adult agencies. (While a discussion of correctional institutions such as half-way houses is beyond the scope of this chapter, it should be mentioned that "most halfway houses are privately operated."[71]) The three services most frequently contracted for that are related to health care are physicians (76%), health services (71%), and mental health services (67%).[72] Although correctional administrators claim that privatization results in improvements in systems operations, improved services and conditions, and cost savings, they also describe problems that have arisen in their use of private services, problems that include difficulties in supervising the contractors' employees, poor quality of services, and the occasional out-and-out failure of the private contractor to provide the promised service; as Levinson notes, "the biggest legal issue in private-sector contracting is clearly defining where the correctional jurisdiction's legal authority and responsibility end, and where the private contractor's begins."[72(p 46)]

In spite of these problems, the American Correctional Association, in their "Public Correctional Policy on Private Sector Involvement in Corrections," has been generally supportive of privatization. As the ACA has pointed out, "Agencies are under great pressure to explore the widest range of alternatives for increasing effectiveness and efficiency of their operations. These alternatives include services and programs provided through the private sector."[73(p 51)] Nonetheless, the general lack of experience with privately operated correctional facilities, particularly secure institutions for adults, that exists makes controversy over this issue both unavoidable and legitimate. Yet Cullen[74] regards the privatization of prison treatment programs as a possible strategy to counter the conservative trend in the country and thus to enhance criminal justice reform in the 1980s. In particular, he suggests that by reaffirming rehabilitation as a humanistic and progressive approach to corrections, it may be possible to link rehabilitation to the ideology of private enterprise.

CONCLUSION

Although mentally ill inmates have a right to receive psychiatric treatment, they have no guaranteed right to correctional rehabilitation.[30] Yet, as Adams[75] has pointed out, contemporary psychiatric theory views criminal behavior as being traceable to some of the same causal factors that lead to mental illness, including stressful experiences in early life that result in maladaptive responses. And because criminal behavior and mental illness represent, at least to some degree, problems of adjustment stemming from early experiences, Adams agrees with Toch's[76] and Halleck's[77] assertion that mental health services aimed at resocialization can benefit the criminal as well as the mentally ill individual. Indeed, a number of factors emphasize the need for and, in some cases, the expansion of mental health services within the corrections system: the general concerns among experts that mental illness comprises a significant health-care problem in prisons, the continuing increase in prison populations, the courts' recognition of inmates' "right to treatment" for mental health problems, and the involvement of professional groups in setting mental health care standards for prisons. But the very concerns that have spurred the development of mental health services to the corrections system have met with retrenchment rather than development of the rehabilitation mission of the corrections system.

A great deal of concern has been expressed about the reduced emphasis on rehabilitation in prisons. Speculating on the possibility of "rehabilitating the ideal of rehabilitation," Allen[78] contends that, if a society is to maintain a rehabilitative ideal in its criminal justice system, "the society as a whole has to have a strong faith in the malleability of human behavior and human character" as well as "a sufficient consensus of values to permit practical agreement on what it means to be rehabilitated."[78(p 151)] Moreover, he warns that the rehabilitative ideal is essential both to the decency of the system, and to society as a whole, for it is society as a whole, as well as the inmates themselves, who ultimately will pay the price of the decline of the rehabilitative ideal within the correctional system. Similarly, in a commencement address at Pace University on June 11, 1983, the then Chief Justice of the United States Supreme Court, Warren E. Burger,[79] lamented the billions of dollars being spent to build new prison facilities that are essentially human warehouses. Burger urged that prisons be changed to become more productive and rehabilitative, to become places where prisoners are not merely incarcerated but are trained, educated, and involved in meaningful work. Only in this way can inmates come to take pride in themselves and their work and thus to consider themselves part of a society in which they too have a stake. Herein lies the most pressing challenge facing mental health workers within the corrections system during the coming years: to work to establish rehabilitation as the goal not only of their work with the corrections system but also as the goal of the corrections system within which they work.

REFERENCES

1. Kruzich JM: Services for mentally ill offenders, in Austin MJ, Hershey WE (eds): *Handbook on Mental Health Administration.* San Francisco, Jossey-Bass Publishers, 1982, chap 23.
2. Halleck SL: *The Mentally Disordered Offender.* Washington, DC, American Psychiatric Press Inc, 1987.
3. Adams K: The disciplinary experiences of mentally disordered inmates. *Crim Just Behav* 1986;13:279–316.
4. Whitmer GE: From hospitals to jails. The fate of California's deinstitutionalized mentally ill. *Am J Orthopsychiatry* 1980;50:65–75.
5. Shervington W: Prison, psychiatry and mental health. *Psychiatr Ann* 1974;4:43–60.
6. *Jail Inmates, 1985: Bureau of Justice Statistics.* Washington DC, US Department of Justice, July 1987, NCJ–105586.
7. *Prisoners in 1986: Bureau of Justice Statistics.* Washington DC, US Department of Justice, May 1987, NCJ–104864.
8. Steadman HJ, Monahan J, Hartstone E, Kantorowski D, Robbins PC: Mentally disordered offenders. A national survey of patients and facilities. *Law Hum Behav* 1982;6:31–38.

9. Carrabba CG: Prisoners' constitutional rights to medical treatment. *N Engl J Prison Law* 1981;7:341–377.
10. Parlour RR, Sperbeck DJ: Mental health services in U.S. correctional facilities. *Med Law* 1986;5:77–87.
11. Steadman HJ, McCarty DW, Morrissey JP: *Developing Jail Mental Health Services: Practice and Principles,* US Department of Health and Human Services. Rockville, Maryland, DHHS Publication No. (ADM) 86–1458, 1986.
12. Roth L: Correctional psychiatry, in Corran WJ, McGarry AL, Petty CS (eds): *Modern Legal Medicine, Psychiatry, and Forensic Science.* Philadelphia, PA, F.A. Davis Co, 1980, chap 28.
13. Monahan J, Steadman H: Crime and mental disorder: An epidemiological approach, in Morris N, Tonry M (eds): *Crime and Justice: An Annual Review of Research.* Chicago, University of Chicago Press, 1983.
14. McCarthy D: Mentally ill and mentally retarded offenders in corrections: A report of a National Survey, in, *Sourcebook on the Mentally Disordered Prisoner,* National Institute of Corrections. Washington, DC, US Department of Justice, March 1985.
15. Bartollas C: *Correctional Treatment: Theory and Practice.* Englewood Cliffs, NJ, Prentice-Hall Inc, 1985.
16. Hirsch AV: *Doing Justice: The Choice of Punishments.* New York, Hill & Wang, 1976.
17. The American Prison: *From the Beginning . . . A Pictorial History.* College Park, MD, American Correctional Association Publishers, 1983.
18. Rothman DJ: *The Discovery of the Asylum: Social Order and Disorder in the New Republic.* Boston, Little Brown & Co, 1971.
19. Rothman DJ: *Incarceration and its Alternatives in 20th Century America,* U.S. Department of Justice, Law Enforcement Assistance Administration, National Institute of Law Enforcement and Criminal Justice. Washington, DC, US Government Printing Office, November 1979, p 71–72.
20. President's Commission on Law Enforcement and Administration of Justice: *The Challenge of Crime in a Free Society.* Washington, DC, February 1967, US Government Printing Office, chap 6.
21. Martinson R: What works?—questions and answers about prison reform. *Pub Interest* 1974;35:22–54.
22. Lipton D, Martinson R, Wilks J: *The Effectiveness of Correctional Treatment: A Survey of Treatment Evaluation Studies.* New York, Praeger, 1975.
23. Palmer T: Martinson revisited. *J Res Crime Delinq* 1975;12:133–152.
24. Kwartler R (ed): *Behind Bars: Prisons in America.* New York, Vintage Books Edition, 1977, chap 6.
25. Bronstein AJ: Offender rights litigation: Historical and future developments, in Robbins IP (ed): *Prisoners' Rights Source Book,* vol 2. New York, Clark Boardman Co Ltd, 1980.
26. *Ruffin v Commonwealth,* 62 Va. (21 Gratt.) 790 (1871).
27. *Monroe v Pape,* 365 U.S. 167 (1961).
28. *Newman v Alabama,* 349 F. Supp. 278, 284 (M.D. Ala. 1971).
29. *Estelle v Gamble,* 429 U.S. 97 (1976).
30. *Bowring v Godwin,* 551 F.2d 44 (4th Cir. 1977).
31. *Vitek v Jones,* 445 U.S. 480 (1980).
32. Cohen F: Legal issues and the mentally disordered inmate, in *Sourcebook of the Mentally Disordered Prisoner,* National Institute of Corrections. Washington, DC, US Department of Justice, March 1985.
33. *Pugh v Locke* 406 F. Supp. 318 (M.D. Alabama, 1976).
34. *Bell v Wolfish,* 441 U.S. 520 (1979).

35. Metzner JL, Dubovsky SL: The role of the psychiatrist in evaluating a prison mental health system in litigation. *Bull Am Acad Psychiatry Law* 1986;14:89–95.
36. Smith RL: Proposed minimum standards for mental health services. *J Prison Jail Health* 1983;3:84–88.
37. Anno BJ, Hornung CA: Health care in jails. *Evaluation Health Prof* 1980;3:365–384.
38. Petrich J: Rate of psychiatric morbidity in a Metropolitan County Population. *Am J Psychiatry* 1976;133:1439–1444.
39. Anno BJ, Hornung CA, Lang AH: An evaluation summary of the American Medical Association's program to improve health care in jails (year three). Presentation at the 1981 Academy of Criminal Justice Sciences Annual Meeting, Philadelphia, Pa, March 11–14, 1981.
40. Singer RG: Providing mental health services for jail inmates: Legal perspectives. *J Prison Health* 1981;1:105–129.
41. McCarthy D: Standards by administrative topic, in *Sourcebook of the Mentally Disordered Prisoner,* National Institute of Corrections. Washington DC, US Department of Justice, March 1985.
42. Correction Care: *84% Retention plus 71% growth.* National Commission of Correctional Health Care, August 1987, vol 1, p 3.
43. James JF, Gregory D: Improving psychiatric care for prisoners. *Hosp Community Psychiatry* 1980;31:671–673.
44. Halleck S: American psychiatry and the criminal: A historical review. *Am J Psychiatry* 1965;121(suppl):1–21.
45. Powelson H, Bendix R: Psychiatry in Prison. *Psychiatry* 1951;14:73–86.
46. Rubin S: Psychiatry and the prison: A negative report. *Int J Psychiatry* 1968;6:218.
47. Tyce FAJ: Psychiatry in correctional systems. *Psychiatr Ann* 1977;7:11–23.
48. Smith CE: Prison, psychiatry and professional responsibility. *J Forensic Sci* 1987;32:-717–724.
49. Halleck S: Psychiatry and the prisoner. *Am J Psychiatry* 1980;137:603–604.
50. Goldstein N: Psychiatry in prisons, in Sadoff RL (ed): *Symposium on Forensic Psychiatry, The Psychiatric Clinics of North America.* Philadelphia, Pa, W.B. Saunders Co, vol 5, 1983, pp 751–765.
51. Roth LH: Correctional psychiatry, in Curran WJ, McGarry AL, Shah SA (eds): *Forensic Psychiatry and Psychology: Perspectives and Standards for Interdisciplinary Practice.* Philadelphia, Pa, F.A. Davis Co, 1986, chap 19.
52. Cormier BM: The practice of psychiatry in the prison society. *Bull Acad Psychiatry Law* 1973;2:156–183.
53. Lamb RH, Schock R, Chen PW, *et al.:* Psychiatric needs in local jails: Emergency issues. *Am. J. Psychiatry* 1984;141:774–777.
54. Danto BL: *Jail House Blues: Studies of Suicidal Behavior in Jail and Prison.* Orchard Lake, Mich, Epic Publications, Inc, 1973.
55. Runck B: Study of 43 jails shows mental health services and inmate safety are compatible. *Hosp Community Psychiatry* 1983;34:1007–1008.
56. Steadman HJ, Morrissey JP, Robbins PC: Reevaluating the custody-therapy conflict paradigm in correctional mental health settings. *Criminology* 1985;23:165–179.
57. Bach-Y-Rita G, Veno A: Habitual violence: A profile of 62 men. *Am J Psychiatry* 1974;131:1015–1017.
58. Jones A: Self-mutilation in prison: A comparison of mutilators and nonmutilators: *Crim Just Behav* 1986;13:286–296.
59. Scarnati RA: Most violent psychiatric inmates and neuroleptics. *J Psychiatry Law* 1986;14(fall/winter):447–468.

60. Lombardo LX: Mental health work in prisons and jails: Inmate adjustment and indigenous correctional personnel. *Crim Justice Behav* 1985;12:17–27.
61. Jails and Prisons Task Force: *Standards for Health Services in Correctional Institutions.* Washington DC, American Public Health Association, 1976.
62. Adams K, Flint GA: Inmate psychiatric history and parole release decisions: A research note. *Crim Just Rev* 1985;10:52–54.
63. Prandoni JR, James GC, Kapit RM, *et al.:* The use of an interagency team approach and mental health referral criteria to improve the effectiveness of pre-parole mental health evaluations. *J Offender Counseling, Services Rehabil* 1985;9:5–18.
64. Baer, AA: *Die Hygiene des Gefängniswesens.* Jena, Germany, G. Fisher, 1897.
65. Dougherty FI: Issues in the provision of mental health care in corrections. *Corrections Today,* October 1984, pp 69,97.
66. Arboleda-Florez J, Chato F: Issues regarding admissions from a correctional facility to a hospital forensic unit. *Int J Offender Therapy Comp Criminology* 1985;29:43–62.
67. Churgin MJ: The transfer of inmates to mental health facilities: Developments in the law, in Monahan J, Steadman HJ (eds): *Mentally Disordered Offenders: Perspectives from Law and Social Science.* New York, Plenum Press, 1983, chap 7.
68. Maier GJ, Miller RD: Models of mental health services to correctional institutions. *J Forensic Sci* 1987;32:225–232.
69. Dix GE: Special dispositional alternatives for abnormal offenders: Developments in the law, in Monahan J, Steadman HJ (eds): *Mentally Disordered Offenders: Perspectives from Law and Social Science.* New York, Plenum Press, 1983, chap 5.
70. Monahan J, Davis SK: Mentally disordered sex offenders, in Monahan J, Steadman HJ (eds): *Mentally Disordered Offenders: Perspectives from Law and Social Science.* New York, Plenum Press, 1983, chap 6.
71. Travis LF, Latessa EJ, Vito GF: Private enterprise and institutional corrections: A call for caution. *Fed Probation* 1985;49:11–16.
72. Levinson RB: The private sector and corrections. *Corrections Today,* August 1984, pp 42, 46.
73. American Correctional Association: *Public Policy for Corrections: A Handbook for Decision-Makers.* College Park, Md, American Correctional Association, 1986.
74. Cullen FT: The privatization of treatment: Prison reform in the 1980's. *Fed Probation* 1986;50:8–16.
75. Adams K: Addressing inmate mental health problems. *Fed Probation* 1985;49:27–33.
76. Toch H: Perspectives on treatment, in Toch H (ed): *Psychology of Crime and Criminal Justice.* New York, Holt Rinehart & Winston Inc, 1979.
77. Halleck SL: *Psychiatry and the Dilemmas of Crime.* Berkeley, University of California Press, 1971.
78. Allen F: The decline of the rehabilitative ideal in American criminal justice. *Clev St Law Rev* 1978;27:147–156.
79. Burger WE: Prisons should rehabilitate. Remarks at the Commencement Exercises at Pace University, June 11, 1983, in Bender DL, Leone B, Szunski B (eds): *America's Prisons: Opposing viewpoints,* ed 4. St. Paul, Minn, Greenhaven Press Inc, 1985.

II

Practical Problems

3

Treatment of Antisocial and Other Personality Disorders in a Correctional Setting

ROBERT WEINSTOCK

We are presently in a very difficult era in regard to the treatment of personality disorders in a correctional setting. During a time when politicians and administrators compete with each other to see who can do less and thereby save more money, it is especially difficult to find funding and support for programs that help unpopular elements in our society. Antisocial personalities and other personality disorders in correctional settings are about as unpopular as possible.

The present time is also an era of relative therapeutic nihilism. Any problem that cannot be corrected in brief therapy or with psychotropic medication is considered generally as not worth even attempting. If it cannot be corrected quickly, the problem is considered as untreatable. The difficult becomes the impossible, the useless, or, even worse in our present era, the ultimate bugaboo—not cost-efficient.

Long-term psychotherapy generally has come into disrepute. Difficulties in doing research in psychotherapy have been interpreted incorrectly as proof that psychotherapy does not work. One of the problems has been the variety of goals for long-term psychotherapy which leads to a variance so large that treatment effects get lost in any analysis of variance which is part of most psychotherapy research. Moreover, it has been rare that extensive therapeutic efforts have been made with such

ROBERT WEINSTOCK • Department of Psychiatry, University of California, Los Angeles, CA 90024-1556.

patient populations. Even under relatively ideal circumstances the therapy offered is less than optimal. The absence of being able to disprove the null hypothesis that psychotherapy does not work often has been interpreted wrongfully to mean that psychotherapy has been proven not to work. A more correct interpretation of such research data would be that psychotherapy has neither been proven to work or not work in these circumstances. The methods of study or the outcome criteria may have been inadequate. In general, however, in most circumstances interventions have been found to be more helpful than no intervention at all even though the specific interventions have not been shown to discriminate between outcomes.[1] Interpretations of psychotherapy research, as stated by Parloff,[2] should be guarded. It is important to realize that different therapists can have differing effects and that therapists who actively do harm can negate the positive effects of helpful therapists in outcome studies.[3]

Despite the current disfavor of psychotherapy, especially with personality disorders, comprehensive reviews have shown psychotherapy generally to be helpful regardless of the patient's condition.[1,4,5] Psychotherapy has been especially difficult to evaluate because of the heterogeneity of conditions for which people want help, the variety of methods claiming effectiveness, the multitude of therapists with varying personalities, as well as differing competencies in the espoused techniques. There is also an art in psychotherapy that is difficult to describe or measure.

Psychoanalytically oriented therapy is widely used, but why it does or does not work is little understood. As with most difficult problems in our current era, there has been a rush to assume that psychotherapy is useless for personality disorders in spite of the experience of many practitioners to the contrary.[6] Kernberg, though pessimistic about treatment of antisocial personalities, does describe them as a primitive form of borderline personality, a condition he finds very treatable.[7]

Studies on the effectiveness of treatment of antisocial personalities have been limited. Martin *et al.*[8] said that research has been flawed by limitations in program evaluation, uncertainty of the degree to which treatments actually were implemented, and the narrow range of attempted approaches. In a review of 295 literature citations,[9] only 10 studies met minimum standards for evaluation: most lacked adequate controls or follow-up. As stated by Madden:[10]

> Over time some violent patients grow in their ability to appreciate how external and internal stresses cause them to act violently or impulsively. Patients with ego strength learn to delay, to verbalize rather than act out, and to seek support when it is needed. Unfortunately, however, the personality of many violent persons greatly limits the hopes for radical change that some thera-

> pists bring to treatment. In working with violent patients, the therapist must settle for less than optimal goals. If patients who formerly assaulted others succeed in getting out of stressful and provocative situations without striking out, this is a major accomplishment. If impulsive patients learn to modulate their behavior to the extent that they can hold a job, this also is a major accomplishment. (p 72)

Robert Kegan[11] has developed an interesting hypothesis in which he claims that there is evidence that sociopathy is a developmental arrest. He hypothesizes that the sociopath is retarded in a developmental stage, corresponding to Piaget's cognitive stage of concrete operations[12] and Kohlberg's moral stage of instrumentalism.[13] There is some empirical data to support his hypothesis.

In the treatment of personality disorders, the first issue to consider is an accurate assessment and diagnosis of the problem. For instance, it is possible that a brief psychotic episode could be present in a patient with a personality disorder diagnosis, and this psychosis might benefit from antipsychotic medication. The *Diagnostic and Statistical Manual of Mental Disorders,* 3rd ed., and 3rd ed. revised, (DSM-III and DSM-III-R) have carefully delineated the criteria for schizophrenia that have come to represent a problem close to dementia praecox and not a problem close to the broad usage of the term *schizophrenia* prevalent in DSM-II. The original borderline schizophrenia described by Knight[14] has been transformed into a personality disorder, that is, a schizotypal personality in DSM-III and DSM-III-R. Again, many of these symptoms might benefit from antipsychotic medication. Borderline personality as described in DSM-III and DSM-III-R utilizes observable criteria that were developed by Gunderson and Singer[15] from symptoms of hospitalized patients with a borderline personality organization as described by Kernberg.[7] Such patients, therefore, exhibit much acting out, as would be expected of hospitalized patients, and are well represented in a correctional-setting population. Antidepressants, as well as antipsychotic medication, have often been useful for patients with such problems.

The diagnosis of antisocial personality is itself complex. The American Law Institute (ALI) criteria for insanity excludes conditions manifested "solely by repeated criminal or otherwise antisocial conduct." Although such a description applies to some hardened criminals, it does not accurately describe even all DSM-III-R antisocial personalities. It certainly does not describe other personality disorders, such as schizotypal personalities who may have brief psychotic episodes. However, since this ALI caveat generally has been applied to all personality disorders, it is important to emphasize and remember that brief psychotic episodes are possible in such persons. Such an independent diagnosis of brief psychosis can be crucial to help counteract an otherwise misleading impression that all personality disorder diagnoses preclude a psychosis. When schizophrenia used to be used in a looser way in DSM-II, personality disorder diagnoses generally did exclude psychoses. It is, therefore, especially important to remember that DSM-III and DSM-III-R personality disorder patients can have brief psychotic episodes.

Results of treatment programs in correctional settings have been difficult to interpret.[16] In the sexually dangerous section at Bridgewater State Hospital in Massachusetts, Kozol reported a re-offense rate of only 6% for those people released on staff recommendation. Those released against advice had recidivism rates of 39%. The initial response of a reader is to be favorably impressed. However, as pointed out by Monahan and Klassen,[17] good as the results may appear to be, there is the problem of false positives. Many people released by the courts against staff recommendation were also not violent. Excessive conservatism could lead to good recidivism rates but also to many people being locked up unnecessarily. There is also the problem of how many actually harmless patients should be locked up, and for how long, to prevent a dangerous person from becoming violent.

Carney[18] in a study of fully treated and released patients at the Patuxent Institute in Maryland found a recidivism rate of only 7%. The indeterminate sentences were for "defective delinquents" or recurrent criminals. There were greater recidivism rates of 46% in those released by the courts against staff advice and without parole status. The Patuxent program consisted of greater freedom in the institution in reward for good behavior. Good behavior would lead to transfer to units with progressively more freedom. Parole supervision was important. Again, the results initially looked good. However, there was once again the problem of false positives.

Overconservatism again could be a problem in that so few people were recommended for release. The ultimate solution of this problem would be a program that hardly released anyone, in that way, the recidivism rate could be made very low. Pollack[19] has described the problem of the prediction of dangerousness in such patients as a problem of a dispositional concept in that the person is potentially violent under certain circumstances, which may or may not actually occur. Dangerousness in this sense is a signal of possible harm. Even though this explanation is partially helpful in explaining the discrepancy, there is the problem of low base rate phenomena, also described by Monahan,[20] and the fact that with rare events, such as severely violent acts, even an excellent test would produce many false positives. There is still, therefore, the ethical question of how many harmless people should be locked up preventively to preclude a violent act.

Another well-known program for people with characterological problems is the program in Denmark at the Herstedvester Detention Center.[21] However, in 1975, a British group found that as a result of objections to the indeterminate sentence, the treatment program at Herstedvester had been modified. Research on offenders who were released from Herstedvester found that the only difference was that those who were released had been reconvicted after a longer interval than those who were released from other prisons. There was, however, disappointingly no significant difference in the reconviction rates themselves.[22]

Samenow[23] has described a kind of cognitive therapy for incarcerated prisoners developed by Yochelson and himself. Although it is a potentially interesting approach, the work is marred by overstatement and hyperbole. Long-term personality change was reported in an evaluation study of his treatment methods in only 15 of the more than 60 men treated. The work was at St. Elizabeth's Hospital in Washington, D.C.

The results of a National Academy of Sciences Panel on Research Rehabilitation Techniques about therapy for antisocial offenders were that:

> Although there is little in the reported literature that demonstrably works, the conclusion that nothing works is not necessarily justified. It would be more accurate to say that nothing yet tried has been demonstrated to work.[8] (p 3)

Other problems include inadequate parole programs for reintegrating offenders into the community. Usually such programs are politically unpopular even though a sudden release into the community of an unprepared patient whose sentence has expired, most likely, is in reality the most dangerous situation possible for the community. However, it is politically much more expedient to keep a prisoner incarcerated until his sentence has expired. No one can then blame an administrator for releasing such a person. Fortunately, not all have given up on rehabilitation despite the recent emphasis of containment, punishment, and deterrence in the prison system.[24] Conditions in correctional institutions are often terrible. States are reluctant to spend money to create humane conditions, and federal court orders have been necessary to correct them.[25] Overcrowding does not help.

It is unclear whether treatment in a correctional institution can ever be therapeutic unless possibly a special unit is created. Some of the goals of such institutions preclude emotional growth. Prisons tend to contain and "break" an inmate, not encourage healthy ego strengths. Paranoia in prison is adaptive because of the danger of brutality at the hands of other inmates or even the prison guards. Paranoia is therefore not necessarily psychotic. Community treatment in a prison setting can be a perversion of the term, unless the treatment is of an offender who is sentenced to a lengthy prison term, and therefore needs to learn to adapt to such an unnatural surrounding.

Monahan and Klassen[17] utilize an approach to treating violent people that can apply in a criminal setting. Attention is given to environmental events that can influence an individual, such as annoyances, frustrations, insults, and assaults. Their approach evaluates how the person interprets the behavior and what he expects or fantasizes. People can be helped to interpret the situation correctly or to develop alternative coping skills. Also, correctional environments can be restructured by enlightened prison officials in order to reduce stresses and provocations for predisposed individuals.

In order to understand violence, Toch[26] had found it necessary to focus on the chain of interactions between aggressor and victim resulting in one harming or destroying the other. Rogers and Cavanaugh[27] have described a community outpatient program for potentially violent offender patients. Valliant[28] has commented on the need for such persons to make new kinds of friendships and form alternative group affiliations in order to prevent antisocial behavior. A wilderness program has also been utilized.[29] Other community-based programs were reviewed by Reid and Solomon[30] and showed that residential rehabilitation programs with a highly structured transition process between one style of life (being a criminal, being an inmate) and another (being responsible, confident, an accepted member of the community) can be successful, both for the individual offender and for the community, difficult as it sometimes can be to get communities to accept such programs.

The essential element in antisocial personality disorders has often been believed to be a lack of true concern for anyone and their use of people solely for manipulative purposes. However, many entrepreneurs have many similar basic characteristics.[31] One essential difference is that entrepreneurs have the ability to stay within the law or not get caught. Less talented entrepreneurs with fewer earlier successes may become antisocial and more impulsive. Although antisocial personalities have childhoods with less successes and more fighting, entrepreneurs may care for occasional peoples, such as family and some friends, but have no concern for people in general. Classically, antisocial persons care for no one. Considering the many similarities, it is curious that our society admires the entrepreneur, yet is ready to punish and even kill the antisocial personality.

In the treatment of patients in a correctional setting, a correct diagnosis is essential. Although most workers are aware of the tendency to malinger and feign illness, the opposite occurrence may actually be more of a problem.[32] Because of the fact that most prisoners, as well as many others in society, consider it preferable and less shameful to be "bad" than to be "crazy," there is often a tendency for patients in prison to hide true mental illness and even delusions or hallucinations. It is even possible to have a defendant feign mental illness in order to avoid being found guilty of a crime when real mental illness, which the defendant is unable to face, is present. Guttmacher[33] called this problem *pseudopsychopathic schizophrenia,* and it is probably as great a problem in correctional settings as is the more readily recognized malingerer of mental illness.

Patients with psychiatric problems that are superimposed on a personality disorder need to obtain treatment for their DSM-III Axis I problem. Probably one of the most difficult problems that needs to be overcome is the negative countertransference toward patients who have committed crimes or who have been violent—natural as such initial reactions may be.

In order to treat such patients, it is crucial that the treating personnel be comfortable. In my experience, fear of a patient is one of the primary precipitants of patient violence. It is impossible and even dangerous to treat a patient in a situation in which the therapist feels insecure and does not know whether adequate help is available.

Additionally, I believe it is important for the therapist to see some potential in the patient and to wish to become the patient's ally in the fight against mental illness. Therapists who see the patients merely as dangerous villains who must be stopped, or as diagnostic entities who must be contained, are correctly perceived by the patients as enemies. However, therapists who see the patient as a person with problems who needs to be helped to contain his own impulses for his own good so that after a testing period, he can manage in society, can be perceived by the patient as a possible ally. Antisocial patients may initially perceive the therapist as someone not to be trusted and who is to be used to further the patient's own ends. The patient may be trying to figure out the therapist's con in order to out-con him. However, if the therapist is realistic about the patient's lack of basic trust and inability to trust and the need to test the therapist, gradually a real therapeutic alliance may begin to develop. The alliance will be tested, and there will be regressions during which the therapist must not give up. I have found it useful to communicate to patients that I know they think they really cannot trust anyone and that people who try to help them are very naïve and dumb, or clever con men, but that I believe the patients have true potential, in spite of the fact that they themselves must doubt it.

It is also a mistake to confront directly a potentially hostile patient and therefore become the enemy. I have seen residents confront a patient's narcissistic entitlement by telling him that "You feel the world owes you everything and you need to do nothing in return." Even though this interpretation may be correct, the timing is egregious. It may be correctly construed by the patient as an angry assault when it is stated in anger. The patient is likely to completely block out the statement or even to become violent. However, after a therapist and a patient have developed a rapport and even partially trust each other, the same statement may be appropriate. It may then be perceived correctly as an attempt by the therapist to convey to the patient that the present manner in which he confronts problems may work against his own interests and alienate people. A correct interpretation can be disastrous if given at the wrong time and out of hostile motivations.

Havens[34] has described a technique of "counterprojection" for use with angry, potentially violent patients. The technique is useful when a patient is either building up to a violent outburst or recovering from one. The therapist does not wish to side against the patient with the other "bad" people; that is the surest way to be assaulted. Instead, the therapist sides with the patient against the other "bad" people with every shred of reality he can find in order to give his statements credibility. The therapist in the acute phase needs to do everything possible to separate himself from the patient's projections and to diffuse them. So-called reality interventions at such a time can just lead to the therapist's being included in the patient's projections with the patient's becoming violent toward the therapist. Clarification, if needed, can be done later when the patient settles down. Moralistic statements can actually be dangerous, as well as antitherapeutic. If the doctor has reason to believe that the patient is favorably disposed to the medical profession, it may be useful to emphasize that he is a doctor and is there to help.

In counterprojection, one might speak negatively about the hated projection or a hated introject and thereby give the patient permission to do likewise. As the therapist takes over the feeling, the patient can give up the feelings that he really did not want anyway and which is why he projected them in the first place. The therapist helps the patient not to bear the feeling alone. Eventually, by successive approximations, the truth will come out. Double statements can explore the other side. The therapist might say, "He is a pain but he has, I suppose, a good side." In my experience, the situation can be especially difficult if the hated people are staff or correction officials, and these people are still suspicious of the therapist. Often those people see the prison as a battleground and can take counterprojective statements to mean that the therapist is against them. Sometimes it is also necessary in such situations to use counterprojective statements for the benefit of the staff, such as stating how difficult and dangerous a hated patient may be, and what a difficult and commendable job correctional staff do in hospitals as well as in prisons. Such problems occur in prison hospitals or hospitals under the auspices of corrections officers, as well as even in general hospitals.[35]

In addition to fear or hate of these patients, another countertransference problem may be the inability to deal with helplessness and hopelessness that may occur in therapists' treating patients who are so unresponsive for such long periods of time.[36] The therapist also may be reacting to the patient's helplessness feelings. Many of these patients have learned to appear tough and independent as a reaction formation against helplessness and dependency, thereby disguising their true underlying dynamics.

Menninger[37] described bravado crimes done with brutality and ruthlessness to prove that the patient is no weakling and that he is a tough man who fears nothing. He stated that Nazi storm troopers were often mere boys trained to stifle all tender emotions and to behave heartlessly, ruthlessly, and brutally. Halleck[38] has indicated that men with serious doubts about their masculinity and with a need to reassure themselves and others in this regard can be prone to violent behavior and, when so driven, can be so desperate that they ignore the consequences of their actions.

Homosexual panic can also lead to violence. Ovesey[39] described pseudohomosexual concerns that are motivated by dependency and power strivings in men who feel inadequate in meeting society's standards for male performance. The man can feel compelled to compete about everything and to have a show of strength. He can counterphobically participate in risky and potentially confrontative situations. He can be overaggressive, exaggeratedly masculine, and try to have men submit to him, sometimes even sexually. He can deny his own dependency at the expense of the weaker man whom he perceives as a woman. However, the homosexual act itself can be disturbing and be a confession of masculine failure, and the defense, therefore, can be inadequate to dissipate the conflict.

A male patient who becomes afraid of dependency feelings on a male therapist can become violent and exhibit homosexual panic. Sometimes gay-oriented groups can encourage such patients to "come out" and accept their being gay, and the resulting panic can lead to these patients' becoming violent or suicidal. It is more useful to be more cautious, and neither to encourage or discourage homosexuality. Sometimes it can be helpful to explore the possibility of pseudohomosexual strivings of power and dependency, or temporary diversions from heterosexuality as a result of a traumatic experience.

Some patients who experience homosexual panic and have fragile ego boundaries may project their homosexual desire onto the therapist.

If the therapist becomes afraid and does not clarify to the patient that it is the patient's increasingly threatening behavior that is making the therapist nervous, the situation can become dangerous. If such clarification does not help, the therapist should excuse himself quickly and get help. Lack of clarification and reality testing could lead to the patient's projecting his sexual desires onto the therapist. He may believe that the therapist is uneasy because he is preparing to rape the patient, and the patient may become violent toward the therapist in what the patient believes is self-defense. I once had a patient who was becoming paranoid comment that the word *therapist* was made up of the two words "the" and "rapist." Woods[40] has described instances of pseudohomosexual panic leading to violence.

Men with sexual insecurity can also exhibit Don Juan behavior as a reaction formation. They can experience a need to score with women in a compulsive and even desperate manner. Sometimes such behavior can even lead to rape, where sex and aggression become fused, and sex can be used in the service of aggression.

Guze[41] and others have found a biological association between sociopathy in men and hysteria in women. One possible explanation of the difference is that they represent the same genetic problem, but that society encourages different expressions in men and in women. Both responses are exaggerations of the societal stereotype. Men who have an underlying dynamic of helplessness and a desire for attention may develop a reaction formation of hypermasculine behavior and appear to be "tough guys." Blacker and Tupin[42] have labeled such people "male hysterics." Chodoff and Lyons[43] have said that women hysterics tend to use exaggerated feminity and passivity in a controlled as well as in a controlling way. Men may be more directly aggressive.

An understanding of the psychodynamics of men with exaggerated male sexual behaviors can show that it is a serious error to challenge directly such a patient's masculinity in an attempt by the therapist to show his own strength. Such a procedure can escalate the problem. It is more useful to understand the underlying insecurity, to be calm with the patient, and to inquire, in a supportive way, as to what has made him uneasy. Such a calm approach is often disarming and can diffuse the situation, as well as calm the patient down. It may be helpful to clarify that the patient is not as weak and helpless as he may think, but that he has a great deal of control over what happens to him. If the patient is out of control, it is important to restrain him and sedate him so that he can calm down enough to converse rationally. In such situations, there should be an adequate show of force so that it is no shame to give in: it is not a display of weakness to surrender to an army. However, when the patient later calms down, it is important to try to reassure him that he is not as helpless as he feels. If the therapist has similar dynamics and has a need to compete with the patient, the results can be disastrous. The continued effort to belittle the patient will produce a reaction either of violence or depression. In being supportive to such patients, it is important not to overly encourage the patient's dependency on the therapist since that can precipitate the homosexual panic that was described earlier.

Intensive psychotherapy should not be attempted unless the patient has the ego strength to cope with his feelings, and the therapist is comfortable with his countertransference. Calm supportive therapists can be much more successful than aggressive competitive therapists who need to challenge and defeat such patients.

Countertransference is a significant problem with antisocial patients. It is difficult to be sympathetic to delinquent, drug-using, and even violent individuals. Such persons are often excluded from hospitals even if they have true psychiatric disorders. *Antisocial personality* can be the name given to the most disliked patients, particularly if they have some history of trouble with the law.[44] Less disliked but still disliked patients are generally called *borderline,* particularly if a borderline diagnosis is also reason at that hospital for exclusion.

Criminal justice systems, in turn, usually try to exclude patients with personality disorders and associated acute psychiatric disorders and send them to hospitals. Neither system likes these patients and feels that they are the inappropriate setting; each system feels dumped on by the other. If a crime is committed, the correctional system may be stuck with the patient and be forced to find some setting in which to contain and possibly even treat the patient. Therapists attracted to such patients may get some vicarious unconscious gratification from the antiauthoritarian attitude of these patients. Repressed therapists may admire the openness of the patient's rebellion and aggression. Therapists need to be able to set limits and be realistic. It is important that the patient not feel he is envied or admired for his "badness." The therapist should not act out vicariously through the patient but encourage the patient to control his impulses. If any of the above desires exist in the therapist, they need to be sufficiently understood in order not to interfere with the therapy. Moreover, the therapist needs to understand the maladaptive aspects of the patient's behavior, even if he has some admiration for the patient's spontaneity and seeming lack of inhibition.

It is also important to avoid splitting—a very ready pitfall in a correctional setting. Insofar as the correctional setting encourages conformity, passivity, and lack of initiative, it may go directly counter to some of the therapist's goals. If the therapist tries to encourage a patient to express feelings verbally rather than physically, such lessons may be untaught by the correctional staff who see any expression of anger as potentially leading to violence in the prison population, often with some validity because of the patient's difficulty in distinguishing between feeling and acting, and his inability to delay action to allow for deliberation. If the therapist wishes to encourage healthy initiative, it may be discouraged by the correctional staff who perceive it as dangerous to allow any inmate to have power or to exert leadership. If the therapist tries to encourage trust in the patient, the correctional staff may attempt to encourage the patient's informing on other inmates, even for minor infractions, as a part of prison security. Such differences may be inevitable but may lead to some irreconcilable differences and place a limit on any possible therapeutic milieu in a correctional setting. However, it is hoped that some work with staff will produce some positive results. Moreover, it is important to be aware of the patient's tendencies to split staff and to be careful not to accept the patient's version as the whole truth. As described earlier, Kernberg[7] has called antisocial personality a very primitive form of borderline personality.

It is also important that the therapist not be grandiose in his expectations. I have frequently seen beginning therapists start with excessive unrealistic optimism, only to be discouraged and give up with a feeling of total and excessive pessimism. The therapist needs to set realistic goals and expectations. He not only needs to be able to see the patient's "badness" but, unlike the borderline patient, also needs to be able to have an integrative whole object view of the patient with good as well as bad points. He needs to be able to see good aspects of the patient. According to Kernberg, the therapist of a borderline patient needs to experience concern in order to overcome the effects of aggression, and he must have a wish to help the patient in spite of transitory "badness."

According to Strasburger, antisocial patients have much to teach about life in general and psychotherapy in particular. Despite the inevitable adverse feelings that are stimulated, "the benefits both to them and to society from their rehabilitation can be most gratifying to those who treat them.[45(p 206)] Lion emphasizes "the need for the clinician to monitor closely his own response to the patient, for the latter is ill-equipped to deal with fantasy and affect and must depend upon the therapist for guidance."[46(p 38)] Madden[47] states that patients must learn that "just talking" actually helps, but limits must be set. Patients must be allowed to talk about anything and even shout, but not strike out. Displays of anger by an angry patient should be viewed as a positive factor. In fact, if anger is never expressed, then either little is going on, or the patient is giving the therapist what he thinks is being expected of him.

It is important to emphasize once again that an accurate diagnostic assessment is crucial. Antisocial patients do have associated psychiatric problems, even if they also have personality disorders. Therapists must not be blind to these very treatable problems merely because of the more striking antisocial behavior. The underlying personality disorders are difficult to treat and resources for them are becoming more scarce. During an era of therapeutic pessimism, it is especially difficult to find resources to treat these patients, but such scarcity of resources should not be confused and equated with untreatability.

The most hardened antisocial personalities may, in fact, be untreatable. However, it is rare to find people who truly meet the literal ALI exclusion of those specific conditions manifested only by repeated criminal activity or antisocial conduct. Even the DSM-III-R definition of antisocial personality is more inclusive than that. Other personality disorders, such as borderline or narcissistic personalities, are frequent, as well as schizoid or schizotypal personalities (who can have brief psychotic episodes despite a personality-disorder diagnosis). Even actual psychoses, such as schizophrenia or bipolar disorders, are possible in patients with antisocial behavior. Some schizophrenic patients have even learned how to use their symptoms to achieve such goals as a bed for the night in a hospital. In my experience in Veterans Administration and in community hospitals, some patients with schizophrenia have learned to say they have command hallucinations if they want to stay in a hospital bed. So even schizophrenics can be manipulative.

Psychotropic medications are efficient and relatively inexpensive for patients who are diagnosed appropriately. Such drugs as lithium, carbamazepine, and beta-blockers have been found helpful in controlling patients with impulsive violence.

In the maximum security section of Bridgewater State Hospital in Massachusetts, where I was Deputy Medical Director and Director of Treatment in the middle 1970s, there was an unusual mixture of patients in this state hospital which was run by the Department of Corrections. The hospital contained patients who became psychotic in prison, who were sent for evaluations for competency to stand trial or for insanity defenses, who were found incompetent to stand trial or not guilty by reason of insanity, or who were too violent to be managed in the Department of Mental Health's state hospitals without being accused of any crime. This section did not treat sexually dangerous persons. One of the first goals was to separate those patients sent for treatment and those sent for a forensic evaluation because of the very differing natures of the two groups. There were difficulties in the disparity between the goals of the corrections people and the therapists, especially for the group of patients who were there for treatment. However, active efforts toward communication helped diffuse suspicions in most cases and enabled some of the more helpful corrections officers to function almost as mental health aides. On occasion, any reluctance of therapists to exclude and scapegoat "bad" patients did lead to difficulty and a tendency to see us as very naïve. Nevertheless, in this setting, corrections people were very helpful in treating the more quiet, docile, and psychotic patients. Because of the lack of physicians with psychiatric training immediately prior to our arrival, significant progress was made as one of our first actions merely by appropriate diagnosis and treatment of patients with the proper antipsychotic medications. Many patients had been on homeopathic doses which needed either to be discontinued or increased. Group and occasional individual therapy was also provided. There were mixed feelings about the changes, however, and some resentment by other personnel about the involvement of Harvard University in the program, especially by the more sadistic personalities or those people who were insecure about their professional competence. Nevertheless, significant numbers of patients were transferred successfully to less restrictive institutions as a result of treatment over a period of several years.

In San Francisco, a different model was employed. Although treatment was provided at the jail, two units at the San Francisco General Hospital were opened in the late 1970s. One unit, which I directed, was devoted to patients who were accused of misdemeanors and had a corrections officer present with high but not maximum security; the other ward with maximum security contained those patients who were accused of felonies or who were believed to be more dangerous. It was felt that it would be preferable to offer treatment in the mental health department and not in the jail because of the differing goals of each, and patients, therefore, were transferred to these units directly from jail. These units were relatively successful and attracted good staff who were interested in working in such a setting.

It is very difficult to have a unit with a therapeutic environment and high security. Halleck[38] has discussed some of the ethical problems and the problems of being a double agent, as when the goals of the patient and the institution conflict, and the therapist has conflicting loyalties and responsibilities. It is ethically important to clarify any limits to confidentiality when working in a correctional setting. In a survey of forensic psychiatrists, a large majority believed it would be unethical to promise confidentiality, yet report marijuana usage to prison authorities.[48] They also believed it would be unethical to do a prearraignment examination before access to counsel unless the sole purpose was treatment. This ethical injunction is also included in the *APA's Annotations to the Principles of Medical Ethics with Annotations Especially Applicable to Psychiatry*. It would be a serious ethical problem to obtain evidence for the prosecution under the guise of treatment or to do an evaluation for the prosecution before the defendant has had the benefit of his counsel's advice.

Another difficult issue in treatment in a correctional setting is the difficulty with the predictions of dangerousness. Studies caused by such situations as the *Baxstrom* decision,[49] which released large numters of so-called dangerous people, showed the extent of overprediction and the difficulty of predicting dangerousness. Monahan[50] has discussed the difficulty in prediction from one setting (e.g., an institution) to another (e.g., the community). Intuitively, if the context of prediction and validation are the same, such as sending an outpatient back home, the prediction likely would be better.

Obviously ethical considerations would preclude such studies with double-blind dispositions of people believed to be dangerous. In addition, if the treating doctor is also the administrator of a program, there can be an ethical conflict between the needs of the patient and the harm done to a program if negative publicity should result from the failure. In my opinion, if such double-agent problems exist, they should be openly discussed with the patient, even though such discussion can complicate the treatment. At least the revelation demonstrates the therapist's honesty. Sometimes a patient who has been found not guilty by reason of insanity is already in remission or under control, but nevertheless the courts and society want some punishment. Such situations can lead to ethical problems because courts and society may pressure the psychiatrist to say that the patient is unable to leave a maximum security setting regardless of the facts or the truth.

Violent patients are only one subgroup of personality disorders in a correctional setting. I have discussed their treatment in detail elsewhere.[51] Other patients with nonviolent personality disorders are also represented, as well as patients with superimposed acute and chronic psychiatric problems.

The goals of the correctional system can be to control inmate behavior at all costs, with total disregard for the psychological state of the offender or the potential of damage to him. Their methods include restraint, seclusion, or even excessive medication for sedation (or even for punishment). The therapist's goal may be the development of internal controls. Correctional staff may have no confidence in anything but external constraint. To the correction officer the worst result is prisoner escape; suicide is even preferable. To the therapist, these priorities are reversed. Such discrepancies in goals can lead to irreconcilable differences. It is hoped that an appropriate balance can be found between security and ego-strengthening activities, and an increased understanding between correctional and therapeutic staff.

Funds for treatment of offenders can be difficult to obtain. The corrections system as well as society have come to value containment, punishment, retribution, and deterrence far above treatment. Some newly trained psychiatrists have come to identify with the punitive aspects of society and have lost any feeling of ethical responsibility to their patients. Some are almost too ready to violate confidentiality or even to use deceptive means in order to get a patient punished.

Sometimes it is very difficult to distinguish between the psychotic and the criminal in a patient who has aspects of both. An interesting case example of this difficulty occurred on the minimum security ward in the San Francisco General Hospital:

> A 34-year-old man was admitted with a history of use of street drugs. He had been arrested for disturbing the peace but denied current drug usage. He said he needed to leave the hospital because there were Russian and Chinese agents who wanted to kill him. The CIA and FBI were also after him. He said he found this out from Russian and Chinese girlfriends, whom he figured out were agents. He declared he had only 30 more days to live and wanted to leave the hospital. He was treated with haloperidol. After a period of several days, he stole a nurse's keys and escaped from the hospital. Approximately one month later, I learned from the police that he had been brutally murdered, gangland style.

Although I still do not believe his story, the best way I can interpret it was that he was involved in drug dealing and/or drug using and had done something which led to the threats and to his eventual murder. He was delusional either because of schizophrenia or a chronic drug-induced psychosis. He knew he would be killed but fit that fact into his delusional system. His story illustrates how difficult it is for such cases to be interpreted with any degree of accuracy.

Treating patients who are psychotic and criminal can be a difficult and complex matter. However, the difficult is not the impossible. It is necessary for forensic psychiatrists to lend some balance and perspective to the situation. Despite the unpopularity and the frequent impossibility of treatment, forensic psychiatrists should combat therapeutic nihilism for these unpopular and difficult patients. Lack of resources is not equivalent to untreatability, and the distinction is important, because resources occasionally can become available. Research needs to be done, including efforts to develop improved research methodologies.

Another area in which forensic psychiatry can be helpful is in the development of outpatient commitment laws that will require patients who become dangerous to remain on medication or else be rehospitalized. Such laws have been adopted in Oregon. The excessive move toward deinstitutionalization, coupled with no community facilities and the unrealistic levels of proof required for involuntary hospitalization, has led to a group of patients who become predictably psychotic without medications, yet who are nevertheless released from hospitals because of the literal interpretations of the mental health law in states, like California, which require that such patients be a danger to themselves or to others, or be unable to provide food, clothing, and shelter for themselves on the day of release. Levels of proof in such cases are totally unrealistic. The U.S. Supreme Court, in *Addington v Texas*[52] stipulated clear and convincing as the required level of proof. However, if this decision were literally interpreted, it would mean that patients should be released if there was only a 50% chance of suicide or homicide, and there was an excellent chance that even a brief hospitalization would be significantly beneficial. But some such patients frequently become antisocial after stopping their medication. They can become involved instead with a much more punitive criminal justice system after they commit an act which is harmful to an innocent person. At times the law is totally unrealistic. Often and unfairly, psychiatrists are held to blame. By being put into these untenable situations, psychiatrists can be asked to be the "janitors" for the criminal justice system,[53] by being expected to make a system work, which has been made impossible by politicians and judges. Psychiatrists have little power but are made to shoulder most of the blame and may even be asked to make impossible predictions.

The treatment of antisocial and other personality disorders in a correctional system is a difficult task at a time when there is minimal support. However, as a profession, it is important for the psychiatrist to remain aware of the problem and to try to confront it when occasional and reasonable opportunities arise—or when society and the correctional system begin again to become less punitive and more humane—and to seek again for solutions that will attempt to accomplish treatment and rehabilitation.

REFERENCES

1. Luborsky L, Singer B, Lubrosky L: Comparative studies of psychotherapies: Is it true that "Everybody has won and all must have prizes?" *Arch Gen Psychiatry* 1975; 32:995–1008.
2. Parloff MB: Can psychotherapy research guide the policy maker? A little knowledge may be a dangerous thing. *Am Psychol* 1979; 34:296–306.
3. Strupp H, Hadley S, Gomes-Schwartz B: *Psychotherapy for Better or Worst: The Problem of Negative Effects.* New York, Jason Aronson, Inc, 1977.
4. Bergen A, Lambert M: The evaluation of therapeutic outcomes, in Garfield S, Bergen A (eds): *Handbook of Psychotherapy and Behavioral Change: An Empirical Analysis.* New York, Wiley, 1978.

5. Smith M, Glass G, Miller T: *The Benefits of Psychotherapy.* Baltimore, Johns Hopkins University Press, 1980.
6. Boyer L, Giovacchini P: *Psychoanalytic Treatment of Characterological and Schizophrenic Disorders.* New York, Science House, 1967.
7. Kernberg O: *Borderline Conditions and Pathological Narcissism.* New York, Jason Aronson, Inc, 1975.
8. Martin SE, Sechrest LB, Redner R (eds): *New Directions in the Rehabilitation of Criminal Offenders.* Washington, DC, National Academy Press, 1987.
9. Levine WR, Bornstein PE: Is the sociopath treatable? The contributions of psychiatry to a legal dilemma. *Wash U Law Q* 1972; 2:693–711.
10. Madden D: Psychotherapeutic approaches in the treatment of violent persons, in Roth L (ed): *Clinical Treatment of the Violent Person.* New York, Guilford Press, 1987, p 72.
11. Kegan R: The child behind the mask: Sociopathy as a developmental delay, in Reid W (ed): *Unmasking the Psychopath.* New York, W Norton & Co, 1986.
12. Piaget J: *The Construction of Reality in the Child.* New York, Basic Books, 1937.
13. Kohlberg L: *The Psychology of Moral Development,* vol 2. New York, Harper & Row, 1984.
14. Knight RP: Borderline states. *Bull Menninger Clin* 1953: 17:1–12.
15. Gunderson JG, Singer MT: Defining borderline patients: An overview. *Am J Psychiatry* 1975; 133:1–10.
16. Kozol HL, Boucher RJ, Garofalo RF: The diagnosis and treatment of dangerousness. *Crime Delinq* 1972; 18:371–392.
17. Monahan J, Klassen D: Situational approaches to understanding and predicting individual violent behavior, in Wolfgang ME, Weiner NA (eds): *Criminal Violence.* Beverly Hills, Sage Publications Inc, 1982, pp 292–319.
18. Carney FL: The indeterminate sentence at Patuxent. *Crime Delinq* 1974; 20:135–143.
19. Pollack S: Purposive concept of dangerousness, in Pollack S (ed): *Forensic Psychiatry and the Prediction of Dangerousness.* Los Angeles, University of Southern California Press, 1980, pp 7–25.
20. Monahan J: The prevention of violence, in Monahan J (ed): *Community Mental Health and the Criminal Justice System.* New York, Pergamon Press, 1975.
21. Sturup GK: *Treating the "Untreatable." Chronic Criminals at Herstedvester.* Baltimore, Johns Hopkins University Press, 1968.
22. British Home Office Department of Health and Social Security: *Report of the Committee on Mentally Abnormal Offenders.* London, Her Majesty's Stationery Office, Oct 1975, p 91.
23. Samenow SE: *Inside the Criminal Mind.* New York, Times Books, 1984.
24. Halleck SL, Witte AD: Is rehabilitation dead? *Crime Delinq* 1977: 23:372–382.
25. Roth L: Teaching violent persons in prisons, jails, and security hospitals, in Roth L (ed): *Clinical Treatment of the Violent Person.* New York, Guilford Press, 1987, pp 207–234.
26. Toch H: *Violent Men: An Inquiry into the Psychology of Violence.* Chicago, Aldine, 1969.
27. Rogers R, Cavanaugh JL: A treatment program for potentially violent offender patients. *Int J Offender Ther Comp Criminology* 1981: 25:53–59.
28. Valliant GE: Sociopathy as a human process: A viewpoint. *Arch Gen Psychiatry* 1975; 32:178–183.
29. Mathews W, Reid W: A wilderness experience treatment program for offenders, in Reid W (ed): *The Treatment of Antisocial Syndromes.* New York, Van Nostrand Reinhold, 1981.
30. Reid W, Solomon G: Community based offender programs, in Reid W (ed): *The Treatment of Antisocial Syndromes.* New York, Van Nostrand Reinhold, 1981, p 93.

31. Parson E: Manipulativeness in entrepeneurs and psychopaths, in Reid W (ed): *Unmasking the Psychopath.* New York, W Norton & Co, 1986, pp 256–274.
32. Diamond B: The simulation of sanity. *J Soc Ther* 1956: 2:1–3.
33. Guttmacher M: Pseudopsychopathic schizophrenia *Arch Crim Psychodynamics* (Special Psychopathy Issue) 1961; 502–508.
34. Havens L: *Participant Observation.* New York, Jason Aronson Inc, 1976.
35. Groves JE: Taking care of the hateful patient. *N Engl J Med* 1978: 298:883–887.
36. Adler G, Buie D: The misuses of confrontation in the psychotherapy of borderline cases, in Adler G, Myerson P (eds): *Confrontation in Psychotherapy.* New York, Science House, 1973, p 154.
37. Menninger K: *The Crime of Punishment.* New York, Penguin Books, 1968.
38. Halleck S: *Psychiatry and the Dilemmas of Crime.* Berkeley, University of California Press, 1967.
39. Ovesey L: *Homosexuality and Pseudohomosexuality.* New York, Science House, 1969.
40. Woods S: Violence: Psychotherapy of pseudohomosexual panic. *Arch Gen Psychiatry* 27:255–258, 1972.
41. Guze S: *Criminality and Psychiatric Disorders.* New York, Oxford University Press, 1976.
42. Blacker K, Tupin J: Hysteria and hysterical structure: Developmental and social theories, in Horowitz M (ed): *Hysterical Personality.* New York, Jason Aronson Inc, 1977, pp 122–123.
43. Chodoff P, Lyons H: Hysteria, the hysterical personality and hysterical conversion. *Am J Psychiatry* 1958; 114:734–740
44. Weinstock R, Nair A: Antisocial personality—Diagnosis or moral judgment? *J Forensic Sci* 1984; 29:557–565.
45. Strasburger L: The treatment of antisocial syndromes: The therapist's feelings, in Reid W (ed): *Unmasking the Psychopath.* New York, Van Nostrand Reinhold, 1981, p 206.
46. Lion L: Countertransference and other psychotherapy issues, in Reid W (ed): *The Treatment of Antisocial Syndromes.* New York, Van Nostrand Reinhold, 1981.
47. Madden D: Psychotherapeutic approaches in the treatment of violent persons, in Roth L (ed): *Clinical Treatment of the Violent Person.* New York, Guilford Press, 1987, p 54–78.
48. Weinstock R: Controversial ethical issues in forensic psychiatry: A survey. *J Forensic Sci* 1988; 33:176–186.
49. *Baxstrom v Harold,* 383 U.S. 107 (Feb 1986).
50. Monahan J: Prediction, research, and the emergency commitment of mentally ill persons: A reconsideration. *Am J Psychiatry* 1978: 135:198–201.
51. Weinstock R: Psychotherapy with violent patients, in Karasu T, Bellack L (eds): *Specialized Techniques in Individual Psychotherapy.* New York, Brunner/Mazel, 1980, p 236–257.
52. *Addington v Texas,* 411 U.S. 418 (1979).
53. Stone A: The ethics of forensic psychiatry: A view from the ivory tower, in Stone A (ed): *Law, Psychiatry and Morality.* Washington, DC, American Psychiatric Press, 1984, p 57–76.

4

The Role of the Forensic Psychiatrist in Jail and Prison Suicide Litigation

BRUCE L. DANTO

INTRODUCTION

Suicide in jail and correctional facilities is a type of death that easily becomes a matter of political charge and countercharge as well as of litigation. It should create an interest for the forensic psychiatrist because, as an expert witness, he will be called on by officers of the court to evaluate that death and render an opinion. An opinion by the forensic psychiatrist may pertain to whether or not appropriate standards of care were followed, or whether wanton and negligent violations of those standards by the holding agency were committed. In this type of litigation, a unit of government automatically becomes involved because it sponsors the creation and management of the facility, sets policy, and creates procedures to be followed by the staff.

In other regards, there may already have been a preexistent litigation against the jail or prison facility arising out of a class action suit. In such an instance, where a death occurs after the court has already intervened, a psychiatrist may then be asked to work as an assistant to the compliance officer to make sure that court-mandated changes in the correctional setting are carried out and have not been violated.

All too often, psychiatrists, and forensic psychiatrists in particular,

BRUCE L. DANTO • Patton State Hospital, Patton, CA 92569.

have sought out too little information or have not had sufficient experience with this type of death and the setting in which it occurs. Thus, few psychiatric experts have attempted to acquire the information or have been in a position to necessarily gain the kind of experience that would make it possible for them to assess death material and render an opinion about its connection and preventability in the jail setting.

It is hoped that the information contained in this chapter will offer the necessary background, provide an introduction to the law, and remedy issues regarding a growing type of death in the American correctional setting: suicide, the number one killer of inmates.

A number of suits have been filed against police agencies and state Departments of Correction since the early 1970s. Such suits have been field against local, state, and federal agencies in terms of suicide as a form of wrongful death action. When a lack of appropriate screening or treatment is involved, the suit can then take on the characteristic of being a violation of civil rights and can then become a federal issue.

Despite the historical position of the government's being immune to litigation for injury and wrongful death in the past, a near avalanche has shown this position to be undergoing considerable change. In point of fact, units of government have been sued effectively for any number of things, including jail suicide. Whenever violations of civil rights or tort actions are involved, government is being held responsible in what appears to be now a long line of cases that have established sufficient precedents. Notwithstanding the swelling tide of litigation against correctional facilities, the agencies that run those correctional facilities continue to resist, or fail to progress toward and develop interest in, an acceptance of learning about the contribution of psychiatry to suicide prevention. The agencies also seem unaware of the contribution of psychiatry to the recognition of signs of serious mental illness in those who are arrested. Compounding their weaknesses in these areas is a failure to recognize the usual signs of foreseeable suicide, notwithstanding the fact that such insights have been published certainly since 1973.

Government politicians seem to assemble all kinds of rationalizations as to why things cannot be done to prevent correctional suicides and the standards necessary to prevent them. Yet the beat goes on, and the deaths involving children, men, women, and citizens of all ages continue to rise at an alarming rate, indicating that something must be done to correct the problem.

It has been estimated, and figures seem to support the view, that jail suicides seem to occur three times more often than the normal population of between 12–13 per 100,000.[1,2] After some 80 cases in which I have personally been involved as an expert witness, the police departments appear to have finally gotten the message that the community will no longer tolerate suicide either in jail or in the police lockup setting. A similar trend can be noticed among prisons. I have participated in correctional officer training programs with the Texas Department of Corrections and the Michigan Department of Corrections, and it is quite apparent that both of these agencies, plus many others throughout the United States, are tightening up their assessment programs and trying to take some steps forward to create a system that will help prevent suicide among the inmates who inhabit their facilities.

I would like to offer some sample cases, with which I have had contact, that have been, or are currently being, litigated against units of government throughout the country. These are cases in which I have appeared as an expert witness. It is not my intention to reveal any and all details of these cases but rather to show the flavor as well as some common factors that underlie all of them. Furthermore, these illustrations do not reflect all of my particular experience in dealing with these situations but rather are intended to offer some idea about all that is involved.

FORESEEABLE SUICIDES

CASE 1

The deceased was a 15-year-old girl who was arrested for aggravated assault in a southwest state. She was admitted to a detention home following her arrest in April, 1981. She began starving herself by refusing food because she was trying to manipulate her way into a detention room that had a toilet. She was taken to the hospital twice for IV feedings and, when out of the detention facility, seemed to improve but threatened to resume her starvation campaign, if sent back, and did keep her word when they returned her to the detention home.

The decision was made not to place her in a psychiatric hospital because she had not been cooperative with psychotherapy in the facility. She was psychologically tested and found to be suffering from a severe oppositional disorder, and residential treatment was recommended. As her behavior continued to be oppositional and she was starving herself, she was placed in the psychiatric annex for observation.

Her psychiatrist felt that she would not take medication. A physician's assistant prescribed for her 30 Norgesic Forte tablets, a one-week's supply, as was the policy of the institution. She received a week's supply of medication, notwithstanding the known history that, in a four-year period, she had attempted suicide seven times, even while she was at a State hospital prior to her arrest. The physician's assistant was advised by the correctional staff that she had ingested the 30 Norgesic tablets. He felt that it was not necessary to do anything. This was at eleven o'clock in the morning.

He recommended that she be watched, and she was watched in terms of vital signs, until she went into convulsions and was taken to the Med unit at 2:10 PM, where she was admitted to an isolation cell and observed every 15 minutes. She expired later that afternoon despite efforts at CPR.

The issues in this case are substantially clear. The staff was totally aware of the girl's previous suicide-attempt history and placed in her hands the agent of her own death—the Norgesic Forte medication. The policy that made it necessary to give a week's supply of medication to a person who was suicidal is, at best, difficult to understand. The physician's assistant, who apparently made decisions on the basis of little information, if any, about suicide-risk assessment, made it impossible for any effective help to be present in order to prevent her death. To this day, that same physician's assistant is adamant in his statement that correctional facility policy was followed and that the deceased was given the proper amount of medication for her back strain.

CASE 2

A 22-year-old white male had a history of depression associated with a psychotic break some two years prior to his death. During a snowstorm in a northwestern state, he became very confused and disorganized and sat, during the blizzard, in the middle of a hospital parking lot without wearing his coat. As his behavior was bizarre and inappropriate, an officer responded to a call from the hospital receptionist, who saw him sitting in the middle of the blizzard. Despite the fact that psychiatric staff were available at the hospital, the arresting officer proceeded to apprehend the suspect without formally arresting him. The boy was placed in a lockup cell despite the protest of the boy's father, whom the officer had called, who verified the boy's psychiatric history and indicated that the boy's brother would be down to pick him up and return him home for medical care.

The officer acted as if he suspected drugs, searched the vehicle without benefit of a search warrant, and found the truck to be free of anything other than the material the boy was driving for delivery for his father.

The boy was then kept in the police lockup. When an officer received a call to go out on the road to take care of an accident, the boy pleaded not to be left alone in his cell as he couldn't stand being locked up. In this boy's cell was a piece of graffiti showing a figure hanging from a printed title underneath that said, "high justice."

The officer never did return to the station, as he was tied up to the end of his shift, and he instructed his replacement that there was a boy awaiting disposition in the jail. When the replacement officer returned to the jail, he found the young man had hanged himself with his shoelaces.

It was very apparent that the officer was untrained with regard to suicide and its prevention, had violated the boy's legal rights in terms of locking him up without a formal charge, had performed an illegal search of the vehicle, and had left this boy in a small completely unsupervised lockup facility.

Of interest in this case is the fact that a near-by sheriff's department was available by way of contractual services to monitor the cell with video. For one and one-half weeks preceding this boy's death, the monitoring equipment was broken down and was never repaired. Thus, the sheriff's department as well as the local police department were sued, and there were sufficient damages assessed to both following the litigation of the case.

CASE 3

In a large prison in a midwestern state, a 40-year-old black male became psychotic and was smearing feces all over the wall of his cell. He had just been sentenced to 40 years in prison following conviction of armed robbery. The man was forcibly removed from the jail cell by correctional staff and sent to a state forensic facility for observation and/or treatment. Some 90 days later, he was returned to the same jail cell, which was on the fourth floor of the prison. Two days later, without benefit of any follow-up psychiatric treatment or continuation of medication, the patient was observed by some inmates as he sat on the railing of the center open space that communicated with the first floor from the fourth tier. He leaned over backward and, as he began his descent down to the ground, smiled and waved at the prisoners on his way down. He died instantly as a result of massive cerebral trauma.

This man had been admitted to prison as a result of a plea-bargained defense of guilty but mentally ill. In this particular state, all this succeeded in bringing about was a single psychiatric interview at the time of his processing through the prison. There was no particular follow-up offered this type of mentally disturbed person, who apparently was psychotic but not considered to be not guilty by reason of insanity.

CASE 4

A 31-year-old white male was observed making an illegal turn by some police officers. When he was stopped, the officers observed that he was highly intoxicated. He refused to exit his van on demand of the officers. They forced entry and extracted him and then began to beat him alongside the van. This situation occurred in a large midwestern city. After the beating, the man fell down and was taken into custody.

Following his arrival at the central police station, he was again beaten. The brother of two other prisoners, who were being held in custody, arrived to pick them up and heard the beating, thinking that it was one of his brothers who was being beaten. He was arrested and charged with interfering with police work when he leaned over the counter to see what was happening. He was placed in a cell opposite the man who had been beaten twice.

A short time later, the visitor who had been recently arrested, thinking his brothers were being beaten, noticed that the man was removing his shirt and attempting to hang himself. Although the shirt tore initially, he repeated his efforts to hang himself and was successful. The newly arrested visitor yelled for an inordinately long period of time, but the police did not respond despite the fact that it was subsequently shown that the door was open between the booking cell and the row of custody cells, and his screams could have been heard through a closed door.

This death cost the city some $4 million in damages.

CASE 5

In a small neighborhood community, a 17-year-old boy was taken into custody for driving under the influence. He was a brilliant young high school student who had already been accepted by a college for a career in aeronautical engineering. He came fom a family which was very close and deeply religious. He and his father were very close.

Following the boy's arrest, one of his companions in the passenger seat vomited because he was so upset at being stopped by the police.

The officer, in investigating the car after it was returned to the police station, got some vomitus on his shirtsleeve. When he talked with the 17-year-old driver, he removed his shirt and gunbelt, leaving them on a chair in a small interviewing room while he went out to check on other prisoners and to offer assistance to the dispatcher, who was new on the job. Less than one minute after he left the room, all present heard the sound of a single gunshot. They returned to find the boy dead.

As a consequence of this tragic death, the police officer was fined 30 days by the mayor of his community. He has been totally destroyed despite the fact that he spent 23 years working as an officer in this community.

The father, who has not been able to come to terms with the death of his son, has been in and out of private psychiatric hospitals ever since.

The court was of the opinion that the negligence here was completely established.

CASE 6

On the West Coast, in a city with a moderate-sized population, a young black male was acting psychotic as he was coming down from a crack trip. At home he began crying and was confused, not recognizing his daughter's voice on the phone. He walked into his mother's room with a knife in one hand and a razor blade in the other, telling her he was thinking of killing himself because he couldn't stand the voices which were bothering him and threatening to kill him.

His mother called the local sheriff's department, which dispatched officers. The family and the man asked to be taken to a mental health facility, but he was taken to the jail instead because there was an outstanding warrant for his traffic offenses.

Following his booking, he began to complain of not being able to breathe and that there was too much noise in his cell, both of which were psychotic symptoms. A nurse was called, but when she finally arrived some 45 minutes later, the inmate appeared to be asleep. Instead of investigating, she apparently thought that this was a good opportunity to take care of some business.

Shortly thereafter, the man was found hanging.

These cases illustrate the fact that mentally disturbed persons do somehow wind up in custody either with the police or in prison. They also indicate that nice people can end up in custody even if the only thing they have done is something foolish, which is particularly applicable to those under the age of 22. From this material, it can be seen that screening forms can be useful in picking up early warning signs and significant history that should raise the suspicion of a potential suicide. Finally, in regard to those warning signs, it should be seen that professional and intelligent follow-up is necessary in order to make the screening form a viable tool in the prevention of suicide in the lockup.

In these police lockup cases, all of the suicides occurred very early following the booking. If anything is critical, it is that short period of time following the booking when such persons should be viewed closely for the first three hours. This would seem to be consistent with what I could consider to be the incarceration crisis. In the majority of the police lockup cases, none of the offenders was arrested because of a major crime, but many were alcohol-related causes and constituted the reason for arrest in the first place.

All the cases seem to show an absolute unawareness on the part of the arresting officers or the prison custody staff about what is involved in mental illness and psychiatric disease. If anything is proven, these cases reflect a total absence of effective training or sophistication on the part of the officers who are being asked to handle mentally disturbed persons without benefit of training or reasonable supervision. A complete lack of psychiatric information regarding the signs and identification of obvious psychiatric disease seems to exist, notwithstanding those officers who have been on the road for years or who have worked the cell blocks of a prison for years.

INFORMATION ABOUT JAIL AND INMATE SUICIDE

The cases that were examined should illustrate that suicide is an omnipresent threat to all staff who are responsible for the health and welfare of inmates. Certainly, one of the few efforts on the part of a national agency to gather such information was seen in the form of a report, published in 1980 by the National Center on Institutions and Alternatives,[3] which was able to establish a profile of lockup suicide. These were suicides in the police lockup. The report found that 73.6% of all prisoners of the suicide group were charged with crimes that were nonviolent. Alcohol and drug-related cases accounted for over 30% of the charges, and 60% of the suicide victims were under the influence of alcohol and/or drugs at the time of arrest and booking.

In terms of this study of some 419 suicides occurring in lockups in 1979, two of every three inmates who committed suicide were being held in isolation. Over 50% of the suicides died within the first 24 hours of incarceration, with 27% occurring within the first three hours. Over 88% of the inmates under the influence of alcohol and drugs at the time of booking committed suicide within the first two days of confinement. Over half of these victims were found dead within the first three hours of confinement. In 63% of the cases, the suicidal inmates were placed in isolation and committed suicide within the first 48 hours of incarceration, with over 30% dying within the first three hours.

In my book, *Jailhouse Blues,*[1] it was determined that, in the jail setting, the profile is a little different. There is a relationship between inmates admitted to the jail for violent personal crimes and suicide. This finding was replicated by other researchers in the same publication. Susan Martin, in her New York study,[4] showed that the vast majority of suicide victims were not charged with violent crimes. Almost all studies are in agreement that a crisis period occurs during the inmate's first three days in jail.

From the bibliography of my book, *Jailhouse Blues,* as well as the publications mentioned thus far in the References of this chapter, it is apparent that two suicide profiles emerge—at least in terms of my experience. The first profile concerns that of a police lockup type suicide. This profile involves a young white male under the age of 22, as a median age, who has been arrested for a relatively nonserious or nonviolent crime. He is intoxicated at the time of his arrest. Not reflected in the literature thus far, but seen in my experience as both a police officer and a forensic psychiatrist, is the fact that many of these suicides involve persons who are arrested because, in addition, they have become very confrontational and belligerent toward the investigating officers and frequently are assaultive as well. Usually, the suicide occurs after they are booked and placed in custody. The death often involves asphyxiation, primarily, as a result of the inmate's employment of some type of ligature material, such as a tee-shirt, regular shirt, shoelaces, or even underwear or socks. Drowning is very rare in the jail setting but is more common in the prison setting, along with jumping from a tier (as was detailed in Case 3 in the introduction) or self-immolation (setting oneself on fire).

Such suicides occur within the first three hours of arrest, following booking in the police lockup, and are more likely to happen if the inmate is placed in an isolation cell with poor supervision. The most likely type of person to commit suicide in the police lockup is the one who does not have a chronic history of criminal behavior and arrests, and who basically may be a very law-abiding person. When he is arrested, he feels impotent as a consequence of his contact with the police, after having discovered that he really cannot fight off efforts at arrest or incarceration. Perhaps, in a state of rage or helplessness, or because he feels great embarrassment over his arrest in terms of what impact it will have on his family, his plight becomes overinvested with more meaning than it should have, and he takes his life in order to end the pressure which he feels as a result of his incarceration. Police agencies should focus their attention on these types of arrested citizens. Unfortunately, the opposite is true, and they rarely receive much interest on the part of the police of the community in which they have been arrested.

The second major suicide profile involves a more serious type of offender, who is arrested by local police or sheriff's officers and confined in the sheriff's holding facility known as the jail. This type of person has committed a serious or violent crime, such as murder, rape, felonious assault, assault and battery, or breaking and entering. He will commit suicide by asphyxiation or hanging, almost always at night, between the hours of 11:00 PM and 6:00 AM, when supervision is at its lowest. Normally, this type of suicide will occur between two and three days following incarceration, or two months after confinement as trial approaches or sentencing has been completed, depending on the length of the court docket. Certainly suicide is an especially critical issue to assess with a high risk when the hope of release is lost. This may mean either a failure to obtain enough money to make bail, or, if sentence is imposed, it appears that the inmate is going to do hard time.

In the jail-setting type of suicide, as is the case with those doing hard time in prison, the most likely candidate is a member of a minority group. He is usually male; in the midwest and in the east, he will be black, and on the west coast, he will be Hispanic. In the southwest, American Indians are predominant among those who commit suicide. Usually, he will be older than the city lockup type of suicide, well over 22 years of age, more likely in his thirties. He will have a history of poor marital adjustment and unemployment as well. He may have a more serious degree of mental illness, including a frank psychosis, and his lifestyle will show a history of instability.

In an effort to deliver a profile of the suicidal inmate in Massachusetts,[6] data were gathered by questionnaire from 386 police departments pertaining to deaths from 1973 to 1984. Some 129 police departments denied having lockups, which seems incredible, as no department functions without some type of holding facility. Perhaps the questionnaire was faulty in not asking whether or not the local county jail was used. In response to this questionnaire, 153 police departments out of the 386 offered information. From this group, there were 69 suicides and 542 suicide attempts. The commission studied 54 suicides from this group.

The commission's profile of their suicidal individual was 32 years of age, white, single, and unemployed. These inmates had a history of criminal arrest, and were natives of the community. They were booked primarily for alcohol-related protective custody holdings, and, at the time of their bookings, seemed to be calm and free from obvious depression or disorientation. They were neat in appearance. No one appeared to be feeling ill at the time of the booking, and they used the phone to call friends and relatives. They suicided within two hours.

The profile of the suicide-attempt group was the same, except the age was 28 and they were hostile, uncooperative, and unkempt in their personal appearance. The suicide group used clothes to hang themselves and, at that time, three staff members were on duty before their deaths were discovered. They were evacuated to a hospital within ten minutes of discovery. The suicide attempts occurred between midnight and 6:00 AM on Saturday. The suicide group was checked between 16 and 30 minutes before discovery.

The commission also felt that if all intoxicated persons were removed from the lockup facility, suicide would be significantly reduced.

It is my feeling that this type of research is rather appalling because it offers no investigation of the deaths, does not examine records of the booking logs, does not contain information that would be available in a screening form or deposition of staff. In addition, it mentions nothing about the inability of the police to recognize suicide risk, particularly when within two hours of their deaths all the suicide cases were calm and appeared nondepressed. My experience as a police officer and a psychiatrist dictates that I absolutely cannot believe such a report. The information offered by way of answers to questionnaires was self-serving and was designed to create a good appearance. I felt that the police themselves answered with superficial insight.

Looking at the issues more closely, with three staff in attendance, how was it that these suicides occurred? It is known that alcohol intoxicated persons are most prevalent among those who commit suicide in the police lockups around the country. Having examined such suicides in three litigations in Massachusetts in particular, I know that such checks are not made within the time frame alleged in this study, that is, 15 to 30 minutes. I also know that those who are booked are often depressed and frequently resist arrest. Furthermore, those who plan suicide attempts do self-injury at all hours of the day, as do those committing suicide in the police lockup. Those who commit suicide between midnight and 6:00 AM are the ones that occur in jail and prison settings. In my opinion, the Massachusetts study is superficial, inaccurate, and worthless.

There are some communities in which the sheriff's department serves as the police lockup. In those instances, it would be important for correctional staff to realize that there may be a fusion, overlap, or even amalgamation of both primary suicide profiles. Either type profile may occur in such a holding facility.

At this point, we all must wonder why it is that persons arrested for crimes for which they may bail out at a low figure in a short period of time should end in their lives with suicide. Why should a person who is arrested for a crime which is nonviolent, and for which he may even be able to expunge the crime following conviction, develop such marked feelings of hopelessness or loss of interest in living that he has to end his misadventure with suicide? The answer to this question requires us to take a look at what impact an arrest has on a basically law-abiding person who has not gone through such an experience before.

When ordinary citizens are arrested, they frequently find themselves in a state of psychological shock, disbelief, and confusion, which to a considerable extent, becomes a form of psychic trauma. During this process, a psychic numbing occurs, and people will walk through the experience of being cuffed, fingerprinted, and assigned to a cell as if they were in the process of sleepwalking. It is a moment of an experience that has little emotional impact, and they function like automatons. At the time of their arrest and also at the time of their booking, many people are read their rights without fully realizing or grasping what the *Miranda* warning means. There are many who have to be led by the sleeve and are encouraged to step into the patrol car or into their cells following their booking. But for many people, filling out the booking questionnaire, if one exists, is very difficult because they are so internally preoccupied. Once they are placed into actual custody behind locked doors, however, it is as if they receive a slap in the face because it is at this point they recognize that their freedom has been lost. They have arrived at the end of the first phase of the arrest crisis.

In the second phase, particularly at the county jail level, the person who is arrested will develop significant anxiety because he is thrown into contact with people whose language is unfamiliar to him. He feels a growing sense of terror because of the possibility of gang rape and exploitation and because of the intimidation offered by other inmates who have more psychopathic or personality disorders and who, having been through the system many times, know how to use power within the incarceration setting. As this new inmate moves toward the preliminary hearing, his anxiety mounts and he makes desperate efforts to reach out for someone who might serve as a rescuer from his plight.

During his court hearing, the inmate will be able to assess his attorney, the judge, the prosecutor, and the witnesses and see evidence of his misdeeds in terms of physical evidence. He will then be bound over for trial and may hear a figure quoted for bail, which he never dreamed was possible to have in his possession at one time.

Following his return to the jail, he may receive further reason for concern from the "jailhouse lawyers" (other inmates), who will be prophets of doom with respect to his chances of achieving a successful defense in due course or in escaping imprisonment.

This stage heralds in the third phase of the incarceration process, where the new inmate begins to feel no sense of hope and may view suicide as his only means of escape from an intolerable circumstance. Up to this point, he may have felt so frustrated and anxiety-ridden that he becomes involved in fights with inmates or with staff and realizes that he is not going to be able to survive well with people who have learned how to fight out in the streets, long before he even considered such a necessity for himself.

And, of course, the fourth and final phase really concerns what happens to the new inmate when he finds himself in prison.

In my book, *Crisis Behind Bars,* I have summarized most of the significant studies regarding prison suicide.[2] In Canadian prisons from 1966 through 1976, the suicide rate was 95.9 per 100,000 inmates, in contrast to a nonprison population figure of 14.2 per 100,000. I also described how *Jerric,* a prison-focused magazine, documented over 400 suicides a year in detention homes, jails, and prisons in the United States. In my book, one study, involving 100 prisons in 28 states, revealed the suicide rate in prisons between 1952 and 1973 as 17.5 per 100,000 inmates. This rate is compared, for the same period, to the nonprison population in the United States of 11 per 100,000.

I also have provided details of a French study that compared suicide rates in prison and the general population from 1852 to 1974. These researchers found that suicide rates increased in the prison population, especially when prison populations decreased. In general, the prison suicide rate was two times greater than the rate for French nonprison male suicides.

I have also included a study from England, in my book, in which it was shown that the rate of suicide in prison in that country is three times greater than the rate for the population at large.

In my first book,[1] I reported that, in the federal prison system from 1950 to 1969, the rate of suicide was 2.1 per 20,000, or 10.5 per 100,000.

In the prison population, suicides are more apt to occur early during the period of incarceration, perhaps the first two months, and the method of choice is hanging. There seems to be no direct relationship between length of sentence and potential for suicide. The fact that federal prisoners may have a slightly lower suicide rate than those in state prisons may be due to the fact that most federal prisoners have sociopathic personalities or show strong sociopathic trends. This type of prisoner has no difficulty acting out aggression and is highly manipulative and survival oriented. Most of the studies of those who have gone through a prisoner-of-war experience, who are not officers, indicate that, among the best survivors of the period of incarceration, are those who have sociopathic personalities or strong traits. They spend their time tolerating pain well, being confrontational and manipulative, and are so opposed to authority that, during their confinement, this strategy becomes a reason for survival, that is to beat the system. Those who suicide in the prisoner-of-war experience are generally those who are the so-called normals, who are sensitive, and who really cannot tolerate the long period of forced isolation and estrangement from their family and friends.

THE LAW*

The forensic psychiatrist must be familiar with the laws and decisions regarding jail suicide if he is to testify. He must know the issues; otherwise, his testimony will be meaningless.

Basically, this section will deal with the case law that has been decided on the basis of both state law involving the legal concept of negligence and federal law concerning constitutional rights. Appropriate citations for each major area of law will be delineated.

In regard to state law, negligence must be something more than simple and must involve the concept of "deliberate indifference." Federal courts have held that mere negligence in providing medical care

*Much of the case law citation, providing actual argument with regard to the plaintiff's position on jail suicide, was generously rendered by Bruce C. Allen of Cleveland, Ohio, an eminent attorney with whom I have worked in behalf of the estates of persons who have committed suicide in the lock-up. His expertise in case law regarding this type of death is remarkable.

is an insufficient charge to create a constitutional violation. However, in some states, simple negligence may be a basis for a claim under state law.

The Eighth Amendment

The constitutional argument is clear: under the Eighth Amendment, prisoners have a right not to receive cruel or unusual punishment. This is interpreted to mean that prisoners are entitled to medical care. However, this amendment does not apply to pretrial detainees, because pretrial detainees cannot be punished at all, since they have not been sentenced.

The Fourteenth Amendment[7]

The courts have interpreted the due process clause of the Fourteenth Amendment to provide equal rights to medical care for pretrial detainees. From this, it can be seen that one can argue that a suicidal prisoner is a prisoner in need of medical care, including psychiatric care as a type of medical care. Failure to provide that care, under circumstances where it is obviously needed and where it is foreseeable, may amount to what has been referred to as "deliberate indifference."

Hirst v Gertzen[8] and *Patridge v Two Unknown Officers*[9]

From the standpoint of filing a lawsuit on behalf of a plaintiff's estate for a lockup or jail suicide, it is important to establish that the deceased was a sick person in need of close supervision. In the event that he has been seriously abused physically or verbally, this is an additional dimension that places those charged with his custody in a particularly bad light. Such abuse, both emotional and physical, may constitute a type of abuse and humiliation that could have provoked the suicide. Aside from the provocative act on the part of the custodial staff, it also should follow that the officers failed to prevent the suicide.

The failure to prevent a suicide may also involve gross deficiencies in jail administration wholly separate from the active misconduct of individual officers. It may be in terms of what was mentioned before: a failure to establish minimally adequate procedures to screen, calssify, and observe prisoners in the custody or holding setting. It may also involve a failure to establish appropriate monitoring procedures or written policies and procedures that would tie up the total package of reasonable standards of care as regards observation and suicide prevention.

Fourteenth Amendment,[7] *Tennessee v Garner,*[10] *Bell v Wolfish,*[11] and *Wilson v Beebe*[12]

If physical abuse has been involved in the arrest of a prisoner and in the care following his arrest, then it can be argued that his right to be free from the use of unreasonable or excessive force during his arrest has been violated. This right is grounded in the Fourth Amendment, which prohibits unreasonable seizures, *Tennessee v Garner,* and in the Fourteenth Amendment, which prohibits the infliction of any punishment of a pretrial detainee, *Bell v Wolfish.* It is also grounded in the due process concept of the right to enjoy the security of life and limb established in *Wilson v Beebe.*

City of Revere v Massachusetts General Hospital,[13] *Estelle v Gamble,*[14] and *Partridge v Two Unknown Officers of the City of Houston, Texas*[9]

When medical care is indicated, either because of a psychiatric condition (for example, the arrested subject fits a well-established suicide profile), or obvious signs of mental illness, or even simple intoxication (as occurs with most arrests), the failure to provide medical care may violate rights based on the due process clause. The latter clause requires government agencies to provide medical care to pretrial detainees, *City of Revere v Massachusetts General Hospital.* These rights are as great as those established by *Estelle v Gamble* and apply to mental as well as physical needs, *Partridge v Two Unknown Officers of the City of Houston, Texas.*[9]

Martin v White[15]

Municipal officials are required to operate a lockup in a manner that reasonably protects the health and welfare of pretrial detainees without regard even to active misconduct on the part of one of its employees. This means that persons arrested on suspicion of some wrongdoing are entitled to the right to be protected as regards body security, freedom from punishment, and to have medical assistance available, *Martin v White.* In the latter case, the court expressed the view that a jail manager must develop policies to classify and observe prisoners, to provide physically safe cells, and to protect them from attack by other prisoners. Liability can be established on the basis to develop such policies and to provide procedures without any involvement of actual misconduct by staff.

Rymer v Davis[16]

In the event that the target of litigation is a police department which provides inexperienced officers without adequate training to basic patrol, the same police agency may find itself charged with circumstances that would lead one to conclude that such officers would predictably overreact to provocation. This issue was discussed in *Rymer v Davis.*

Marchese v Lucas,[17] *Black v Stephens,*[18] and *Herrera v Valentine*[19]

In the event that it can be demonstrated that a police department gives tacit approval of the use of excessive force, by failure to adequately investigate or supervise officers who are offending citizens in this manner, then the department may be held liable also under *Marchese v Lucas, Black v Stephens,* and *Herrera v Valentine.*

Dewell v Lawson,[20] *Soto v City of Sacramento,*[21] and *Watson v McGee*[22]

If the police agency in question maintains any policy of assigning jail personnel without benefit of training in suicide prevention or any other aspect of jail administration, they may have to face the charge of negligence on this basis, as seen in *Hirst v Gertzen.*[8] Not uncommonly, there is, in most states, an agency that oversees the administration of corrections at the state, county, and local levels. Periodic inspections are conducted, and reports are issued to the administrator of the lockup facility. If such findings reveal the failure to provide a reasonably safe environment for pretrial detainees, then responsibility may be established, as was the decisions in *Martin v White*[15] and in *Dewell v Lawson,* a case that involved the failure to establish procedures to train jail personnel to recognize symptoms of diabetic coma. In *Soto v City of Sacramento,* the issue of suicide-proof cells was raised, and fire hazards with regard to jail assignment and safety were discussed in the case of *Watson v McGee.* These cases also apply to situations involving the failure on the part of a police agency to establish health-screening procedures and to ensure adequate communication in a physically remote cell block, either by audio monitoring or of video monitoring of the catwalk.

McKinnon v City of Berwyn[23]

The case law in regard to liability derived from the failure to supervise and train is seen as a measure of negligence and was discussed in *Marchese v Lucas,*[17] *McKinnon v City of Berwyn,* and in *Hirst v Gertzen.*[8] It is important to understand that negligence constitutes an appropriate standard by which to evaluate the breakdown of a system, even when an individual staff person within the system has no evil intent to violate an incarcerated person's rights.

Oklahoma City v Tuttle,[24] *Brandon v Holt*[25]

In the case of *Oklahoma City v Tuttle,* the Supreme Court held that a municipal liability could not be based on a single isolated incident of police brutality without proof of any failure as regards supervision or training. A similar finding was held in *Brandon v Holt* (especially footnote 6). In both cases, the Supreme Court held that negligence was established on the basis of failure to achieve standards of supervision and training.

In *Marchese v Lucas,*[17] it was held that governmental authorization for illegal acts may be seen when there is a failure to adequately investigate and punish employees responsible for the very incident in question.

Drake v Handman[26]

At times, a court may decide on bifurcation of the trial of individual defendants from the trial of the city. Some city jurisdictions press for settlement of the basic question of excessive force so as to resolve the issue of the city's responsibility for a suicide. In a brief submitted by Bruce Allen in regard to a case, he urged the court to try all issues in one proceeding. He cited *Drake v Handman,* in which it was held that a single trial was more desirable when there are multiple claims involving different people doing different things but all of which arise out of the same underlying events.

The United Mineworkers v Gibbs,[27] *Posen v ABC Motor Court Hotel,*[28] and *Falkenstein v City of Bismarck*[29]

Relevant to the above point is the fact that, in *The United Mineworkers v Gibbs,* the court has undisputed jurisdiction to hear and resolve claims because they arise from the same set of facts. Each state has citations bolstering the idea that the city will be liable for the torts of its employees committed within the scope of the employment. Such a decision was verified in the case of *Posen v ABC Motor Court Hotel.* Admittedly, suicide is a novel application to negligence principles. However, these principles have been well covered by case law and may be seen in such cases as *Falkenstein v City of Bismarck.*

In the same vein, the case of *Partridge v Two Unknown Officers of the*

City of Houston, Texas,[9] plus the host of other cases already cited, very clearly recognizes the cause of action when a prisoner's death occurs by suicide as a result of the negligence or deliberate apathy on the part of jailers.

Wesley Roberts v City of Troy and Forrest Fisher Jointly[30]

In a case with which I was intimately connected as an expert for the defense, *Wesley Roberts, in behalf of the estate of David Roberts v City of Troy and Forrest O. Fisher jointly*, it was decided that the mere failure of a jailer to comply with the state regulation is not a constitutional violation. The latter point was cited in terms of 42 United States Code Annotated, and it has one of those legal sections in 1983. In addition, the court felt that, despite offers on the part of the Michigan Department of Corrections to provide a training course in suicide detection and prevention, some six months before Roberts' death at the City of Troy County Jail, the police department had no required pretrial detainee screening for suicidal tendencies. Thus, the failure to screen Roberts was consistent with a nonscreening policy. It was felt that the failure to screen Roberts could be deemed random and unauthorized.

It should be pointed out that the Roberts case opposes most other decisions and, in regard to the need for screening newly booked inmates, violates all recommendations of those in the field of suicide prevention, including the recommendations of the American Medical Association, the American Corrections Association, and the American Jail Association. Opposing this case, as well, is the National Institute of Corrections.

Metzner and Dubovsky[31] offered a very comprehensive set of guidelines regarding the evaluation of a prison mental health system involved in litigation. They said that such litigation basically can be viewed in three different stages. The first stage involves proving the alleged constitutional inadequacies of the current mental health system in prison. The second stage is a remedial one; the state is ordered to develop a constitutionally adequate mental health program for inmates. The third stage is an evaluation of the state's compliance with implementing the remedial plan. Testimony by experts assumes a significant role during all three stages.

In order for an expert to make an assessment of mental health care for a correctional institution, he, first of all, must be familiar with the various published standards and manuals regarding mental health care for a correctional institution. He must be aware of the fact that little is published directly on what the role of a psychiatrist is within the mental health system.

A variety of different models can be used to create a constitutionally adequate psychiatric treatment system for inmates. Such models should include provision for: (1) psychiatric or other mental health services as a part of a general medical care delivery system; (2) mental health services by a psychology department that is administratively independent of the medical department; (3) mental health services through a psychology department as well as a psychiatric division of a general medical service; the policies and procedures differentiate mental health services through the medical department from the correctional and/or rehabilitative services through a psychology department; and (4) mental services through a separate mental health department but closely coordinated with the medical department of the institution.

A system that is centralized, wherein the health care authority works at the departmental level, is more administratively sound than having the director of a mental health services directly responsible to the superintendent of the institution. It provides more power and independence to negotiate for an adequate budget at the departmental level.

The expert or psychiatric consultant needs to be familiar with the constitutional deficiencies in the prison's psychiatric services and must review all reports of previous evaluations of the medical and mental health systems. His review of records should focus on issues of housing, procedures for prescribing and administering psychotropic medications, administrative organization of the mental health system, and psychiatric liason issues involving the medical department. The proposed mental health plan, which is really a proposed remedy to the pertinent constitutional deficiencies, needs to be carefully reviewed. The expert should assess the particular mental health needs of the prison population, and adequate study is required to insure that projected staffing patterns of the mental health system are reasonably sound.

Remedial mental health planning should include reference to the goals of the mental health system, reliable and valid plans for identifying the severely disturbed inmate, as well as providing appropriate treatment. They should address the issue of confidentiality of information obtained during the diagnosis and treatment, the issue of involuntary treatment—including the use of restraints and seclusions—and the administrative organization of the mental health system. Along with this material, there should be job descriptions of the mental health staff and provision for a formal training program of the correctional staff regarding mental health issues. Anything less than these levels of focus, in my judgment, represents an inadequate plan. This would certainly be true of any of us in the field who have done such assessments.

The medication distribution system should be in compliance with legal and professional practice standards, and provision should be made for treatment plans to address appropriate housing and work assignment limitations.

In matters of evaluating issues of compliance, it should be emphasized that the consultant, who is evaluating such issues, should repeat many of the steps already recommended before visiting the prison. He needs to be thoroughly familiar with the accepted mental health plan. Evaluating compliance requires several different site visits in order to become familiar with the functioning of the prison system and the mental health system within it. Visits should not be limited to daytime activities, and there should be contact with the system at night to assess the crisis services available to inmates.

If it should happen that there are barriers to the evaluation, then this in and of itself is a frequent sign that the system is not in compliance with the court-ordered mental health plan. Such barriers include having a planned site visit cancelled with very little notice because of scheduling conflicts or visits that require official clearance.

Key people should be interviewed and among these should be the chief of psychiatry, the superintendent of the prison, the medical director, the head nurse, selected inmates, and correctional officers. Contact with the superintendent should help clarify some of the administrative efforts related to the effective operation of the mental health system.

Getting the other side of the program can only come by way of interviews with inmates, and this should be done on both a random and preselected basis. Metzner and Dubovsky recommend that inmates should be questioned about the kind of treatment they receive individually, their knowledge of inmates who appear to be mentally ill and who are not receiving treatment, and their general impressions regarding the availability and quality of the mental health services in the prison.

Since this can be very useful, the consultant should walk the tiers of the cell blocks in order to attempt to talk to every inmate on that tier. Also, it is important for the consultant to assess the administrative segregation and the protective custody as a result of such walks. The consultant should make very clear the purpose of the discussion, and, once this is done, inmates are usually willing to answer questions openly.

Informal discussions with frontline security staff and with various shift captains are also beneficial. Such staff will frequently help pinpoint areas of noncompliance and will describe their working relationship with the mental health staff.

I have found my reviewing the mental health records to be very helpful when such records involve inmate care. It helps to show something about the professional level of treatment as well as the quality of the recording, and also helps to verify stories that may be shared by inmates in order to achieve a level of credibility about what is being recorded and what is being told. Particular attention should be given to documentation of the treatment plans and the confidentiality of the reports.

Finally, the compliance assessment for prison mental health systems should include a comparison of the operating budget of the mental health system with the originally proposed budget. This information can be very important and may show discrepencies, which again will help pinpoint areas of noncompliance. Generally, the originally proposed budget is a reflection of what was felt to be minimally required to achieve a mental health service. If the true budget falls short of this, it means that services will fall short of what is required and what has been proposed.

SUICIDE PREVENTION PROGRAMS IN JAIL AND PRISON

Having been involved in some 80 cases of litigation regarding suicide in jail and prison, I have arrived at a point where I feel that it is vital for the institutions in question to have written policies and procedures concerning those citizens who are kept in their custody. This is not only my experience but is also what the courts have decided at the class action and compliance level regarding jail and prison suicide. This basic factor is in compliance with the standards written by the American Medical Association in September, 1981, which has also been approved by the National Sheriffs' Association, the American Corrections Association, the Commission On Accreditation for Corrections, and the American Medical Association House of Delegates.

Of importance has been the need for medical autonomy to assure a quality and well-organized medical intervention in those instances in which health issues are presented by incoming and regularly maintained inmates. It is also felt that there should be administrative meetings and reports relative to the way the health unit is conducting its activities.

Incarceration agencies, such as prisons, jails, and police lockups, present an extremely unprofessional image if they omit developing a written set of guidelines in reference to policies and procedures. Furthermore, such essential policies and procedures regarding training, screening, booking, and referral for health assessment and classification should be kept in a book, which can be passed out to members of the correctional staff.

Because I have been active in teaching such guidelines to correctional agencies, I feel that any training syllabus should contain the following points: (1) an introduction to suicide facts and theory; (2) the psychological impact of arrest; (3) the value of the booking procedure;

(4) a screening for suicide risk; (5) the importance of classification; (6) the crisis intervention techniques; (7) the need for training of correctional staff; (8) what happens after the suicide in terms of the survivors usually involving friends, family, and officers; (9) suicide litigation and the correctional setting, issues and standards; and (10) the clinical case presentations and the psychological autopsies.

I would recommend regular refresher courses for supervisory personnel in the correctional setting, because there is a promotional and retirement turnover of supervisors, and each new group should be well oriented toward the cause and management of potential suicide among inmates.

The booking phase of the initial contact by the corrections agency with the inmate is of consequence in the jail and in the prison settings, because it is the most important screening opportunity. At this time, a screening should be done on a form which requires the inmate to answer questions, either by writing out the answers or by having the booking officer circle the correct answers on a preprinted sheet. I feel that the form, which is adopted for this purpose, should be standardized, so that each member of the booking staff covers the same basic ground with each inmate. The form should also provide an opportunity to circle standardized observations of the inmates. I have devised such a form, and it was made a part of the court order for the Santa Clara County Jail in California.

In my opinion, it is not enough to have a screening form without some opportunity to elicit information from the arresting officer, if a jail is involved, or from the jail staff, if the inmate is transferred to a prison. There should be another sheet attached, which can be stapled to or become a part of the screening form, in which the referring officer answers a few questions regarding his observations about the mental state of the arrested person; whether that person had verbalized thoughts about suicide or whether some family member or witness had heard some comment by that person to the effect that he would commit suicide or has attempted suicide in the past. It is important for the referring officer to know if the subject was physically confrontational and challenged the authority of the officer during the arrest or the transfer to prison. This information is particularly significant for those inmates, in the police lockup suicide profile, who have shown resistance, who feel impotent following their arrest, and who then commit suicide as a way of achieving potency through death.

Once sufficient criteria have been established by way of the inmate's response to the screening form, the supervising officer of the day, usually a sergeant, should be alerted so that the inmate can be classified into an area of the lockup where very close monitoring will take place and be maintained with absolute regularity. Correctional staff should be alert to the risk of suicide if the inmate shows an uncooperative attitude or is very belligerent in the booking area and refuses to give any information or will not talk at all. When people do not talk following an arrest or a transfer to a prison, they should be watched very closely as they may attempt to commit suicide.

A classification system with procedures and policies should be spelled out in the departmental manual concerning the placement of persons who are considered to be a high-risk suicide. The classification regarding this type of inmate should be closely coupled with another important aspect of the entire process, namely, monitoring.

Along with the crisis of arrest, there is also the crisis of transfer to a prison. Inmates are often filled with anxiety about the possibility of homosexual assault as well as their loss of contact with family and their social isolation. Particularly, if they have not been chronic offenders and are unfamiliar with the criminal justice system, this can become a very crucial interval in their introduction to the facility, where they will be housed for a given period of time.

Anybody who is considered to be a suicide risk should be placed in a mental health unit, regardless of whether it is in the jail or in a prison. If the person is going to be bonded out in the jail setting, he can be kept under close scrutiny or can be placed in a cell, with an audio monitor or a video camera focused on the catwalk side of the cell where the bars are, so that officers can see if anything is tied to a bar—a possible portent of a self-destructive gesture.

It is apparent to most of us who have been in the corrections field that electronic surveillance is not very reliable. Monitoring units malfunction and are not repaired, and those whose ears and eyes are supposed to be tuned in to either an audio or visual monitor soon become insensitive to the noises as they concentrate on performing other chores. Thus, there is no substitute for eyeball monitoring, where the officer who is responsible for this duty not only visits each cell holding a potentially suicidal inmate, but also records the time of the visit. In my experience with suicide lawsuits, there has been substandard eyeball monitoring prior to the inmate's suicide. Subsequent to that suicide, the jail staff may scurry around trying to falsify records with regard to the frequency of visits. Invarriably the officers make mistakes on these cases, in which the log otherwise clearly reflects the properly recorded time, which can look very bad in court. If the jail has been substandard in most of its operations, the jury has no trouble with the idea that there has been an effort to try to obstruct justice in this manner.

Once the judgment has been made by a mental health professional that a given inmate is a suicide risk, then the next remedy should be the availability of mental health staff or mental health-oriented personnel, for example, psychiatric nurses, who should immediately interview the inmate. A considerable number of lawsuits have been successfully filed and litigated around this very point; namely, resource staff were available but were delayed beyond what is considered to be a reasonable time period in getting to the inmate to conduct the evaluation. One recent example of this problem was seen in a jail, in a western state, where an inmate was observed by a correctional officer to be crying. The inmate was placed in a security room and the officer went to the medical module to request a psychological evaluation for the depressed inmate. For reasons not quite clear, the evaluation was delayed for one hour, and when the nurse arrived at the security cell, she found that the patient had hanged himself.

If the person assigned to do the mental screening feels that the inmate has significant psychopathology, then there has to be some arrangement for either a staff psychiatrist or a community mental health facility, or a general hospital emergency room that has a psychiatrist who can perform a professional review of the inmate's history and behavior regarding treatment and/or custody.

Consistent with the historical tradition of the medical profession, it is then a longstanding policy to conduct autopsies following the death of an inmate, particularly one that has occurred under rather suspicious circumstances. In keeping with that tradition, I would recommend a psychological autopsy to see if it is possible to reconstruct the events and factors that may have been known or missed, which might have led to that inmate's death. Through the psychological autopsy, it may be possible to see if some new factor, which has some predictive factor regarding suicide, can be identified properly.

Not uncommonly, correctional staff who have experienced a suicide of an inmate should have an opportunity to receive emotional support from the mental health staff to help them with feelings of guilt or resentment they may feel toward the person who has committed suicide under their supervision. All too often, correctional officers are left bereft of any support of this type, as it is generally assumed in most correctional agencies that officers do not have feelings and it is enough to be a well-disciplined person operating within the terms and structures of a paramilitary agency. I have worked with many officers who have experienced significant stress as a consequence of dealing with suicide, sometimes more than one with their background.

Audio and video monitoring must be kept operational. Video monitoring can offer problems because of the blind spots in the corner of the room that may be dark. Thus, an inmate may asphyxiate out of view of the camera because he chooses an area that is not well lighted. Similarly, hanging is not always noisy, and auditory monitors can miss this action of self-destruction. In addition, because inmates are rather noisy, correctional staff may turn off the audio monitoring because it interferes with their thinking about the other routine assignments they have to complete.

Staff who operate audio and video monitoring equipment must be mindful of the fact that, after a period of time, the officer assigned to watch this equipment may begin, unconsciously, to tune out significant noises, such as cries for help, or may even tune out viewing an inmate attempting to tie a towel or a T-shirt to a bar of his cell. The more duties this officer is assigned during his shift, the less likely it will be that he pays careful attention to his monitoring assignment.

Some attention needs to be paid to the suicide-proofing of the architecture of the facility that houses inmates. Plastic shieldguards should be added to the top portion of the bars so that inmates cannot reach up to these high levels to attach something to the top of the horizontal locking bar. There should be repair and sealing off of all water pipes and heating ducts so that they do not appear in the cell to serve as something around which to attach a ligature. Restraining screens or plastic shields above the guardrails should be present to prevent jumping, and laundry chutes should have locked doors or covers. The cells should be well lighted, have cheerful colors on the wall, preferably with some artwork. The artwork should possibly be done by inmates themselves who have some interest as well as talent in this type of decoration. The themes of such artwork should convey a mood of hope and humanization.

From a broad administrative standpoint, good and effective prison and jail architecture should be complimented to efforts to reduce overcrowding, because crowding can spread a negative physical and psychological effect on the whole inmate population. Large institutions produce more psychological and physical stress than do smaller ones.

Wards or blocks broken up into smaller dormitories with private cubicles have a marked effect in reducing the stresses of psychological and physical symptoms that are associated with self-destructive behavior. When inmates are alloted spaces of at least 50 square feet each, they get along better, and stress factors are reduced. It should be emphasized that, notwithstanding the importance of architecture, for the inmate who is admitted to a jail or a police lockup during a crisis period, more is needed than simply architecture and screening forms. There has to be an active interest and skill on the part of the correctional officers to maintain dialogue with the newly arrived inmates to insure, not only what they have watched, but also what they feel is a level of interest on the part of those who are charged with their care. There has to be more of an interchange, not simply having a man fill out a questionnaire, and this is part and parcel of an effective suicide prevention program.

CONCLUSION

It appears that suicide in jail and in prison is a form of death that has many determinants. The emotional impact of incarceration is often significant in bringing about this type of death. Suicide is also associated with a background of social isolation on the part of the offender, guilt feelings about the crime, hurt to the family, and an inability to adjust to the world in general.

Juveniles in an adult facility not only run the risk of homosexual rape but such stress factors as guilt for letting their parents down, which may ultimately be dealt with through suicide. Furthermore, it is important that correctional officers stand by a policy, which should be in writing, concerning the prohibition of the use of handcuffs for juveniles, unless they are unruly or unmanageable. Juveniles should not be placed in a jail cell and should not be left alone, without rather constant supervision during the booking, because they tend to be more volatile and impulsive in regard to suicide, as a means of coping with feelings of hopelessness about the future and with fear of facing their family, even in light of a minor crime.

Jail inmates have not been able to deal with stress on the outside, and it is no less true that, once they are in a holding facility or prison, they cannot contend with that stress either. This is a factor that, in itself, makes suicide in jail or prison almost predictable.

Certainly, the suicide profile regarding those most likely to commit suicide was covered in this chapter. Once the inmate is admitted who fits the profile, whether it be jail or prison, appropriate monitoring should be employed to insure that the inmate survives the crisis experience of his arrest.

Unquestionably, in the absence of electronic monitoring, such a potential suicide risk should be kept in a holding cell, in full view of the booking officer, during his stay in jail, or upon his entrance into the classification system in prison. That he should be checked every 15 minutes is a reasonable standard, which is not only my recommendation but also has the backing of the American Corrections Association and the American Jail Association, as well as orders issued by the courts in class-action lawsuits.

The entire correctional staff and inmate population can work toward an effective suicide prevention program if all parties can achieve an understanding of the agreement to preserve all lives. Better career hopes may be helped by developing skills to render suicide prevention services to inmates. The jail administrative staff and the prison administrative staff can maintain a better public image if the community and the bodies governing those agencies know that the lives of all inmates will be protected. Suicide prevention helps the jailer realize the goal that he sought by choosing law enforcement, namely, helping others and saving lives.

Regardless of the plaintiff's or the defendant's position, to successfully litigate a jail or prison suicide case from the presence of records and witnesses is not enough. Professional opinion from a forensic psychiatrist, concerning the dynamic factors in the case before the bench, and what can be done versus what was done to prevent the suicide are the major issues.

It is essential that a forensic psychiatrist possess the experience and knowledge about jails and prisons, law enforcement, and the incarceration setting for his opinion to carry any weight in a courtroom. Such an expert must know about inmates and the emotional impact of an arrest, especially for the citizen who has not been exposed to the criminal justice process before.

All of this information, regardless of the legal issues involved, is almost meaningless, as an opinion of value for either plaintiff or defendant, unless it is rendered within the appropriate legal concepts. No expert besides the forensic psychiatrist is capable of working on such a case as this, because the forensic psychiatrist possesses all the attributes of the expert witness who has skills and responsibility to aid the court in rendering a judgment about the cause of jail or prison suicide. He knows what standards of care are required in jails and prisons to prevent suicides, and whether gross or wanton negligence was shown by the jail or the prison staff in breaching an acceptable standard of care for such police-custody programs.

REFERENCES

1. Danto BL (ed): *Jail House Blues—Studies of Suicidal Behavior in Jail and Prison.* Orchard Lake, Mich, Epic Publications, 1973.
2. Danto BL: *Crisis Behind Bars—The Suicidal Inmate.* Troy, Mich, The Dale Corporation, 1981.
3. Hayes LM Kajdan B: *And Darkness Closes In . . . National Study of Jail Suicides.* Washington, DC, National Center on Institutions and Alternatives, 1981.
4. Martin S: *Prison Suicide Study.* New York, Health Services Administration, 1971, p 3.
5. *Suicide in Massachusetts Lockups, 1973–1984.* Commonwealth of Massachusetts Special Commission to Investigate Suicide in Municipal Detention Centers, 1984.
6. U.S. Const. amend. XIV.

7. *Hirst v Gertzen,* 676 F.2d 1252 (9th Cir. 1982).
8. *Partridge v Two Unknown Officers of the City of Houston, Texas,* 751 F.2d 1448 (5th Cir. 1985).
9. *Tennessee v Garner,* 105 S. Ct. 1694 (1985).
10. *Bell v Wolfish,* 441 U.S. 520, 99 S. Ct. 1861 (1979).
11. *Wilson v Beebe,* 743 F.2d 342 (6th Cir. 1984).
12. *City of Revere v Massachusetts General Hospital,* 103 S. Ct. 2979, 2983 (1983).
13. *Estelle v Gamble,* 429 U.S. 97, 104, 97 S. Ct. 285 (1976).
14. *Martin v White,* 742 F.2d 469 (8th Cir. 1984).
15. *Rymer v Davis,* 754 F.2d 198 (6th Cir. 1985).
16. *Marchese v Lucas,* 758 F.2d 181 (1985).
17. *Black v Stephens,* 662 F.2d 181 (3rd Cir. 1981).
18. *Herrera v Valentine,* 653 F.2d 1220 (8th Cir. 1981).
19. *Dewell v Lawson,* 489 F.2d 877 (1974).
20. *Soto v City of Sacramento,* 567 F. Supp. 662, 682 (E.D. Cal. 1983).
21. *Watson v McGee,* 527 F. Supp. 234 (S.D. Ohio, 1981).
22. *McKinnon v City of Berwyn,* 750 F.2d 1383, 1391 (7th Cir. 1984).
23. *Oklahoma City v Tuttle,* 105 S. Ct. 2427 (1985).
24. *Brandon v Holt,* 106 S. Ct. 873 (1985).
25. *Drake v Handman,* 30 F. R. D. 394, 397 (S.D.N.Y. 1962).
26. *The United Mineworkers v Gibbs,* 383 U.S. 715, 86 S. Ct. 1130 (1966).
27. *Posen v A.B.C. Motor Court Hotel,* 45 Ohio St.2d 427, 740.0 2d 427 (1976).
28. *Falkenstein v City of Bismark,* 268 N.W. 2d 787 (N.D. 1978).
29. *Wesley Roberts, in behalf of the estate of David Roberts v City of Troy and Forrest O. Fisher jointly,* No. 83–1134–773, Federal Reporter, Second Series (1985).
30. Meetzner, JD, Dubovsky SL: The role of the psychiatrist in evaluating a prison mental health system in litigation. *Bull Am Psychiatry Law* 1986; 14(1):89–95.
31. *American Medical Association Standards for Health Services in Jails.* American Medical Association, 1981.

5

The New York State Model of Suicide Prevention and Crisis Intervention with Local Jails and Police Lockups

GERALD LANDSBERG, JUDITH F. COX, DENNIS W. McCARTY, AND M. PETER PARAVATI

INTRODUCTION

Jails and lockups function primarily to address the immediate detention and/or short-term detention needs of the host community. Nevertheless, these facilities are among the most neglected community institutions within our nation. This lack of attention is surprising because jails serve as the central intake point for the entire criminal justice system and are a virtual microcosm of the problems faced by society as a whole. In that role, these facilities hold persons with a multitude of problems and needs. Typical populations include the homeless, the mentally ill, the intoxicated, and runaway juveniles. These people are at high risk for committing suicide.

GERALD LANDSBERG • New York City Department of Mental Health, Mental Retardation and Alcoholism Services, New York, NY 10038. **JUDITH F. COX** • Bureau of Forensic Services, New York State Office of Mental Hygiene, Albany, NY 12209. **DENNIS W. McCARTY** • State Law Enforcement Accreditation Program, New York State Division of Criminal Justice, Albany, NY 12207. **M. PETER PARAVATI** • Medical Review Board, New York State Commission of Correction, Albany, NY 12207. The material in this chapter does not reflect the official policy of the authors' agencies.

During recent years, the incidence of jail and police lockup suicides has grown significantly. This trend has greatly heightened concern among correctional and police officials. It has also clearly reinforced the need for enhanced linkages between jail and lockup facilities and local mental health service providers.

This chapter describes the problem of jail and police lockup suicides and presents a cooperative interagency model that has been developed in New York State specifically to address this issue.

THE PROBLEM OF SUICIDE WITHIN LOCAL JAILS AND LOCKUPS

There are approximately 16,000 local jails and police lockups scattered throughout the counties, cities, towns, and villages of the United States. In 1983, there were over 8 million admissions to these facilities.[1] Police lockups detain persons who have been arrested and are awaiting arraignment. The detention period within a police lockup does not typically exceed 48 hours. Jails, by contrast, hold individuals who have been arraigned and are awaiting trial or sentencing and individuals who are serving sentences that are usually less than one year in duration. Because lockups and jails tend to be small-sized facilities, it is not uncommon for a lockup to have just one or two cells; over half of all jails have fewer than 21 cells. This large number of jails and lockups combined with their dispersed locations, high volume of admissions, and rapid turnover are all factors that make suicide prevention within our nation's jails and lockups a complicated problem for any state.

Suicide is the leading cause of death among jail inmates. In 1983, suicides accounted for 55% of the deaths of adult males, 79% of the deaths among adult females, and 100% of the juvenile deaths in county or municipal jails.[1] Although similar data are not available for police lockups, many states (e.g., New York and Massachusetts) report that the suicide problem in these facilities is at least equally as serious.

The jail suicide rate is three and one half times greater than that of the general population according to Danto, 1983.[2] The high rate of suicide among jail inmates is not surprising because the average jail population tends to be much more "suicide prone" than the community at large (Maffucci, 1986).[3] Concentrated within the hostile, nonsupportive environment of a jail are many persons who would have to be considered as being very high risk:

- Individuals who by virtue of their age characteristics (20–24) are wihin the highest overall suicide risk group (40% of the local jail population is between 20–24 years old);

- Persons with psychotic and depressive disorders;
- Individuals undergoing major life changes, such as divorce or the loss of a significant other;
- Persons who are about to lose a respected status within the community because of the nature of the charges pending against them; and
- Individuals who are intoxicated or under the influence of drugs at the time of their arrest.

The widespread practice of incarcerating suspected criminals who are under the influence of drugs and/or alcohol is especially problematic. A recent study found that 70% of all inmates who committed suicide in Massachusetts jails during 1984 had been charged with driving while intoxicated or with other alcohol-related crimes. Almost 90% of these suicides were committed within the first four hours of confinement. The study concluded that there is a "direct correlation between the advent of tougher drunk-driving laws and the incidence of local suicides and attempts."[4 (p 48)] This study complements a finding by the National Center on Institutions and Alternatives (1981) that 63% of the jail inmates who committed suicide within the first three hours of incarceration were charged with drug- or alcohol-related offenses.[5]

Independent of the detainee's mental health status or use of drugs and alcohol is the fact that incarceration is, of itself, a very stressful experience. The sudden shock of being separated from families and other sources of social support, the anxiety over trial or sentencing outcomes, and the doubt about one's ability to meet self- or peer-imposed standards of behavior can all induce feelings of intense helplessness or hopelessness. Shame over one's past and despair for one's future have driven mentally ill and nonmentally ill prisoners alike to view suicide as the only feasible way of ending the mental anguish that they are experiencing.

Communities face many obstacles in identifying and serving the suicidal detainee. Approximately 50% of all jail and lockup suicides occur within the first 24 hours of incarceration. Many of these incidents, which occur after the first 24 hours, are associated with critical periods or losses in the inmate's life, such as divorce or loss of job that jail officials may not even know about. Effective identification requires a structured screening process at the entry point into the jail or lockup and a continuous postintake screening process that ends at the detainee's release.

Implementing such a screening process is more difficult than it may first appear. The issue of who will be responsible for the screening must first be resolved. Jails and lockups cannot rely on the mental health system for this critical service because the mental health system will never have the resources to provide 24-hour on-site coverage at over 16,000 jails and lockups. Resolution to this problem rests with the utilization of local officers to provide the screening function.

Officers are responsible for booking all detainees and for maintaining their safety and custody throughout the confinement period. Utilizing officers to identify suicidal inmates creates other obstacles that must be overcome. First, most jail officers have received inadequate mental health training. Such staff have not been prepared to recognize obvious signs of depression, hopelessness and/or other indicators of suicide risk. Second, most jails have not developed procedures for officers to follow during intake and postintake screening. A third problem is that intake screening has to be completed within a relatively short time frame (less than 10 minutes). A lengthy screening process would cause unacceptable delays in the general jail-booking process. Finally, in order for screening officers to solicit appropriate responses from a detainee about his or her background and current ideation, a relatively private area is required for the screening. Most jails and lockups, however, do not have a suitable place for intake screening.

Postintake screening requires that officers be well trained to observe signs of suicidal intent during routine supervisory rounds and during other important periods, such as sentencing and family visits. The process also requires that officers communicate their observations across shifts. For example, by knowing an observation made by an officer on the day shift, an evening officer may be able to identify a mood swing or confirm an earlier impression that the inmate seemed depressed. Operationalizing this intershift communication is not inherently difficult. Rather, officers need only make frequent log entries regarding inmate behavior and read the entries of their fellow officers. Nevertheless, many officers resist such mundane tasks.

Once the suicidal inmate is identified, jails face the problem of arranging appropriate supervision and treatment services. This task frequently entails overcoming the jail's lack of internal resources and its general detachment from existing community services. Most jails rely on their local jurisdictions for funding to provide needed services. Generally, the types and quality of jail services are dependent on the economic level of the community jail and the level of priority that the community places on such services. Frequently, however, the jail is largely ignored by community administrators, and adequate resources to address the treatment and supervision needs of detainees are not allocated. In 1980, the National Coalition for Jail Reform (NCJR) reported, for example, that half of our country's jails have no medical facilities and that three fourths have no rehabilitation or treatment services whatsoever.[6]

Other problems that must be overcome involve the level of supervision that is given to prisoners generally and to suicidal inmates in particular. Providing adequate supervision is especially difficult in police lockups, where the priority is public safety, and staff are not permanently assigned to detention areas. In many rural areas, for example, a patrol officer (often the arresting officer) must be reassigned to the detention area when a person is arrested in order for the department to provide any supervision at all. Even when officers are assigned to the lockup, efforts to provide quality supervision are sometimes hampered because the cells are located apart from the booking or in an isolated area of the building. County and municipal jails are in a better situation because they have regularly assigned staff to provide supervision, but even jails often cannot provide sufficient supervision during the evening and night shifts. This staffing pattern is potentially tragic because most suicides occur between midnight and 3:00 A.M. Finally, it should be noted that supervision in both jails and lockups is often weak even for detainees who have been identified as suicidal. Most facilities simply do not have the staff for one-to-one supervision and seldom have special observation sections.

In summary, the task of identifying and serving suicidal inmates represents a very serious challenge. Many obstacles must be overcome before this challenge can be met. In effectively addressing these obstacles, communities must utilize a structured interagency approach. Certainly neither the mental health nor the correctional systems have the resources to resolve the challenge independently. Agreements must be developed to link the lockup or jail with existing local and state mental health service providers, and officers charged with the care and custody of prisoners must assume increased responsibility for identifying and referring inmates in need of crisis mental health care. Finally, personnel from both systems will need to be oriented to each other's operational constraints and, as appropriate, be trained to provide specific services required by this population.

NEW YORK STATE JAIL SUICIDE PREVENTION EFFORTS

Background

In 1983, in response to the problem of jail suicides in New York State, the New York State Office of Mental Health Bureau of Forensic Services and the New York State Commission of Correction Medical Review Bureau initiated the Local Forensic Suicide Prevention Crisis

Service Project. This project resulted in the design, demonstration, and implementation of a model that provides a clear framework for operationalizing interagency efforts in jail suicide prevention.

The project was structured in a way that had three distinct stages. The Developmental Phase occurred between March 1 and December 31, 1984. During this phase, the New York State Office of Mental Health Bureau of Forensic Services, the New York State Office of Mental Health Bureau of Evaluation Research, the New York State Commission of Correction Medical Review Bureau, and Ulster County Mental Health Services collaborated with a statewide advisory committee in the initial design of the crisis model for jails, lockups, and mental health agencies. The statewide advisory committee had representatives from the following agencies:

- New York State Association of Chiefs of Police
- New York State Sheriffs' Association
- New York State Division of Criminal Justice Services—Bureau for Municipal Police
- New York State Division of Alcoholism and Alcohol Abuse
- New York State Office of Mental Retardation and Developmental Disabilities
- New York State Division of Substance Abuse Services
- Governor's Task Force on Alcoholism and Criminal Justice

The first step involved reaching an agreement on the basic principles that formed the conceptual and operational basis for the model. During this development phase, broad organizational and personal areas of responsibility were outlined. These assumptions became key to defining the characteristics and parameters of what was considered to be an appropriate overall service-delivery strategy utilizing existing resources. These assumptions were as follows:

1. Administrators and line officers of both lockups and jails are legally and morally responsible for assuring the physical safety of all prisoners in their custody.
2. Local government units have the responsibility for assuring that mental health services are both available and accessible to all people living within their catchment areas.
3. For suicide prevention and crisis intervention services to have maximum impact, there must be a systematic, interagency effort to identify, manage, and refer prisoners who may be at risk.
4. The identification and referral process can only be effective

when local correctional facility administrators support it and when line staff have been trained to implement the necessary procedures.

5. The criminal justice and mental health systems must be integrated to be effective in providing suicide prevention/crisis intervention services.
6. It is neither practical nor appropriate to expect officials of lockups and rural jails to develop the capability to deliver all mental health services internally.
7. The state has an important role to play in assisting local government units in addressing the problems posed by mentally ill/suicidal prisoners being held in county correctional institutions, police lockups, and detention facilities.
8. The delivery of effective suicide prevention and crisis intervention services is beneficial to the prisoners in custody and to the jail where the services are offered.

Five counties demonstrated the model during a Demonstration and Evaluation Phase, which lasted from January 1985 through June 1986. The five counties had markedly different population sizes and demographic characteristics: Erie—an urban county with a population of over 1 million: Nassau—an urban county near New York City that also has a population of over 1 million; and the primarily rural counties of Ulster, Oswego, and Greene. The latter three counties have populations of 160,000, 80,000, and 40,000, respectively. Participating within these counties were all five county jails and a total of 16 police lockups. The jails ranged in size from 1,000 beds in Nassau County to 40 beds in Greene County. Training was provided at each facility, new policies and procedures were developed and implemented, and a detailed evaluation documented both the successes and deficiencies of the crisis service program. This evaluation included pre- and posttesting of officer training, in-depth site-visit evaluations, comprehensive interviews with project participants, an analysis of intake screening procedures, and a review of data on actual and attempted suicides.

Significant revisions were made in the model following the initial demonstrations. The program then entered the Statewide Implementation Phase, which was completed July 1987. The objective of this phase was to ensure the implementation of the model in every county throughout New York State. Seven regional contractors, working under the direction of the State Office of Mental Health with the assistance of the State Commission of Correction, and the State Division of Criminal Justice Services trained and worked with staffs of jails, police lockups, and mental health agencies in all 62 counties in the state.

Model Components

The revised model consists of four major components: policies and procedures, a training program for correctional/police staff, screening guidelines, and a mental health practitioner training manual.

Policies and Procedures. Separate manuals were developed for county correctional facilities, police lockups, and mental health agencies. These manuals describe the crisis service model and specify detailed procedures for both administrative and on-line staff. The procedure manuals have been designed to serve as a template for local officials who can then adapt the various provisions in a way that best conforms to their individual needs and circumstances.

Training Program for Correctional/Police Staff. Training materials developed for the program include: (1) a Trainer's Manual of more than 100 pages that outlines the specific training contents of an 8-hour training program for correctional/police officers. The manual not only identifies the specific topics to be covered but also provides teaching strategies, training exercises, and information on how to integrate the project videotape into the curriculum. (2) A four-part 45-minute videotape addresses basic issues on the identification of high-risk inmates, demonstrates the use of the screening guidelines, and offers suggestions for effective interviewing and communication. The videotape presents information on the signs of suicide shown by newly admitted inmates and inmates who have been in the jail for a substantial period of time. (3) An Officer's Handbook provides an executive summary of the training program and that was written in a manner that is easily understood by the police and correction officers.

Screening Guidelines. A one-page form, consisting of questions and officer observations, was designed to provide officers with a quick procedure for identifying high-risk suicidal inmates and inmates with other problems. Booking officers administer the form to all inmates during intake to identify those who should be considered high-risk during hours of incarceration.

Mental Health Practitioner Training Manual. This manual is a comprehensive document for on-line mental health staff who provide clinical services at jails and lockup. Part I provides mental health staff with information on the criminal justice system, jail, and police lockup operations and the role of crisis intervention services in jails/lockups. Part II describes the various psychiatric hospitalization options and the appropriate actions and responses that are available to mental health workers under New York State laws and regulations. Overall, the manual represents a useful how-to guide for the mental health practitioner.

Operationalizing the Model

Operationaling the model requires close cooperation between mental health agencies and local detention/correctional facilities. Successful implementation involves the coordination of skills from multiagency personnel encompassing three disciplines (security, medical, and mental health) to localize the model procedures and to provide critical crisis services. Local policies and procedures are developed jointly by mental health and jail administrations in a manner that clarifies the independent and shared responsibilities of each agency and discipline.

Following the development of facility-specific policies and procedures, training is scheduled for mental health, medical, and security personnel who serve the jail population. Through the training, mental health personnel are familiarized with the operation of the jail, the criminal justice system, and appropriate inpatient commitment procedures. Officers are trained to identify, manage, and refer inmates who are suicidal or seriously mentally ill.

The actual provision of services is begun as soon as staff training is completed. Security officers are primarily responsible for identification, referral, safety, and supervision. These responsibilities were assigned to security personnel because only the officers remain within local correctional facilties on a 24-hour basis. The utilization of trained officers to provide these services maximizes resources and provides a solution to the problem of timely identification of high-risk inmates. Significantly, these service roles are consistent with the classification, observation, and general inmate management functions that officers typically perform as part of their normal duties. In the jail setting, facility medical personnel are expected to assist security personnel with the identification and referral services. Medical staff are usually available to provide such assistance, however, during routine working hours.

The treatment and consultation services required by this model are the responsibility of medical and mental health personnel. It is customary for police lockup populations to receive these services through general hospital inpatient and emergency room clinics. Nevertheless, police chiefs and community service directors are required to establish clear linkages between all lockups and existing community agencies that provide emergency mental health services. In addition, police chiefs are expected to establish similar linkages for the emergency medical services required by the model.

Treatment and consultation services for county jail populations will usually be provided through multiagency coordination of general hospital inpatient units, emergency room clinics, state psychiatric facilities, county mental health outpatient programs, and county jail medical personnel. The model requires correctional administrators and community service directors to establish linkages among these multiple programs and the jail. Similar to the police lockup requirements, the community service director and the county sheriff/correctional administrator are responsible for the medical program linkages.

In addition, administrators from both agencies must collaborate to assure appropriate service coordination between mental health staff and jail medical personnel. Such coordination is especially critical under this model because jail medical staff are utilized to provide some of the mental health treatment services. Specifically, medical staff are expected to dispense and monitor psychotropic medications and to help mental health personnel provide emergency coverage for the jail.

IDENTIFYING HIGH-RISK INMATES

A cornerstone of the Suicide Prevention Crisis Service Model is the screening process that was developed to help jail or police staff identify high-risk inmates. This process focuses on three groups of risk variables: (1) the personal characteristics of the inmate; (2) such factors as intoxication that enhance the level of risk at the time of intake; and (3) high-stress situations, such as court appearances, including sentencing that occurs in the weeks and months following intake. Operationally, the identification process has two central components: formal, structured screening during intake, and ongoing observation on the tiers.

Risk Variables in Identifying High-Risk Inmates

Personal Characteristics of the Inmate. As with the general population, the personal characteristics of individual inmates have much to do with determining who will commit suicide. Among the various significant factors we would include age, sex, lack of close family or friends, recent significant loss, drug and/or alcohol abuse, psychiatric history, history of previous suicide attempts, and criminal history.

Age. The National Center on Institutions and Alternatives (NCIA) states emphatically that "age is a significant factor in jail suicide."[5 (p 20)] Authors of several studies have reported that suicide victims in local correctional facilities tend to be much younger than suicide victims in the general population. The importance of this finding is considerably diminished, however, when the age distribution of jail detainees as a group is taken into account. Thus, it should come as no surprise that, according to the NCIA,[5] 75% of the detainees who kill themselves are under the age of 33, whereas 76% of all inmates are under the age of 35 according to the U.S. Department of Justice.[1] At the other end of the spectrum, the NCIA reports that 2.4% of all inmates who killed themselves in 1979 were aged 54 and over. The U.S. Department of Justice[7] figures for 1978 indicate that "about 2% of the inmates were aged 55–64."

Sex. A similar analysis will account for the preponderance of males among jail suicide victims. Ninety-seven percent of all jail/lockup suicides involve males. This number is only slightly disproportionate because 94% of all jail inmates are also male.[7]

Age and sex are thus significant, but they are weak predictors when one considers the nature of the jail population. Although the high-risk factors of being young and male apply to two thirds of all those who are admitted to jails and lockups, their value as predictors is very limited.

Lack of close family or friends. Inmates without close family or friends are isolated from important sources of emotional, social, and financial support. Having someone to turn to in times of crisis can be absolutely essential in helping an inmate to overcome depression and hopelessness. Inmates without these close supports are often much less able to cope with the many stressors associated with incarceration.[2,8,9]

Experience of a significant loss. Significant losses recently experienced by the inmate can affect the individual in a way that greatly heightens the risk of suicide. Incidents that fall into this category include the loss of a job, the dissolution of a marriage or close relationship, and the death of a close friend or family member.[5,8,10,11]

A history of drug or alcohol abuse. A history of drug and/or alcohol abuse is another high-risk indicator. A recent unpublished study by the New York State Commission of Correction[12] found that 43% of the inmates who committed suicide between 1977 and 1981 had known histories of drug abuse and that 50% had histories of alcohol abuse.

Prior psychiatric history. In three retrospective clinical studies of suicides, all[13,14] or nearly all[15] of those who killed themselves were judged on the basis of clinical history, independent of the suicide, to have been psychiatrically ill. Within correctional environments, Danto[2] reports that 7 of the 10 detainees who committed suicide at the Wayne County Jail between 1967 and 1979 had a suspected history of mental illness. In an unpublished report, the New York State Commission of Correction[16] has similarly found that 55% of all inmates who committed suicide in New York State and in local facilities during 1979 had been hospitalized for treatment of a mental disorder on at least one occasion.

History of suicide among relatives. Several studies have demonstrated that "there are generations of suiciders in families, almost as if it were a kind of family thing."[2 (p 6)] Farber[17] and Dublin [18] are two of many researchers who have documented the relationship between suicide and prior familial suicide in the general population. Danto[3] cites the research of Koller and Castanos who felt that 65% of the suicide attempters in their study of prison inmates came from families in which one or both of the parents committed suicide when the prisoners were 10 to 15 years of age.

Previous suicide attempt. Several studies have documented that inmates who have attempted suicide in the past are more likely to do so again rather than those who have never tried.[2,19,20]

Criminal history. Research suggests that offenders who are arrested for the first time are high-risk because the initial entry into a correctional facility is extremely frightening and because the inmate may feel intensely fearful and helpless. Research also shows that chronic offenders (four or more arrests) may try to commit suicide following an onset of hoplessness or desperation about being arrested yet again.[2,5,19]

Factors That Enhance the Level of Risk at the Time of Intake. As previously noted, the first 24 to 48 hours are particularly critical for the purpose of suicide prevention. There are a number of factors that markedly heighten the risk during this period. These risk factors include alcohol/drug intoxication, acute psychiatric symptoms, shame about one's arrest, and serious personal problems.

Alcohol/drug intoxication. The relationship between alcohol intoxication and suicide is clear and unmistakable. A national survey conducted by the NCIA showed that:

> Almost 60% of the suicide victims were under the influence of alcohol and/or drugs at the time of their incarceration. Of these victims, moreover, a full 90% committed suicide within the first 48 hours of confinement. Almost 94% of the detainees who committed suicide within the first 3 hours of incarceration were under the influence of alcohol and/or drugs at the time of arrest.[5 (p iii, p 39)]

A more recent study that was conducted in Massachusetts[4] indicates that the relationship between jail suicide and alcohol intoxication is increasing. According to the authors, "there is a direct correlation between the advent of tougher drinking/driver measures and the incidence of lockup suicide attempts."[4 (p 50)] The study found that 70% of the reported suicides and attempts occurred among persons charged with driving while intoxicated or with other alcohol-related charges. It also found that 90% of those suicides were committed within four hours of admission to confinement.

Acute psychiatric symptoms. Numerous observers have noted the relationship between jail suicide and various aspects of mental illness. Esparza[21] and Fawcett and Mars,[22] for example, have reported a high incidence of severe depression among inmates who have attempted suicide. Not all mentally ill persons are suicidal, but the appearance of overt psychiatric symptoms is an important consideration to keep in mind. It is similarly significant to note that many jail suicide victims are believed to have experienced feelings of intense despair prior to taking their lives. Fawcett and Mars, for example, studied 13 suicides and 8 high-intent suicide attempts at the Cook County Jail and reported finding "significant hopelessness beneath a surface of apparent confidence and arrogance."[22 (p 105)] Danto likewise found hopelessness to be highly problematic in his study of ten suicide victims at the Wayne County (Detroit) Jail.[2 (p 8)]

Shame about arrest. Overt anxiety and shame about one's arrest is another high-risk factor. Frequently, this sentiment is expressed in statements, such as "I'll never be able to face my boss or family or friends again" or "This will kill my mother if she finds out." During demonstration period, we observed one suicide and several suicide attempts involving respected members of the community who were arrested for such crimes as child sexual abuse and who felt intense embarrassment about the nature of the pending charges.

Serious personal problems. All prisoners probably experience at least some stress following their detention and pending incarceration. For some, however, an arrest might constitute the proverbial last straw if they are already very worried about other problems. These problems may be related to any number of issues, such as health, finances, and job security. The compounded effect of many pressing concerns can cause at least some individuals to think very seriously about suicide.

High Stress Situations That Occur in the Weeks and Months Following Intake. There are several events that can occur during an inmate's incarceration that can heighten his or her risk of suicide. These events include experiencing significant personal loss (e.g., where a spouse decides to terminate a long-standing relationship), receiving a much longer sentence than had been expected, developing a severe physical illness, and suffering sexual or other types of physical assaults that greatly affect the inmates's sense of self-esteem. Holidays and family visits have also been known to induce intense depression that ultimately contributes to the inmate's decision to commit suicide.

Screening Components Utilized in the New York State Model

Intake Screening. Research conducted during the development of the New York State model clearly showed that a formal, structured approach to assessment at booking would be essential for several reasons. It has already been noted that most suicides occur within the first few hours of incarceration. Even if booking officers realize this, however, they may not always consciously assess a prisoner's risk of suicide, unless procedures require that they complete a protocol that will show that they have addressed all risk factors. The risk that the screening will be overlooked is especially great when the officers are rushed or when a detainee presents no overt symptomatology. A screening form is also useful because it may reveal information, such as a pending divorce, that officers should be aware of during the person's incarceration.

The screening guidelines being used in New York State were developed in various stages covering nearly a 2-year period of time. Ulster County Mental Health Services initiated the process by conducting a detailed review of the suicide literature. Ulster County faced a considerable challenge in this regard because the suicide literature, in general, is marked by "much semantic confusion, lack of clarity and definition of terms . . . even contradictory use of terms by the same author" (Pokorney, cited in Beck).[23 (p 30)] According to Dr. Edwin Schneidman:

> There are no universals, absolutes or "alls" in suicide. The best one can reasonably hope to discuss are the most frequent ("common") characteristics that accrue to most committed suicides and to make this discussion in as reasonable or as ordinary a language as possible.[24 (p 22)]

Although there are many unresolved questions about suicide in general, information on the nature and etiology of suicide in local correctional settings is even more unsettled. Virtually the only book-length studies of inmate suicide currently available are *Jail House Blues,* the collection of essays edited by Bruce Danto[2] and *And Darkness Closes In,*[5] a national study of suicides that occurred in jails and lockups during 1979.

The lack of information specific to jail and lockup settings is highly problematic. It is widely believed that the signs or groups of signs effective in predicting suicide in one group of people are not necessarily generalizable to either the entire population or to all varieties of special populations (prisoners, housewives, medical students).[25] No suicide rating scale yet devised is applicable to all populations.[26,27]

Ulster County clinicians drafted an initial screening form based on the literature and their best collective judgment. The form was then reviewed by the staff of the Office of Mental Health Bureau of Forensic Services and the Commission of Correction Medical Review Bureau. After revision, a semifinal version was forwarded to the project advisory committee, and their feedback was incorporated into the form. Committee members reemphasized the importance of designing a form that was brief and easy to use, but not so brief that it contained an inordinate number of false positives. A modest pretest of the form was then conducted at one jail and one lockup. The form was revised one more time, and this version was employed in the demonstration phase of the project.

During the demonstration phase, the Screening Guidelines were subjected to intense scrutiny. The evaluation included: (1) a visual review of over 9,700 completed forms to study officer comments and to determine if the forms were generally being filled out in the proper manner; (2) a computer analysis of a 25% random sampling from the three largest facilities and a 100% sampling of the remaining facilities; and (3) interviews with a variety of on-site officials who were in a position to comment on the forms and suggest ways to improve them. Finally, the guidelines were reviewed by recognized experts in the field of suicide prevention. These experts, who generously agreed to donate their services, were: Dr. Edwin Schneidman, founder of the American Association of Suicidology and Professor of the UCLA Neuropsychiatric Institute; Dr. Aaron Beck, Professor of Psychiatry at the University of Pennsylvania School of Medicine and Chief of the Department of Psychiatry at Philadelphia General Hospital; Dr. Allan Reichman, Medical Director of Forensic Services for Nassau County, New York, and one of just 180 board certified forensic psychiatrists in the United States; and Dr. Bruce Danto, the psychiatrist and accredited Certified Social Worker who edited *Jail House Blues.*

The screening guidelines (Figure 1) that emerged from this evaluation were compiled in a one-page form that can be administered in 5 to 10 minutes by a trained intake officer. The form is divided into three major sections. The first part contains general administrative information, inmate demographics, and data regarding symptomatology during previous incarcerations at the facility. This information is obtained by posing direct questions to the inmate and by consulting special files prepared for this purpose.

The middle section contains items that require the officer to ask the inmate additional questions and to make several observations regarding the inmate's behavior/appearance. The officer records all of this information by checking a yes/no column. Five of these items are especially significant and are set apart by shading in the boxes that the officer checks. Space is left on the right hand side of the form for the officer to record any additional information that may emerge when asking follow-up questions.

The first item in this middle section is a question that focuses on the transporting officer's impressions of the inmate. Sixteen additional items address high-risk factors that were discussed earlier.

The bottom section of the form contains six dispositional questions that are completed by the officer and, as applicable, by medical/mental health staff who may be asked to evaluate the inmate. The officer must record, for example, the level of supervision initiated (routine, active, or

Form 330 ADM(CC) (3-86)

State of New York
Commission of Correction
Office of Mental Health

SUICIDE PREVENTION SCREENING GUIDELINES

DETAINEE'S NAME	SEX	DATE OF BIRTH	MOST SERIOUS CHARGE(S)	DATE	TIME
NAME OF FACILITY		NAME OF SCREENING OFFICER		**Detainee showed serious psychiatric problems during prior incarceration.** Yes ____ No ____	

Check appropriate column for each question.

	Column A YES	Column B NO	General Comments/Observations
OBSERVATIONS OF TRANSPORTING OFFICER			
1. **Arresting or transporting officer believes that detainee may be a suicide risk.** *If* **YES**, *notify Shift Commander.*			
PERSONAL DATA	No Family/ Friends		
2. **Detainee lacks close family or friends in the community.**			
3. **Detainee has experienced a significant loss within the last six months** (e.g., loss of job, loss of relationship, death of close family member).			
4. **Detainee is very worried about major problems other than legal situation** (e.g., serious financial or family problems, a medical condition or fear of losing job).			
5. **Detainee's family or significant other** (spouse, parent, close friend, lover) **has attempted or committed suicide.**			
6. **Detainee has psychiatric history.** *(Note current psychotropic medications and name of most recent treatment agency.)*			
7. **Detainee has history of drug or alcohol abuse.**			
8. **Detainee holds position of respect in community** (e.g., professional, public official) **and/or alleged crime is shocking in nature.** *If* **YES**, *notify Shift Commander.*			
9. **Detainee is thinking about killing himself.** *If* **YES**, *notify Shift Commander.*			
10. **Detainee has previous suicide attempt.** *(Check wrists and note method.)*			
11. **Detainee feels that there is nothing to look forward to in the future.** (expresses feelings of helplessness or hopelessness). *If* **YES**, *to 10 and 11, notify Shift Commander.*	Nothing to Look Forward to		
BEHAVIOR/APPEARANCE			
12. **Detainee shows signs of depression** (e.g., crying, emotional flatness).			
13. **Detainee appears overly anxious, afraid or angry.**			
14. **Detainee appears to feel unusually embarrassed or ashamed.**			
15. **Detainee is acting and/or talking in a strange manner** (e.g., cannot focus attention, hearing or seeing things which are not there).			
16. A. **Detainee is apparently under the influence of alcohol or drugs.**			
B. **If YES, is detainee incoherent, or showing signs of withdrawal or mental illness?** *If* **YES** *to both A & B, notify Shift Commander.*			
CRIMINAL HISTORY	None		
17. **No prior arrests.**			

TOTAL Column A ____

ACTIONS
If total checks in Column A are 8 or more, notify Shift Commander.

Shift Commander notified: **Yes** ____ **No** ____

Supervision Instituted: **Routine** ____ **Active** ____ **Constant** ____

Detainee Referred to Medical/Mental Health: **If Yes:**

Yes ____ **No** ____

EMERGENCY	NON-EMERGENCY
medical ____	medical ____
mental health ____	mental health ____

Medical/Mental Health Personnel Actions: (To be completed by Medical/MH staff)

Figure 1. Suicide prevention screening guidelines.

constant) and whether the inmate was referred to mental health staff for evaluation.

The screening guidelines are used to identify detainees whom booking officers consider to be at risk. High-risk individuals are identified in three ways: (1) if a detainee gets eight or more check marks in the high-risk column; (2) if a detainee receives even a single check in the shaded high-risk categories; and (3) if the officer notices anything that he or she feels warrants further action or observation. This last category is particularly important because of what the officers are told repeatedly during training; that is, that, even if the guidelines indicate that a given inmate does not appear to be a high risk, the inmate should be referred to the shift commander anyway if the officer has a "gut feeling" that the person may be suicidal.

The detainee's overall risk score is usually brought to the attention of the Shift Commander prior to any housing assignment. The Shift Commander then has a key role in determining whether any action is needed. He or she may, for example, order that closer than normal supervision be given or that the inmate be referred to medical or mental health staff for evaluation. These dispositions are not made totally at the discretion of individual shift commanders. Rather, jail and lockup administrators are required to write detailed policy and procedure manuals that are consistent with the requirements of the New York Crisis Model.

Post Intake Screening and Observation. Officer screening and observation do not end after intake. As many as 50% of jail suicides occur *after* the first 48 hours, so officers must remain vigilant during the inmate's entire length of confinement. The New York State Model promotes this ongoing vigilance in several ways. First, officers are trained to observe inmates for behavioral and verbal indications of suicidal intent and/or mental illness during routine security checks. High-risk indicators commonly found among correctional populations include: periods of crying, insomnia, and sluggishness; extreme restlessness, pacing up and down; sudden drastic change in mood, eating, or sleeping habits; giving away personal property; loss of interest in activities or relationships which an inmate had previously enjoyed; and a refusal to take prescribed medication or a request for an increased dosage of medication.

A second way that officers monitor inmate behavior is by interviewing them as indicated following sentencing or during other critical periods (e.g., following a death in the family). Officers specifically look for signs of depression and/or hopelessness at these times.

Finally, officers who supervise the visiting areas are expected to watch for possible disputes or problems that emerge during the visiting period. Many facilities encourage visitors to report any signs of suicidal ideation by posting a sign near the entrance that specifically solicits information from family and friends. Promoting communication with those who know the inmate best is an aspect of the model that was added following a suicide in which the victim's family had failed to tell jail officials that the victim had informed them of his plans to hurt himself.

Supervising officers in the visiting room and on the tier are required to record mental health related observations in a jail log that is accessible to all shifts. This recording process is a critical part of the postintake screening process. It facilitates intershift communication regarding high-risk inmates and enables officers to become aware of behavior changes regarding inmates in crisis.

The screening guidelines form is laid out so that next to each item is a Column A—Yes and a Column B—No, with the officer's needing to check one of the boxes on each line. For the higher risk ideas, with yes, the officer must notify the Shift Commander. The yes box is in a dark shade.

The left side of the screening guidelines form has open space with the title "General Comments/Observations," and offers the officer an opportunity to make notes and comments.

CONCLUSION

Data from several sources clearly demonstrate that the problem of jail and lockup suicides has become extremely serious. This trend is likely to continue growing as states increasingly enact legislation that directly or indirectly results in the incarceration of drunk drivers, drug abusers, and other high-risk individuals.

Concerned officials in many communities have already taken initial steps to reduce the risk of inmate suicides at their facilities. The potential impact of such efforts is often diluted, however, by the fact that the administrators do not always take the time to implement prevention and risk management programming in a comprehensive manner. Many sheriffs and police chiefs, for example, have introduced new intake screening procedures, but this process has limited value if officers have not been adequately trained or if linkages are not in place to arrange timely mental health evaluations and other services.

The model developed by New York State was specifically designed to address significant facility, systematic, and interagency factors that tend to impede timely identification of risk factors, problems involving special supervision, and service delivery. The model also integrates the responsibilities of administrative and on-line staff in a manner that provides direction and greatly enhances personal accountability. It is unrealistic to think that all inmate suicides are preventable; however, the strategies being proposed in this model appear to have a great deal of potential in managing the risk. The five jails that first demonstrated the model experienced only one suicide during the 12-month demonstration period, whereas five were reported from these same facilities the previous year. The feedback is certainly encouraging and is a testamonial to the potential for positive results when conscientious and comprehensive efforts are applied.

REFERENCES

1. US Department of Justice, Bureau of Justice Statistics; *The 1983 Jail Census.* Washington, DC, Government Printing Office, 1983.
2. Danto BL (ed): *Jailhouse Blues: A Study of Suicidal Behavior in Jail and Prison.* Orchard Lake, Mich, Epic, 1973.
3. Maffucci JJ: Jail suicide: An unsolvable problem in corrections and law enforcement. *NY Law Enforcement J* 1986; 3:19–26.
4. Special Commission to Investigate Suicide in Municipal Detention Centers of the Commonwealth of Massachusetts: *Suicide in Massachusetts Lockups 1973–1984.* Boston, MA, Special Commission, May 1, 1984.
5. National Center on Institutions and Alternatives: *And Darkness Closes In . . . National Study of Jail Suicides.* Alexandria, VA, National Center on Institutions and Alternatives, 1981.
6. National Coalition for Jail Reform: *Fact Sheet on America's Jail,* Washington, DC, National Coalition for Jail Reform, 1980.
7. US Department of Justice: *Profile of Jail Inmates.* Washington, DC, Government Printing Office, 1980.
8. Fawcett J, Leff M, Bunney W Jr: Suicide—Clues from interpersonal communication. *Arch Gen Psychiatry* 1969;21:129–137.
9. Burtch BE, Ericson RU: *The Silent System: An Inquiry into Prisoners Who Suicide and Annotated Bibliography.* Toronto, University of Toronto, Centre of Criminology, 1979.
10. Hogarth D: *Manual of Suicide Prevention—What to Look for, What to Listen for, What to Do.* Boston, Mass, Suffolk County Jail Lifeline, March 1984.
11. Danto BL, Eubank J: *Suicide in Jail and Its Prevention.* Boulder, Colo, National Institute of Corrections, US Department of Justice, 1980.
12. New York State Commission of Correction: Risk factors relating to suicides in state and local correctional facilities, 1977–1983. Albany, NY, 1982.
13. Dorpat T, Ripley H: The relationship between attempted suicide and committed suicide. *Comp Psychiatry* 1967; 8:74–79.
14. Barraclough B, Nelson B, Sainsburg P: The diagnostic classification and psychiatric treatment of 25 suicides, in Faberow N (ed): *Proceedings of the Fourth International Conference for Suicide Prevention Centers.* Los Angeles, Delmar Publishing Co Inc, 1968.
15. Robins E, Murphy G, Wilkinson R, Gassner S, Kayes J: Some clinical considerations in the prevention of suicide based on a study of 134 successful suicides. *Am J Public Health* 1959; 49:888–898.
16. New York State Commission of Correction: *Suicide Study: 1977, 1973 and 1979 Systemwide.* Albany, NY, January, 1981.

17. Farber M: Factors determining the incidence of suicide within families. *Suicide Life Threatening Behav* 1977; 7:3–6.
18. Dublin L: *Suicide: A Sociological and Statistical Study.* New York, Ronald Press, 1963.
19. Beigel A, Russel H: Suicide attempts in jails: Prognostic considerations. *Hosp Community Psychiatry,* 1972; 23:361–362.
20. Gaston A: Suicide prevention in the New York City corrections system. Read before the American Medical Association Fourth National Conference on Medical Care and Health Services in Correctional Institutions, Chicago, IL, Oct. 19, 1980.
21. Esparza R: Attempted and committed suicide in county jails, in Danto B (ed): *Jail House Blues.* Orchard Lake, Mich, Epic, 1973, pp 27–46.
22. Fawcett J, Mars B: Suicide at the county jail, in Danto B (ed): *Jailhouse Blues.* Orchard Lake, Mich, Epic, 1973.
23. Beck A, Resnick H, Lettieri D (eds): *The Prediction of Suicide.* Bowie, MD, Charles Press Publishers Inc, 1974.
24. Schneidman E: *Definition of Suicide.* New York, John Wiley & Sons, 1985.
25. Diggory J: Predicting suicide: Will-o-the-wisp or reasonable challenge? in Beck A, Resnick H, Lettier D (eds): *The Prediction of Suicide.* Bowie, Md, Charles Press Publishers Inc, 1974, pp 59–69.
26. Neuringer C: Methodological problems in suicide research. *J Consult Psychol* 1962; 26:273–278.
27. Rose A: Detection of suicidal patients: An example of some limitations in the prediction of infrequent events. *J Consult Psychol* 1954; 18:397–403.

6

AIDS in Prisons

Recommended Policies and Procedures

THOMAS A. COUGHLIN III

INTRODUCTION

It has been seven years since the first AIDS (acquired immune deficiency syndrome) diagnosis in the country was made, and, in the intervening years, our collective societal consciousness, with its underlying fears, has been raised to an intensity and a fervor seldom asserted by a new disease. Institutional hospitals and prisons have been at the vanguard ever since in dealing with new problems associated with this disease. The first of what is now 500 confirmed AIDS inmates appeared in the New York State prison system in Novemter of 1981, a scant six months after the Center for Disease Control established the existence of the disease. By mid-1987, there had been over 2,000 confirmed AIDS cases in prisons across the country, making the most concentrated population of this diagnosis in any setting. The problems created by this emerging population subset constitute a new chapter in the annals of correctional administration. In an extraordinarily short period of time, under the microscope of public attention and scrutiny, hospitals and correctional systems have had to develop policies and procedural guidelines to address a multitude of new medical and administrative issues. To the extent that correctional systems have been able to meet this scrutiny and cope with the myriad of problems associated with AIDS in the middle of unprece-

THOMAS A. COUGHLIN III • New York State Department of Correctional Services, Albany, NY 12226.

dented overall population growth, those correctional administrators and medical staff are to be commended for a job well done.

The focus of this chapter is an attempt to document the steps necessary to meet this emerging crisis in the correctional setting and to demonstrate the importance of developing an integrated approach to administering equitable, judicially sanctioned AIDS policies and procedures. As other crises, such as population growth, budget shortfalls, and judicial scrutiny, make demands on an administrator's time and attention, this issue is certain to add to that load, but it need not deter correctional administrators from implementing sound management of AIDS matters. I am not a medical professional or a criminologist but a manager, and I have based my management decisions on the sound advice of those who are experts. The measures we have put into place in New York State have withstood the legal and budgetary tests of the past six years and have succeeded in addressing the operational concerns advanced by inmates and staff. Throughout the course of this chapter, I will refer frequently to the experiences I have gained dealing with administering AIDS-related issues in New York, as well as to the practices we have put into place to deal with the problems we have encountered.

POLICY AND PROTOCOL DEVELOPMENT

An integrated approach starts with policy input from all the relevant control agencies, including such agencies as health departments, executive control agencies, as well as the correctional agency's own medical, administrative, and institutional staff. Of primary concern should be the medical definitions recommended by health departments. In the policy and protocol developed by the New York State Department of Correctional Services, the definitions conform to the Federal Centers for Disease Control, with the concurrence of the New York State Health Department. The 11-page *AIDS Specific Policy and Procedural Guidelines* acknowledges in its Preface that AIDS has a far-reaching impact on the system's health care delivery as well as other institutional systems because of the multifaceted and unique problems associated with AIDS. The policy statement notes that it is in the interests of uniformity of procedures and definitions that the protocol *Guidelines* are published and distributed. The goal of uniformity insures the intent of fairness and consistency, which is good policy and procedure, and also insures favorable consideration in subsequent judicial proceedings.

Although AIDS in the context of this chapter is a management problem, management's first line of defense is to rely as much as possible on medical professionals to identify, evaluate, and treat inmates with

AIDS. The medical definitions contained in a good policy statement or protocol can be understood by administrators and nonmedical personnel and should be fully comprehended, but the diagnosis and treatment regime should be physician directed. Management's overall purview calls for a balanced approach to security interests, population movement, and bed-space issues, as well as a logistical review of medical determinations, but the medical recommendations must be considered first and the policy and protocol must adhere foremost to the medical considerations. For example, the protocol followed by the New York prisons calls for acute cases of either AIDS or AIDS-related complex (ARC) to be transferred to the nearest available hospital capable of handling AIDS or ARC cases. Upon discharge from the hospital, the inmate is to be returned to the institution where facility management, in consultation with medical staff, determines either placement in the institutional infirmary or back to population if medically suited. If the doctors say that the inmate is fit to return to general population and if the inmate meets security qualifications for that facility, then policy and protocol dictate that the course of action should follow the medical advice.

Identification and Movement

Identification of inmates with AIDS or ARC is a management and a medical problem. Because of the stigma and the fear associated with the disease, many inmates will avoid coming to sick call for treatment until their debilitation reaches a point that such a visit becomes unavoidable. Although good medical practice will have dictated that a clinical evaluation be made of all incoming inmates at reception, symptoms may develop at some later point, and the practice of inmates failing to appear for treatment, until absolutely necessary, makes the job of identifying and diagnosing potential cases of AIDS and ARC problematic. Short of mass testing, there is no available administrative procedures to bring such cases to the administrator's attention. Whatever the case may be for small or large numbers of latent AIDS or ARC cases out in population, neither the medical professionals nor an administrator can deal with the disease until the diseased inmate makes his or her medical condition known by coming in for treatment.

Once an inmate's symptoms are brought to the administrator's attention, infection control for AIDS and ARC cases should follow the Federal Centers for Disease Control's guidelines for AIDS/hepatitis B that dictate extraordinary caution and care for handling materials possibly contaminated with AIDS-related waste and that call for extra precautions in avoiding accidental wounds or lesions from patients or materials.

Precautionary measures should also be taken in handling laundry and food for patients with AIDS or ARC in infirmaries or hospitals. Laundry should be stored in the quarantine unit with the AIDS patient. It should be collected in a soluble linen bag and laundered weekly, after normal hours, in a specified dilution of household bleach. Similarly, food should be served to inmates in disposable dinnerware. If a tray is used for serving purposes, it should be cleaned with bleach. Leftover food items and disposable ware should be bagged in an impervious bag prominently labeled "Infectious Disease Precautions" and disposed of in the same manner as medical specimens or articles. The imposition of these measures should not cause undue stress or dislocation because, in all likelihood, staff working in close proximity with "infectious disease" inmates, whom they suspect to have AIDS, will be prepared to incur extraordinary measures in handling these inmates. Our experience in New York with these precautions supports this contention.

Security precautions normally followed for transporting inmates should be adhered to in moving inmates with AIDS or ARC. If handcuffs and leg irons become contaminated with blood or other body materials, they should be washed with a solution of bleach. When an inmate has had an AIDS diagnosis confirmed by the Centers for Disease Control, any staff coming into possible physical contact with the inmate should be advised that the inmate has an infectious disease. Security personnel transferring or moving this inmate should be advised of the infectious disease condition and warned to take extra precautions to avoid allowing direct body-fluid contact with the inmate. Both staff and the inmate should be advised that they may wear a surgical-type mask to avoid crossinfection while under transport. Upon informing staff that the inmate they are moving requires special treatment, the appellation *infectious disease* should be used to describe the inmate's condition rather than the words *AIDS* or *ARC* in order to protect confidentiality and to avoid the legal prohibition against labeling an inmate AIDS or ARC.

Placement and Programming

As the number of inmates with AIDS and ARC increases, correctional administrators are increasingly faced with the problem of where to place these inmates in the institution without jeopardizing, on the one hand, either the inmates' needs for medical care or programming opportunities or, on the other hand, the overall system needs for security and absence of conditions that might allow the spread of contagious or infectious diseases. For inmates or staff who harbor strong fears of the disease, the issue may be viewed as them versus us. Fear and paranoia of the disease are always present. Equally strong should be management's resolve to adhere to sound legal and management practices that call for following medical advice for hospitalizing inmates with AIDS or ARC and that also resolve to follow a protocol dictating that placement decisions should not be made on any basis other than strictly medical advice. Following those assumptions and presuming a return of the inmate to a facility, management is then faced with several choices for placement, when the inmate's medical condition is stabilized and the inmate is returned to a facility from a hospital. The practice in New York State has been that, upon return from acute care in an outside hospital, a returning inmate is placed in one of three levels of care defined by medical staff in keeping with the inmate's medical condition. The first and typically initial level is a return to the facility infirmary. Here the inmate may stay several days or weeks, or may never return to a level of fitness allowing a return to general population in the facility. If an inmate is determined to be medically fit and able to be returned to general population in the institution and if a suitable program is available to that inmate in general population, the inmate should be placed back in population. Generally, inmates in the New York State facilities who have AIDS-Related Complex and are physically fit are placed in population. Only the inmates themselves and the medical staff know of the diagnosis. As long as there is no outward evidence of symptomatology, ARCs, suspected ARCs, and even occasionally AIDS patient inmates should be housed in population. The policy and protocol developed in New York State clearly states this approach as normative. By comparison, the Federal Bureau of Prisons segregates all AIDS cases, but presumptively houses HIV (human immuno virus) seropositives and ARC cases in general population. These cases are subsequently segregated on a case-by-case basis upon the display of high-risk behavior or the onset of medical conditions that dictate separate housing. In further contrast, California's segregation policy calls for housing all HIV seropositive cases away from the general population.

Identification of new AIDS and ARC cases typically occurs in New York State when an inmate, who is not known to medical staff as a suspected AIDS or ARC case, chooses to come in for medical attention because his or her medical condition has deteriorated, and the effects of the disease can no longer be suppressed. The decision to take the inmate out of population is made in concert by medical and facility management staff. In practice, inmates invariably delay coming to sick call until the very last possible moment, going to great lengths to disguise their condition from other inmates and their families. Facility staff may suspect a particular inmate of AIDS, through observing weight loss, skin discoloration, or other symptomatology, but until the inmate shows up for treatment or suffers a physical lapse out in the facility, staff are severely hampered in treating the disease. An inmate can be escorted to sick call or even an outside hospital and still refuse treatment. Short of a court order, there is no practical means of ensuring treatment.

A third option for placement of inmates with AIDS or ARC is the creation in a facility, usually in a part of the hospital or infirmary, of a discrete special-needs unit. This option allows facility management and medical staff the option of offering longer term care than is normally available in infirmaries and with a level of programming greater than is available in infirmaries. Inmates in this placement may not need nursing-level care associated with infirmaries. This option may be exercised as the numbers of AIDS and ARC patients accumulate to the point that normal infirmary operations are impacted.

Congregating all AIDS or AIDS and ARC inmates from a prison system into one facility is an option rejected by New York State for a variety of reasons. Primarily, it has been the advice of our State Health Department that congregate care is neither medically nor legally appropriate. From a medical point of view, the disease is to be treated as any other medical condition that develops with an inmate, to be dealt with by facility staff at the infirmary level of care or at outside hospitals on contract with the department. Legally, there is a potential liability associated with congregating all of any class or category of inmate. To congregate all AIDS or AIDS and ARC cases into one facility would jeopardize the program options and the security level classifications of some inmates, as well as certainly the geographic options open to such inmates. As the disease progresses, the importance of location in proximity to home becomes paramount to an inmate. As common as the occurrence is now of an inmate with AIDS dying far from home or relatives, the move to consolidating all inmates with the disease into one location would have the effect of exacerbating the problem. Also, as a practical matter, no one facility in our system has sufficient medical capacity to accommodate the 225 AIDS and ARC patients we have in our 50 prisons at any one time.

As a large correctional system, such as New York's, matures in its capacity to handle growing AIDS and ARC case loads, another option to housing this population is contracting with a metropolitan hospital for larger quantities of beds. There are several advantages associated with this option: a metropolitan location allows readier access to families for inmates; economies of scale offer savings to the prison system and the hospital; and congregating in this setting provides significantly reduced security coverage costs compared to normal hospital coverage. We anticipate this institutional relationship will cover acute, skilled nursing, and hospice level care. The inclusion of all three levels of care under one roof also offers operational benefits, inasmuch as AIDS inmates typically progress and regress between levels of care.

Education Efforts

From the onset of this disease, the most conspicuous and effective response to the disease taken by public managers has been their leadership in educational efforts. The intensity of the society's fears about AIDS is exacerbated and abetted by the continuous media attention, some of it factually inaccurate, and this underscores the importance of education efforts by public institutions like hospitals and prisons. Prison administrators should embark on an early and often multifaceted approach to educating staff and inmates about all aspects of the disease, including definitions, numbers affected by the disease, training curriculum modules, and multimedia systemwide material distribution.

The emphasis on education begins by articulating the importance of education efforts in a department policy statement on AIDS. The policy and protocol developed for New York State states that such efforts are an integral part of the curriculum offered to new staff as well as in-service training for existing staff. Brochures and pamphlets are distributed to all institutional staff as well as to the entire inmate population. Because of New York's large Hispanic population, printed materials are also made available to inmates in Spanish. Furthermore, seminars should be offered at facilities for selected staff members and selected inmates as a means of reaching a broader audience with a greater level of detail. In New York State, the AIDS Institute has assisted us in conducting these seminars.

The content of the material contained in the pamphlets and brochures as well as the seminars should be explicit and detailed. The material should cite the Federal Centers for Disease Control's definitions and explain, for example, that someone who exhibits a sustained high fever, enlarged lymph glands, unexplained weight loss, diarrhea, or other classic signs of HIV infection is possibly suffering from AIDS-related complex. The material should explain that technically no one dies of AIDS and that all of us carry infections that, if not for our immunity systems, would kill us. The material should explain that when someone exhibits ARC symptoms, an infection lying dormant in the body may take advantage of the opportunity presented by reduced immunity and that, after, and only after, the onset of that opportunistic infection, can an individual be tested to be medically confirmed as an AIDS case.

Educational materials should answer the often asked question, "Is AIDS spreading among staff or inmates?" The answer should be, "No, there are no confirmed cases of anyone contracting AIDS while in prison in our state or in any other state prison system." And the information should reiterate the medical fact that blood to blood and semen to blood contact are the main routes of transmission. It does not hurt to reiterate the basic facts over and over again.

The most effective educational tool we have found in New York is a film made by our inmates of inmates who were slowly dying of AIDS over a period of many months. This film, entitled "AIDS: A Bad Way to Die" is shown to all incoming inmates in our system and has proven its effectiveness as a powerful tool for portraying a graphic and emotional message. The impact is underscored by the fact that the film was made by inmates, for inmates, and about inmates and their families. The response we hear from our facility staff tells us that this approach, without medical jargon, is by far the most effective educational tool we are using.

Our labor-management meetings at all levels now include frequent discussions of AIDS issues. Together, with the Governor's Office of Employee Relations, all three of the labor unions have addressed training and educational efforts for staff in an attempt to educate and allay staff fears of AIDS.

Testing, Condoms, Needles, and Tattooing

In a statement recently released, the Department of Correctional Services has made clear its position that there is no test for AIDS. That assertion is based on the medical evidence and advice given to date. The commonly ascribed AIDS HIV test is designed to screen the nation's blood supply for evidence of AIDS antibodies, just as blood is commonly tested for the presence of tuberculosis. It indicates exposure to the antibody, not who will develop the disease. The latest figures indicate that approximately 20% to 30% of those exposed to the AIDS virus have actually developed the disease. Contrary to public perception's linking prisons as the fastest growing segment of the affected population, the statistics indicate a leveling off in the rate of increase of inmates with AIDS and ARC. In the New York State system, the infection rate has stabilized at 3 per 1000 inmate admissions for the past 2½ years. In addition, we have incurred no confirmed transmission of the disease for inmates to staff in 5 years of dealing with the disease. And, in fact, the Centers for Disease Control statistics indicate that nationally the rate of increase of disease confirmations in prisons is below the rate of increase of the disease in the overall population.

To those who would still push for mass testing for AIDS, notwithstanding the medical facts, my response is that, because the virus is not passed through any form of casual contact, there is no need for prison officials to know if an inmate is infected unless the inmate becomes ill and needs care. As the manager of the prison system, I am also concerned that the confidentiality of the results of any type of mass testing might be violated and that those testing positive would be stigmatized on the basis of a test designed to screen blood, not people. Just what does a commissioner or a warden do with all of the inmates who test positive—segregate them somehow? I submit that the information as to who tests positively would lead to many more management problems than an approach that takes each positive AIDS or ARC inmate as they come along and deals with them one at a time as medically indicated. None of the four large states, with 70% of the national total of inmates with AIDS, currently does mass testing, and, of the three smaller states who do mass test, one has stopped the testing.

Similarly, the availability and use of condoms in prison will create more problems than they will solve. In the New York system, as in all corrections systems, homosexual relations among inmates, the possession or use of intravenous (IV) needles, and the practice of tattooing is against the rules for inmates. The approach I take on these activities is to remind inmates that, not only are these activities against the rules, but all three can now kill you because of AIDS. Allowing condoms is an incentive that could be interpreted as an endorsement of homosexual activity. It makes no practical sense to allow condoms in prisons—period.

Given the predominance of the use of single cells in our system, I am not as concerned over the issue of homosexual practices as I am over the practice of tattooing. Consequently, our education efforts toward inmates emphasizes heavily the danger of tattoos.

Legal and Confidentiality Issues

Public administrators are increasingly driven in their management practices by judicial considerations. It is a fact of life. Nonetheless, administrators can still steer the issues and their practices by carefully adhering to their own carefully crafted policies and regulations. It has been my experience that most judges do not want to run prisons, but what they are interested in is ensuring consistent compliance with specific factual administrative practices. For example, they are interested in assurances that quality medical and dental care be available to all inmates on a timely basis. Thus, it is the administrator's job to ensure that such is the case.

In the area of AIDS related issues, judges are interested in assuring the quality of care, access to programming and other normally available inmate privileges, access to grievance mechanisms, and the assurance that confidentiality is maintained. Administrators who honor these interests stand a good chance of winning litigation. Clearly, all affected staff should be thoroughly attuned to a policy that states that there should be no equivocation to a hard-and-fast rule protecting the confidentiality of an inmate's medical information, especially any serological test results indicative of AIDS or ARC. Inmate patients' medical charts should be safeguarded by placing the chart in a sealed envelope marked "Confidential." Other inmates, correction officers, and medical personnel not in direct care of the inmate should not have access to this information. This is our legal mandate. In addition, many inmates do not want even their families to know of the specifics of their illness and display a great deal of anxiety at the thought that other inmates or their families might learn of their diagnosis. As administrators, we need to stress to staff the priority of honoring confidentiality for legal reasons as well as respect for an individual's dignity.

Centralized AIDS Case Review

Because of the extraordinary nature of the AIDS illness, correction departments should initiate a centralized review and monitoring of all cases. Decisions regarding placement and treatment should be determined jointly between facility and central office staff with final sign off by central office staff. It has been our experience in New York that, at the discretion of the central office staff, all functionally related staff should be involved in placement decisions for AIDS and ARC cases. In addition to facility health staff, including a physician, placement review input may come from mental health staff, support operations, security, ministerial services, parole board, and by the inmate's family or significant others. In New York, the protocol we follow calls for primary responsibility for systemwide coordination of AIDS and ARC cases to be directed by the central office Division of Health Services staff, including matters concerning external community hospitals, clinics, Parole, Mental Health, Mental Retardation and Developmental Disabilities, Social Services, and Department of Health. Furthermore, facility level coordination of services for AIDS and ARC inmates is the responsibility of the facility Superintendent or Warden and his or her Executive Team. Thus, although the condition is medically defined, the management of the facility as a whole is involved with these cases, not just the medical staff. Identification and definition of the illness begins with medical staff, but because of the extraordinary nature of the logistics and the broad spectrum of affected agencies and divisions involved, some redundancy in management review is called for.

Coordination with Parole

For the most part, parole decisions regarding inmates with AIDS or ARC follow the same procedural guidelines that are in place for any other inmates leaving prison, sick or healthy. However, in view of the overlay of concern and attention occasioned by the Departments of Health and the Centers for Disease Control, special attention should be given to the procedures followed in paroling inmates with AIDS or ARC. To date, in New York State, we have paroled over 90 inmates with this disease.

Coordination with Parole entails the sharing of information on identified AIDS or ARC inmates and on scheduled parole hearings. As spelled out in our Policy and Procedure protocol, the agreements we have reached in New York State with our Division of Parole include Corrections sending a confidential monthly listing of all AIDS and ARC inmates to Parole. Parole in turn provides the department with a schedule of hearing dates for listed inmates. We provide an updated medical report on each listed inmate to Parole 60 days prior to the scheduled hearing date. The report includes a recommendation for postrelease treatment, including hospitalization where indicated. If postrelease hospitalization is recommended, facility health services staff assist Parole with preliminary arrangements for placement in a community hospital. If the recommended plan includes outpatient treatment, such treatment should be clearly indicated so that Parole can tailor a treatment plan that includes such treatment. As a policy footnote, it should be noted that, unless legislative authorization is specifically given, there should be no special consideration given for early release for AIDS or ARC inmates simply because of their debilitation from the disease. Notwithstanding that debilitation, such an early release would be illegal.

Budgets

I have purposely avoided addressing budget concerns as they relate to AIDS and ARC issues because, in fact, budgetary concerns become secondary in dealing with this disease. If it follows, as I have argued, that our management practices should be guided by medical considerations and that appropriate levels of placement, along a continuum of care, should be provided for inmates with AIDS or ARC, then it also follows that administrators would incur whatever appropriate costs are associated with that level of care. Beyond incorporating whatever efficiencies we can in transporting, or congregating, or guarding these inmates, we cannot impose our managerial fiscal judgments on the physician who makes the decision for placement. We would not be legally justified in doing so.

Notwithstanding this basic position, I would add that there are staffing efficiencies to be gained by congregating skilled nursing-level care placements, concomitant with the added benefit of proximity of families, if the setting is in the urban area where most inmates come from. In New York State, we have developed a relationship with a hospital that now accommodates ten AIDS inmates and that will expand to up to 60 beds by 1989. The efficiencies for us include significantly reduced security costs. Inmates now in hospitals throughout the state, sometimes with individual one-on-one security coverage, will be sent to this hospital. All of these AIDS inmates are in advanced stages of the disease, a time when family visits become increasingly important. Although from a strictly cost-based analysis such congregated care may be cheaper in a geographic setting further away from the major urban areas, a compassionate policy dictates that the setting should be closer to the families of the dying patients. For inmates who are in earlier phases of the disease, facility infirmaries throughout the system are the appropriate placement.

If the experience of other commissioners of large correctional systems mirrors my own, budget and fiscal concerns can pose an obstacle in a manager's efforts to provide optimal care to inmates with AIDS, but our best efforts should be extended to overcome those obstacles and to address the problems of these human beings, who are caught in a traumatically painful and socially debilitating death sentence.

7

Competency to Be Executed

CHRISTINA B. CASALS-ARIET AND
HARVEY BLUESTONE

The legal system defines standards of competence for a variety of civil and criminal activities. Some of these include competence to make contracts, to make a will, to consent to research, to stand trial, and to consent or refuse medical or psychiatric treatment. In arriving at determinations of various competences, the legal profession often seeks the expert opinion of psychiatrists. One particular area of competence that has come under recent scrutiny is that of competence to be executed; indeed, the medical literature has increasingly addressed this topic.

A recurring note in the literature discussing competency to be executed is the increasing number of people sentenced to death row and the increasing number of executions. In itself this might be expected to lead to an increase in the number of instances in which an inmate's competency to be executed is questioned. Correspondingly, the issues raised for psychiatrists by the requests for involvement in the competency evaluation and treatment process will increasingly be forced into consciousness. Soon, the various roles that psychiatrists can play will have to be defined with greater precision, and perhaps a consensus will have to be reached by the profession with regard to its stand on these issues.

This chapter will survey a sampling of literature from the disciplines grappling with these concerns and will suggest further questions that appear to require efforts at solution. It will look at some background

---

CHRISTINA B. CASALS-ARIET • Department of Psychiatry, Albert Einstein College of Medicine, Bronx, NY 10456. **HARVEY BLUESTONE** • Department of Psychiatry, Albert Einstein College of Medicine, Yeshiva University, Bronx, NY; Department of Psychiatry, Bronx-Lebanon Hospital Center, Bronx, NY 10456.

facts about capital punishment and at some of the work done on the stresses of confinement. Then, it will briefly review some aspects of the legal background, with specific reference to competency to be executed. Some views of the psychiatric community will be examined, as well as ethical questions that have so far been identified. This survey is not meant to be a comprehensive review but rather an introduction into this important area.

BACKGROUND

Capital punishment has existed for as long as human civilization has.[1] In Biblical times, heretics were stoned, and, in Roman times, criminals were crucified. Death was a mandatory sentence for murderers in England. The death sentence came with the colonists to North America, and the first legal execution in the territory destined to become the United States took place in 1622.[2]

Since then, at least 11,000 people are known to have been executed.[2(p122)] Nonetheless, in the years after the initial colonization of North America, the use of capital punishment was restricted to the most serious crimes, such as rape and murder. The framers of the Constitution accepted capital punishment, but in the Fifth Amendment wrote that "no person shall be held to answer for a capital crime without an indictment, that no one shall be twice put in jeopardy of life and limb," and that no one shall "be deprived of life" without due process of law.

Historically, American executions were public, and the last was in 1936 in Kentucky.[3] For 200 years, through the 1800s, hanging was standard. Even in the 17th century more primitive methods were rare. Until 1900, local jurisdictions performed most executions, though lynchings were frequent. State authorities took over by about the 1920s. Even by the 1850s, a number of states had abolished the death penalty. In 1846, Michigan eliminated capital punishment, Rhode Island in 1852, with Wisconsin in 1853. Iowa followed in 1872, and Maine in 1876.

This movement to eliminate capital punishment was halted by the Civil War, and then, by the 1900s, increasingly sophisticated methods of execution were used. New York, for example, electrocuted its first convict in 1890. Executions peaked in the 1930s, at which time an average of 150 criminals were electrocuted yearly. This number began to decline in the 1940s and 1950s, with a sharp drop in the 1960s, as the concern about the constitutionality of capital punishment grew.[1(p48)] In 1962, 46 executions took place, in 1964, there were 15, and in 1966, there was one. In 1967, an unofficial moratorium began. Presumably, this suspension of executions occurred to give the Supreme Court a chance to consider the constitutionality of capital punishment. The moratorium was widespread but unofficial. Ten years after it began, the moratorium ended with the execution of Gary Gilmore, a convicted murderer who was shot to death by a firing squad in Utah.

Within the larger framework of execution, there exists a tradition surrounding the specific question of competency to be executed. There was a common-law requirement, which has been incorporated into statute in many states, that prisoners be competent before they are executed. This prohibition has existed since the medieval period, although its rational is unclear.[4] Various explanations have been offered. Sir William Blackstone suggested that the state of insanity itself served as sufficient punishment.[5] Lord Coke had stated nearly a century earlier that the deterrent effect of execution would not be served by execution of the insane, but instead would provide a spectacle of "extreme inhumanity and cruelty, and can be no example to others."[6] Sir John Hawles, the Solicitor General in the time of King William III, argued that executing insane criminals was inconsistent with principles of Christian charity because it deprived a man of his life before he could make his peace with God.[7] Finally, another common-law rationale was that an incompetent inmate was unable to assist his attorney in pursuing issues that might still be present in his case.[5]

A modern rationale or explanation is based on the theory of retribution. One view holds that killing an insane person does not have the same moral value as killing a sane one, and, therefore, does not satisfy the requirements of retribution that a wrong be offset by a punitive act of the same quality, a killing. "Executing an insane prisoner would not satisfy retribution because society wishes to take a life of equal value to the one taken."[8(p 536)] Another view of this rationale is that the prisoner is required to "perceive the expression of society's moral outrage."[9] If an inmate is incompetent to comprehend the relationship between his conduct and the execution, this goal is frustrated. According to Radelet and Barnard, retribution does not simply extend to comprehension of punishment but requires an element of mental suffering on the part of the condemned as well.[10]

With this historical information as background, a closer examination of current trends is possible. One impetus to the more careful examination of the question of competence to be executed is that, since the resumption of executions, their pace has accelerated rapidly. Constitutional barricades have been erected and knocked down, which has quickened the pace. In the 1986–1987 term, the Supreme Court considered what may be one of the last major questions on the constitutionality of capital punishment: whether statistical evidence that killers of whites are 4.3 times more likely than killers of blacks to be sentenced to death will support claims that the punishment is being administered in violation of the Equal Protection Clause and the Eighth Amendment. In an opinion issued in May, 1987, the Court held that the statistical evidence did not support such a claim.[11]

The most recent figures on capital punishment issued by the Department of Justice's Bureau of Statistics, including 1985 as well as prior years, indicate that since 1930, when data were first collected, 3,909 executions have occurred.[12] From 1971, the year after the Supreme Court reinstated the death penalty, through 1987, a total of 3,404 persons entered prisons under a sentence of death. Of these, the state executed 58 people:

1974 : 4	1978 : 3	1982 : 6	1986 : 4
1975 : 3	1979 : 7	1983 : 3	1987 : 1
1976 : 4	1980 : 9	1984 : 4	
1977 : 1	1981 : 7	1985 : 2	

Of the 37 states that have the death penalty, a total of 12 have carried out executions since 1977. Thirty-two states reported 1,591 persons under sentence of death on December 31, 1985, an increase of 171 or 12.2% over the count at the end of 1984. States with the largest number of prisoners under sentence of death were Florida (226), Texas (206), California (170), and Georgia (107).

It is noteworthy that for persons executed since 1977, the average time between sentence imposition and execution was 6 years. For the 11 prisoners executed between 1977 and 1983, the average time elapsed was 5 years; in 1984, it was 6½, and then in 1985, it was 6 years. This long period of time is one of the factors adding to the relentless stress of existence under sentence of death. As such, if the time period does not begin to be shortened and if the number of people convicted and awaiting execution continues to increase, it is entirely likely that more cases of competence to be executed will present themselves.

Indeed, time is just one of several factors that has been noted in a number of studies of death row stress. These studies consistently show that psychological deterioration of death row inmates occurs.

Bluestone and McGahee, in their study of death row inmates at Sing Sing, detailed various symptoms and psychological defense mechanism observed in the inmates.[13] They studied 18 men and one woman and correlated the mental illness not just to the prison setting but also to the unique stress of anticipating both the manner and time of one's death. The authors identified various symptoms and three major defense mechanisms displayed by the inmates: denial, projection, and obsessive rumination. Of interest, several of these defenses reached psychotic proportions, which may have implications later for the discussion of the psychiatrist's role in treating these inmates. One form of denial described was the delusional belief that a pardon had been granted. Also, regarding projection, this was described as typically taking the form of persecutory delusions, by which prisoners converted themselves into martyrs. Finally, the obsessive preoccupation described bordered on the psychotic. There was endless rumination about appeals or the development of hyperreligiosity. This innovative study demonstrated the unique stress of the inmates' situation and may give some guidance for the role psychiatrists could play.

Ten years later, Gallemore and Panton studied individuals confined to death row in North Carolina.[14] In an effort to learn the effects of extended confinement, the authors evaluated eight individuals living under sentence of death for two or more years. Five men appeared to adjust adequately over time, whereas three became significantly less functional. In contrast with the earlier findings by Bluestone and McGahee of the use of denial as a defense, this study showed that as a group these men were more apt to use projection and to identify with each other and to an antisocial life-style. Overall, their potential for adjustment in a new environment, if that were to become necessary, was felt to be diminished.

A methodologically different study, Johnson's *Condemned to Die: Under Sentence of Death,* based on tape-recorded interviews conducted in 1978 with 35 of 37 prisoners then on Alabama's death row, focused deliberately on encouraging introspective descriptions of stress. "The prisoners were asked to reconstruct their thoughts and feelings in relation to various grievances. . . . The condemned prisoners' subjective perceptions were sought."[15(p 13)]

Although not a scientific study, Johnson's work highlights the paradox that exists with regard to capital punishment. There is an ambivalence about actually executing a death sentence once it has been pronounced. In order to ensure that the condemned prisoners truly deserve death, they are allowed to spend years on death row waiting for the state to decide whether or not to kill them. They live year after year in small cells near the machine that will execute them. They may be required to endure conditions worse than those found to be unconstitutionally cruel. They live between hope and dread. "The prisoners must fight for their lives through the exercise of their legal rights, and it is reprehensible that their legal rights are asserted at the expense of their emotional and psychological well-being."[15(p 122)]

Johnson estimates the human costs: the palpable deterioration and decay of death row prisoners stands as proof that they have suffered real harm far in excess of that required by sentence, and that they have been victims of real brutality.[15(p 129)] Thus, for all intents and purposes, a death row sentence amounts to death with torture in a society that has explicitly renounced torture as a remnant of barbarism. In the end, Johnson found that normal psychological defense mechanisms do not suffice to manage the stress of death row confinement.

In addition to these studies, detailed examination of individual inmates documents overwhelming stress and dehumanization. In *Waiting for It,* a study of a condemned inmate on death row in Georgia, Davis states that in "dealing with the threat of their imminent extinction . . . [t]hose with natural balance and strength of mind survived more arrests intact until they are killed. The rest failed visibly from month to month and are destroyed in effect before the state can do its work."[16] In *Sentenced to Die,* a collection of eight case histories of murderers convicted to death, Gettinger concludes that the main feature of life on death row is "the intense psychological stress." The author quotes a study by Dr. Lewis J. West, a psychiatrist who described death row as a "grizzly laboratory . . . the ultimate experimental stress, in which the condemned prisoners' personality is incredibly brutalized."[17(p94)]

As these studies indicate, if conditions are not improved on death row and if the time to execution is not shortened, the cumulative effect of the stresses of such confinement will lead to increasing deterioration of inmates. If, in addition, the number of people convicted and awaiting execution continues to increase, as has been the case, it is entirely likely that more cases of competency to be executed will be presented to psychiatrists. The role of psychiatry must be more clearly defined for the individual psychiatrist and for the profession as a whole.

THE LEGAL BACKGROUND

Before examining some of the literature about competency to be executed and ethical considerations, it is helpful to have a view of the most recent legal case, *Ford v Wainwright.*[18] In an article in the *American Academy of Psychiatry and the Law Newsletter,* Zonana has clearly and succinctly detailed the background and the role of the American Psychiatric Association. He raises some of the questions that must be faced by the psychiatric community, as well as reiterates some of the legal questions. The following is a summary of his article.[19]

Almost every state, either by statute or through case law, requires that a person not be "insane" at the time of execution. The statutes by and large do not define the term *insane,* although a few states, such as New Mexico, do provide a more explicit standard:

> If the prisoner has not at the present time, from the defects of his faculties, sufficient intelligence to understand the nature of the proceedings against

> him, what he was tried for, the purpose of his punishment, the impending fate which awaits him, a sufficient understanding to know any fact which might exist which would make his punishment unjust or unlawful, and the intelligence requisite to convey such information to his attorneys or the court, then he would not be sane and should not be executed.[20]

This standard is similar to the standard used to determine competency to stand trial, with the additional requirement of an understanding of the crime and the punishment to be faced.

As noted above, this competency requirement stems from common-law prohibitions against executing insane prisoners. The question of competency to be executed as a constitutional right arose in *Ford v Wainwright.*

Earlier, in 1950, the issue first arose in *Solesbee v Balkcom,*[21] in which a man scheduled for execution argued incompetency. He was examined by a governor-appointed panel of psychiatrists and was found to be competent for execution. He appealed, based on violation of due process safeguards, including a hearing on his competency to be executed and the right to offer his own psychiatric experts and to cross-examine the psychiatrists opposing him. The Supreme Court denied the claim, saying that the competency examination was under the state governor's clemency power, and thus not subject to constitutional due process constraints. The issues are raised again in *Ford v Wainwright,* but, in the interim, the Supreme Court has applied the due process safeguards to the states.

Alvin Ford killed a wounded police officer on July 21, 1974, by shooting him in the back of the head. Ford was convicted and sentenced to death.[22] His mental state was not an issue until late 1981, after his trial, sentencing, and appeals had taken place. At that point, he developed hallucinations and delusions, and his speech became disorganized. This florid psychosis led his attorneys to have him examined by two psychiatrists, both of whom concluded that he was suffering from paranoid schizophrenia. Under the Florida statute, one psychiatrist decided Ford was not competent to be executed. Section 922.07 (1) of the statute states:

> When the Governor is informed that a person under sentence of death may be insane, he shall stay execution of the sentence and appoint a commission of three psychiatrists to examine the convicted person. The Governor shall notify the psychiatrists in writing that they are to examine the convicted person to determine whether he understands the nature and effect of the death penalty and why it is to be imposed upon him. The examination of the convicted person shall take place with all three psychiatrists present at the same time. Counsel for the convicted person and the state attorney may be present at the examination.

As a result of Ford's deterioration, the Governor appointed the three psychiatrists required by the statute. Together they examined Ford for about 30 minutes in a courtroom before attorneys and correctional officials. Two psychiatrists thought Ford was psychotic but competent; the third thought he was malingering. The Governor would not hear from the defense's psychiatrists and concluded that Ford was competent. The case was appealed to the Florida Supreme Court and the U.S. Court of Appeals for the 11th Circuit.[23] These appeals were denied, and the case was reviewed by the Supreme Court.

The American Psychiatric Association filed an amicus curiae brief that focused on the procedures specified by the Florida statute, rather than on the substantive questions of whether a constitutional right defined in these circumstances should be supported by psychiatry, and what legal standards should be applied. The brief identified a number of areas in which procedures afforded to a defendant under capital sentence by the Florida statute were deficient, failing as they did to allow for adequate psychiatric assessments and also for proper judicial procedures. A lack of fundamental fairness was identified in the refusal of the Governor to allow any advocacy on the part of the defense.

The Supreme Court rendered its opinion on June 26, 1986. Execution of the insane violates the Eighth Amendment prohibition against cruel and unusual punishment. As noted by Justice Marshall, writing for a divided court with a 5 to 4 majority, the earlier cases considering competency to be executed, *Solesbee v Balkcom*[21] and *Caritativo v California*,[24] were decided before the time when the Eighth Amendment was made applicable to the states by the Fourteenth Amendment. The Court held that whatever the aim of the competency to be executed restriction, "restriction finds enforcement in the Eighth Amendment."

As Zonana states toward the conclusion of his article, the Court was not sufficiently in agreement to be able to adopt definite guidelines to be employed in competency hearings. It did accept a number of the principles outlined in the APA brief, but neither the Court nor the brief discussed the difficult ethical questions for psychiatrists. The article reclarifies what some of these are. Current American Medical Association guidelines only mention the giving of lethal injections and state that it is unacceptable for physicians to participate, except for the pronouncement of death. The APA standard regarding execution is: "A psychiatrist should not be a participant in a legally authorized execution."[25] At what point does the psychiatrist, when participating in execution competency proceedings, become involved in the infliction of death? Psychiatrists have evaluated competency to go to trial, criminal responsibility, competency to be sentenced, competency to waive appeals, and competency to be executed. Is the last phase too close? Should the line be drawn at an earlier point?

Also, once the finding of incompetency to be executed has been made, the state requires that the prisoner be treated. Is it ethical for a psychiatrist to treat this prisoner? If the psychotic pain is very severe? If the patient objects? To what level of health?

As the article indicates, the Supreme Court rejected the Florida procedure, which failed even to allow the defendant to challenge the state's psychiatrists' findings, and left it to the states to develop procedures for fair hearings. Perhaps the states will try to establish panels of psychiatrists to be the ultimate arbiters. Zonana expresses the belief that this is an inappropriate function for the medical profession as it renders the psychiatrist a decisionmaker, rather than a consultant to the legal system.

ETHICAL QUESTIONS FOR PSYCHIATRY

With the foregoing survey providing the context, it is possible to focus on ethical questions. A number of articles have begun this investigation and will be summarized in some detail.

Applebaum, a leading authority in the field of law and psychiatry, discussed the ethical questions briefly in his column in *Hospital and Community Psychiatry* in July, 1986, followed by a lengthier treatment in 1987 (personal communication, 1987).[26] In the article, Appelbaum describes the rationales given for the common-law requirement of competency to be executed and summarizes the issues in *Ford v Wainwright.* He then identifies the two separate dilemmas that exist for mental health professionals, involvement in the competency evaluation and involvement in treatment.

Three positions are described regarding competency evaluation. One is that there is no problem and that this evaluation is no different from any other competency evaluation performed for the legal system.

The second position acknowledges that there are some differences between evaluations for competency to be executed and other evaluations, but would allow the execution competency evaluations, if adequate protections for the prisoner were in place.[26(p13)] In essence, psychiatrists supporting this position require that the prisoners be afforded a fair hearing if contesting the evaluation, and that standards be defined. This view was expressed by the APA amicus brief in *Ford.*

Finally, the third position is one espoused by psychiatrists who reject the idea of any participation in the evaluations. The difference between these evaluations and other forensic evaluations is critical, according to this view. Most other evaluations aid the administration of justice by facilitating the determination of guilt or innocence, or by finding an appropriate disposition. Execution competency evaluations, on the other hand, only facilitate the administration of punishment. According to this view, involvement in such a process threatens to compromise the healing role of physicians.

Turning to the second problem, treatment participation, Appelbaum finds this to be perhaps even a more troubling issue. He again discusses three views, not necessarily congruent with the three above. The first position is that of clinicians who maintain that they have responsibility to treat severe mental illness regardless of the consequences. The pain of severe psychosis cannot be ignored. The National Medical Association, an organization of black physicians, subscribes to this view.[27] As they express it:

> The treatment of a 'death row' inmate's mental illness does not imply that the treating psychiatrist agrees with capital punishment but rather is committed to the adequate health care of the correctional population.[27(p 3)]

The second position is an intermediate one. Prisoners may be treated, according to this view, if they themselves request or want treatment. Appelbaum states that, although this partly relieves the dilemma theoretically, in practical application the likelihood is high that a person incompetent to be executed will also be incompetent to make an informed judgment about the desirability of treatment. (Although if the standard of competence for these were defined differently, this would not necessarily be the case.)

Finally, at the other extreme, is the position that psychiatrists should not at all be asked to treat prisoners incompetent to be executed. Treatment at this point is done for the sole purpose of inflicting greater suffering, and, as the article states, it might well be more humane to allow a person to suffer the ravages of psychosis than to treat with the goal of execution. Also, this view distinguishes treatment by a psychiatrist at this stage from acute treatment by medical specialists. The latter are attempting to prolong life, rather than to enable an execution to take place.

Appelbaum concludes with mention of a possible partial way out of the dilemma: commuting the sentences of incompetent prisoners to life imprisonment. This position was adopted by the Florida State Hospital Human Rights Committee.[28] Alternatively, it might be possible not to require that a prisoner be competent before execution. The rationales given for the requirement for competency to be executed can be questioned, as Appelbaum does. Few people would avow the punitive explanation for the requirement, and the dignity-of-man rationale is possibly too vague a concept to be meaningful. The notion of helping one's attorney becomes too farfetched at the extreme end of the litigation process, and the religious explanation is difficult to maintain in a secular society. "It is unclear why a society that accepts the legitimacy of putting people to death for the crimes they commit should feel any differently about doing so when the condemned are psychotic."[26(p 683)]

Alan A. Stone, another leading psychiatrist in the area of psychiatry and the law, has written on this topic in the September 1986 edition of the *Psychiatric Times*.[29] In addition to discussing several cases, Stone touches on other issues. He considers the recent emergence of these competency to-be-executed cases as apparently understood as part of a larger effort by the opponents of capital punishment to pursue all legal means against the death penalty. He sees irony in the fact that:

> Civil libertarians who on other fronts have insisted on the right to commit suicide and have attacked psychiatric paternalism and psychiatric expertise are on this front prepared to sacrifice their client's autonomy on any psychiatric pretext.[29(p16)]

To pose some of the ethical questions that he identifies, Stone uses the example of Dr. Grigson, a Texas psychiatrist who has testified for the prosecution on many occasions. Rather than looking at the criticism levelled against Dr. Grigson and his testimony on dangerousness that was rendered without benefit of an examination, Stone sets forth what could be said in defense of Dr. Grigson. These points include his extensive clinical experience with criminal offenders diagnosed as having antisocial personality disorder, and his apparent belief that the available research on clinical psychiatric predictions of dangerousness are not based on the kind of criminal antisocial population he knew. Also, regardless of one's personal views, Texas law allows capital punishment. Thus, the prosecution must make its case and be entitled to the assistance of experts. To this end, psychiatrists ought to be able to do thorough psychiatric examinations before offering professional opinions, but this is not always possible due to legal constraints. Finally, there is nothing unethical in an expert's offer of testimony stemming from clinical expertise that has not been documented by accepted standards and methods. Indeed, for psychiatrists in other contexts, for example, in prediction of suicide or determination of the best interest of the child, often opinions are offered lacking a basis with good scientific documentation.

Stone says that although these defenses may not be completely convincing, they do suggest that psychiatrists in Dr. Grigson's position may conclude that no professional obligation prevents them from offering testimony of this sort in death penalty cases. Other psychiatrists, troubled by the ethical difficulties raised by the offering of testimony that seems to favor the death penalty, should consider what Dr. Stone calls the crucial question. Namely, are they disturbed about Dr. Grigson's participation on the basis of personal moral objections to the death penalty, or based on professional reasons grounded in some accepted principle of medical ethics. For Stone, the personal moral objection is a valid one, but the professional objections are not convincing. He sees the objections as based on the ethical injunction to do no harm and says that this principle is no longer part of medicine's official code of ethics, because it has, in any case, been compromised by the medical profession's acceptance of abortion. The AMA, nonetheless, has continued to apply the injunction narrowly to the proscription against physicians' administration of lethal injections at executions. Stone points out that despite this injunction against participation, physicians have traditionally been present at executions to declare the person dead. If the executee is alive, then more drugs might be ordered by the authorities. An inconsistency is apparent to Stone:

> Is Dr. Grigson's testifying for the prosecution in favor of the death penalty more like the expert function of determining that the person is dead? Can the weakened and unofficially abandoned ethical injunction, do no harm, be resurrected and stretched far enough to guide forensic psychiatrists involved in the death penalty?[29(p26)]

More troubling still is the argument that because of the "do no harm" principle, it is unethical even to participate in capital sentencing competency determinations. Also troubling are the possible consequences of any decision on this question, some of which have been enumerated above. Additionally, one consequence is that if psychiatrists refuse to participate, then a psychotic person might be executed. Another is that the people on death row in need of psychiatric care will be untreated.

Stone sees difficulty for the profession in resolving this issue. On personal moral grounds he can understand and support a refusal to treat a person to render him competent to be executed, but he asks "in a society which considers the death penalty just retribution, should clemency hinge on the psychiatrist's ethical obligation to do no harm?"[29(p26)] Perhaps the execution competency requirement will become the new insanity defense, whose purpose years ago was identified by the Chicago law professor Norval Morris as being only to avoid capital punishment. Although these issues are similar to those identified by Appelbaum, they are viewed from a slightly different perspective.

Another view has been provided by Radelet and Barnard.[10(p39)] After reviewing the background of increasing requests for competency examinations, legal requirements for competency, rationales for the requirements, and the Florida statutes, they addressed the ethics of physician participation, in the body of their article.

Radelet and Barnard do not try to resolve the conflict but raise issues for individual consideration, beginning with the need for clarity of definition in statutes, including the definition of competence. As they see it, participation can still happen despite vague statutes if certain pragmatic safeguards are in place. If written reports are very detailed and the examinations performed are meticulously done, then evaluations of this sort are probably not problematic. The premise is that "the unnecessary death of an incompetent person is a stake that many will find too high to refuse participation."[10(p46)] An approach to an overall solution in this situation is suggested in the form of a panel of physicians, prosecutors, and defense attorneys (among others) to attempt to reach a definitional consensus on what competency to be executed should involve and how it should be evaluated.

A second, and, as they see it, more fundamental, ethical problem is that under present rules opinions by participating physicians about competency to be executed cannot be challenged in adversarial processes. The decision in *Ford v Wainwright* will have an effect in this area, as the flaws in the Florida statute were addressed by the Supreme Court. What will result is still in the process of being determined, as Justice Marshall left the development of procedures to satisfy the newly established constitutional right to the states.

A final ethical problem area identified involves the implications of a finding of incompetence. Two issues arise, the ethics of treating an inmate to restore him to competence to be executed, and the problems involved in the psychiatric assessment when it is believed that competency has been restored. The treatment problem includes economic issues (use of a state's limited resources to treat condemned persons), as well as informed consent and the inmate's right to refuse treatment. The problem of assessment includes who makes the determination of when competency is regained, and what criteria are used to determine competency. The authors argue that rather than refusing to participate, a psychiatrist might espouse the more pragmatic position that involvement that requires a finding of competence simply places more responsibility on the physician for clarity, certainty, and comprehensiveness.

Finally, Radelet and Barnard note that the participation by psychiatrists might increase the number of people sentenced to death. This could occur if jurors are reassured by psychiatrists' participation, and thus the psychiatrists might be seen less as neutral participants than as active agents in the legitimation of death. A result, then, could be that the medical participation might make the act of sentencing to execution more palatable, as well as increasing the general legitimacy of capital punishment in the public's mind.[10(p50)]

Radelet and Barnard, in their unpublished manuscript that is cited by Ward,[30] had further contributed to the clarification of thinking about the ethics of psychiatric participation. They identified four positions useful for analyzing the ethical dilemmas: the principled, the consequentialist, the empirical, and the psychological approaches. Each is controversial and ultimately none provides a ready solution to the problem.

Very briefly, the principled approach holds to the view that the area of execution competency is one in which psychiatrists should refuse to participate. The consequentialist position is that, because statutes and procedures already exist, it is better for right-thinking clinicians to participate rather than to surrender to "hired guns." The third position, the empirical, is that the psychiatrist should examine the prisoner and report on the degree of mental impairment, yet the clinician should avoid the ultimate question of execution competency. Finally, under the psychological approach, the psychiatrist should examine the prisoner, arrive at a DSM-III-R diagnosis, and then state an opinion on competency.

As stated, each of these positions is ethically (and pragmatically) problematic. Apparently Radelet and Barnard lean to the consequentialist approach, whereby psychiatrists participate to avoid interpretation of refusal as abdication of their professional responsibility. Alleviation of the ethical dilemma comes in part by adherence to strict procedural safeguards. If the profession used this approach, then due process would require careful avoidance of language suggestive of opinion on the ultimate question of competence for execution. From the work described, one thing becomes clear, as indicated by Ward[30]: Opinions on the many issues pertaining to competency to be executed are directed not only by one's position on the death penalty but also by perceived political realities. The more pro-death penalty psychiatrists there are in a particular area, the more appeal there is to a consequentialist approach.

Similar issues are discussed by Sargent in a December 1986 Hastings Center Report.[31] Sargent highlights slightly different aspects of the questions, pointing out, for example, that failure to warn the patient that the therapist is colluding with the state in removing the last barrier to execution is dishonest. His view is that any therapy not grounded in the patient's welfare is inherently dishonest. Patients have a long-standing trust in physicians, and this trust is betrayed when psychiatrists treat patients so that they may be executed; this is like "treating the patient to death."

A further issue analyzed by Sargent is the inmate's ability, or lack of it, to consent to or to refuse treatment. Because informed consent is not possible under these circumstances, the therapist who complies with the order to treat can only be acting as a double agent in the service of the patient and the state. Refined objections to diagnosing and treating the condemned, which amount to participation, are superfluous if the entire process lies beyond the scope of medical activity. To address the detail of acts that are forbidden is likened to an executioner's concern for the niceties of sterile technique. Sargent advocates psychiatrists' nonparticipation.

Most of the foregoing points are also covered by Salguero in a *Yale Law Journal* article entitled "Medical Ethics and Competency to be Executed."[32] In careful and clear detail, she sharpens conceptualization of the interests to be weighed.

The dilemma is set forth to clarify how it is that the physician cannot make an ethical choice. Procedures that require psychiatrists' participation, yet violate medical ethics, assume that the state interest in executing the condemned overrides concern for the ethical integrity of the profession. To comply with the state's interest and treat, the psychiatrist is forced to violate a professional ethical prohibition; namely, participation in an execution. By refusing to treat, though, the psychiatrist must violate the professional duty to heal.

Further aspects of the dilemma present themselves. Total physician abstention may adversely affect individual rights, for example, the right to a fair trial. If a psychiatrist refused to evaluate an inmate for competency to stand trial, the defendant's right to defend himself or herself might be in peril. At this stage the connection with execution is rather distant. In contrast, the connection when the psychiatrist treats a death row inmate is quite close; indeed, the restoration of sanity is the only condition precedent for the execution of the individual. As Salguero concludes, but for the state exoneration of the action, similar to the privilege afforded soldiers in battle, the physician is taking life in violation of his or her ethics. This exemption may insulate the physician from legal liability, but it in no way diminishes the ethical violation.

A tension in the state's interests is also identified: the rights of the state in using psychiatrists for their professional skills and the humane appearance infused into the proceedings by their presence versus the competing state values in protecting the integrity of the medical profession from the executioner's role. Arguments in favor of this physician participation are discussed. One is that given the state's legitimate interest in executing a criminal (as the Supreme Court has done in *Gregg v Georgia*),[9] the state has an interest in ensuring that competent prisoners do not frustrate the process with false pretensions of incompetency. A second argument for using psychiatrists is to implement a statute in a fair, scientific, and reliable manner. Finally, an argument for participation is that physicians have an obligation to fulfill their duty to the state, which the state deems legitimate and necessary.

A countervailing state interest is in protecting the integrity of the profession. This interest undermines the state interest in using psychiatrists to treat the condemned. Also, there is a state interest in protecting public health. This requires a trust by the public in physicians, which trust is undermined by use of psychiatrists in the execution process, or by the appearance of medical participation in the death penalty.

From the premise that it is not legitimate for the state to enact statutes that invite the medical profession to breach its ethics, particularly given the strength of the interest involved, possible resolutions to the ethical dilemma are suggested. The state might conclude that the exception for the insane from execution is a policy that is no longer relevant. Alternatively, the state could accord a psychiatrist the status of a conscientious objector. This, though, does not rescue the physician from the dilemma; it simply allows the psychiatrist to make the choice without sanctions. The conflict set up by the state remains. Finally, the state can involve physicians after sentencing to treat the condemned. Salguero proposes that this must not be done at the expense of the profession's integrity, and thus the state should defer to medical ethics. The only way to do so is to specify in advance that subsequent to a finding of incompetence to be executed, and before treatment by a psychiatrist, the sentence would be commuted to life imprisonment.

CONCLUSION

After examination of all these facts, what questions remain? More will be brought to view as the discussion continues within the medical profession, as well as between psychiatrists and members of other disciplines. Individual psychiatrists will increasingly face these issues with regard to personal choices.

Appelbaum has noted (personal communication, 1987) that further questions for study include: what should a psychiatrist do if treatment of an inmate is begun before the issue of incompetence arises? Does the psychiatrist raise the question? Report the concerns? Wait? Also, he suggests further clarification and refinement in the thinking about the point at which participation in evaluation becomes unacceptable. This will include consideration of the view that by allowing an inmate to go forward, or treating him or her to the point of competency, the psychiatrist is perhaps helping to afford the prisoner a chance for self-defense and exoneration. Finally, further explanation needs to be undertaken of the role psychiatrists should play in treatment. How much suffering is too much, and what is humane?

Appelbaum has also indicated (personal communication, October 1987) that, since the lively debate on the question of competency to be executed at the May 1987 meeting of the American Psychiatric Association, a topic under much discussion has been psychiatry's choice of position on treatment. The four basic positions on treatment participation are:

1. A psychiatrist should not treat unless the death sentence is commuted.
2. A psychiatrist should not treat unless the patient or a substitute decision maker makes a competent decision that the patient accepts treatment.
3. A psychiatrist may treat only until the patient reaches a level of competence.
4. Treatment should be undertaken because (a) it is a psychiatrist's job to treat and treatment is beneficial to the patient and diminishes suffering, regardless of the consequences, or (b) it is a psychiatrist's job to treat, and treatment serves the interest of the state, which requires that prisoners be returned to competency for execution.

Appelbaum subscribes to the first position. We also subscribe to this position: a psychiatrist should not treat an incompetent death row prisoner unless the sentence is commuted to life imprisonment prior to the commencement of treatment.

Besides these, another question among many for consideration is the role that psychiatrists as a group should play vis-à-vis a position about capital punishment. Perhaps if the consensus were that capital punishment *per se* should not be practiced, then the profession could work vigorously toward that end, while still, in the interim, providing reasonable, humane, and caring services for the condemned.

APPENDIX

The authors strongly believe that psychiatrists should not participate in competency to be executed evaluations under current conditions. In the interest of scholarship, however, this brief section is included to summarize some of what has been written on the subject of the performance of competency examinations, in general, and with specific reference to competency for execution.

In *Forensic Psychiatry and Psychology*, Curran, McGarry, and Shah outline broad considerations applicable to the performance of any type of competency.[33] Rather than giving a detailed procedure, they describe larger issues. First, one must define the question that is asked. They mention that it is helpful to consider Morse's analysis of the logical requirements of mental health, in general, outlining the competency question as follows:

1. Is there evidence of current mental disorder, and if so, what is the nature and extent of the disorder and its general symptomatic consequences?
2. Does the defendant manifest some specific, functional inabilities that are of special concern to the legal standard for competency (to be executed)?
3. Given evidence for both of the above elements, is there a logical causal connection between the disorder and the legally relevent inabilities?[34]

If answers to these three questions suggest that a court might find the defendant incompetent, a fourth question will arise in many jurisdictions:

4. Is there a substantial likelihood that treatment can bring the defendant to a state of legal competence?

This last question, of course, is the thorniest for the psychiatrist with regard to competency to be executed.

The next step is to collect background information about the case and the defendant. The type of information sought, in addition to general background information needed for any psychiatric diagnostic evaluation, should consider the particular needs of the situation. For example, consideration should be given to a defendant's ability to withstand emotional stresses specific to the circumstances (e.g., death row).

Next, it is important to remember that, at the outset of the competency examination, the defendant must be informed about the nature of the examination. The interviewer must make an explicit statement about the aim of the conversation, and the fact that it is not confidential. The evaluation is neither confidential nor is it voluntary.

Appropriate assessment tools must be used for a full evaluation. This would include a range of physical, psychometric, and psychological tests.

Finally, after all the information is amassed, the psychiatrist must form conclusions and report them appropriately. In their proposed Criminal Justice Mental Health Standards, the American Bar Association endorsed the following content for written evaluations:[35]

1. Identify the specific matters referred for evaluation;
2. Describe the procedures, tests, and techniques used;
3. State clinical findings and opinions on each matter referred for evaluation and indicate specifically those questions, if any, that could not be answered;
4. Identify the sources of information and present the factual basis for the clinical findings and opinions;
5. Present the reasoning which was used to reach the clinical findings and opinions. A report issued by the Group for Advancement of Psychiatry (GAP) cogently stated a majority opinion that the ultimate legal question should not be addressed in the reports.[36(p 853)]

Other clinical issues that must be considered with regard to competency examinations generally are described by Appelbaum and Roth.[37] The authors stress that, in assessing competency, the examiner must not fail to consider five factors:

1. The psychodynamic elements of the defendant's personality;
2. The accuracy of historical information conveyed by the defendant;
3. The accuracy and completeness of the information disclosed to the defendant;
4. The stability of the defendant's mental status over time;
5. The effect of the setting in which the evaluation is performed.[37]

The article addresses competency to consent to treatment, but the issues are applicable generally.

In addition to these clinical issues, other questions must be addressed before performing a competency evaluation. These include consideration of what is the generally agreed upon standard of competency, and what tests are to be used in the assessment. Appelbaum and Roth[38] discussed these issues and state that competency has lacked a clear and generally agreed upon standard. The various standards that have been used are found usually to fall into one of four groups. These categories, if arranged hierarchically, furnish a progressively more demanding standard for the assessment of competency. These four standards are briefly described below, as well as the psychiatric considerations that Appelbaum and Roth find to be clinically relevant to each.[38] This discussion is followed by the tests described for each standard to assess a patient's abilities. Finally, there is a short summary of the issues that Appelbaum and Roth consider important in shaping the particular standard to a particular situation.

The first standard is evidencing a choice. This is the least-demanding standard and consists of the patient's actual communication of a decision. Psychiatric states impinging on this ability to indicate a choice include mutism, catatonic excitement, profound psychoses, word salad, and marked ambivalence.

The next standard is factual understanding of the issues relevant to the question under consideration. As Appelbaum and Roth state, a typical formulation requires that the subject have "the cognitive capacity to consider the relevant issues."[38(p953)] The person must know "who he is, where he is, what he is reading, and what he is doing in signing the paper."[39] The authors indicate that the rigor of the standard increases as the complexity of the issues increases. "Factual understanding" subsumes two different standards: One can require that the patient have "ability to understand," or more stringently insist that he or she manifest "actual understanding" of the material.[40] Relevant psychiatric aspects include intelligence, language skills, orientation, brain damage, toxic states, and possibly memory impairment resulting from chronic schizophrenia.

The next standard is rational manipulation of information. This requires measurement, beyond factual understanding, of the individual's ability to use the information in the decision-making process. The standard has been described as measuring "judgement, rationality, rational weighing of risks and benefits, reality testing, and decision-making capacity."[38(p954)] Psychiatric difficulties affecting this test include delusions, hallucinations, loosening of associations, severe thought disorder, phobia, anxiety, depression, anger, and obsessive preoccupation, among others.

Finally, the fourth and strictest standard is appreciation of the nature of the situation. "Appreciation is distinct from factual understanding in that it requires the subject to consider the relevance to his immediate situation of those facts he has understood previously in the abstract."[38(p954)]

One alternative description is that the patient recognize "in a mature fashion, the implications of alternative courses of action and appreciate both cognitively and affectively the nature of the thing to be decided."[41] The major psychiatrically relevant condition impinging on appreciation is denial. Others include the capacity for abstract thinking and psychotic distortion or hopelessness.

Appelbaum and Roth include for each standard the usual methods employed to make the appropriate assessment. For evidencing a choice, generally what is required is that the patient be asked to make the choice. Only instances of a patient's extreme ambiguous behavior will be very problematic. Deferral is appropriate in that case. For the second standard, factual understanding, demonstrating the patient's actual understanding, can be accomplished by asking the patient to repeat the information provided, to paraphrase it, and to put it to practical use. For rational manipulation of information, a frequently used test is to ask if the patient is experiencing hallucinations or delusions. Alternatively, inquiry might be made about the rationality of the person's decision-making outside the formal psychiatric examination. A problem with assessment of ability to meet this standard is the difficulty in drawing the required causal links between the presence of the delusion and the patient's decision. Finally, for the standard of appreciation of the nature of the situation, the usual techniques are to assess the patient's insight and to look for the presence or absence of psychotic-level defenses.

After delineating standards, clinical issues, and tests, Appelbaum and Roth turned to a discussion of the factors influencing choice of standard for particular situations. A detailed summary of this critical material is beyond the scope of this Appendix but is of importance to any clinician involved in competency determinations. In brief, Appelbaum and Roth state that, where the line is drawn, which standard is chosen ought to be determined by policy-oriented goals. The difficulty is that generally more than one policy goal is sought, and often these conflict. The standard chosen is usually a compromise, one that seeks to serve various societal values. Some of these values include respect for individual autonomy, the promotion of rational decision-making, an effort to protect others from harm (beneficence), respect for persons, and justice. Which values are served ideally should be determined by the achievement of public consensus on policy goals.

The summary above indicates competency issues in general. Although little has been written specifically about competency to be executed in terms of the performance of the examination, Radelet and Barnard have provided the fullest discussion.[10(p45)] Rather than enter the argument of participation or not by psychiatrists, the authors "raise issues that individual psychiatrists should consider in determining the proper course of action." These issues are the need for professional standards in the examination and the problem of due process.

The need for procedural standards relates to the vague definition of competency that is generally found in statutes. The definition is a legal one, and yet, because of vagueness, often considerations other than legal considerations are brought to bear on the assessment process; for example, the psychiatrist's opinion of the death penalty, or the nature of the offense. Radelet and Barnard suggest that two pragmatic steps be taken by psychiatrists before making a competency evaluation of this nature. One is that written reports be sufficiently detailed so that readers can follow the assumptions, facts, and reasoning process used in the evaluation. This requires reports of an extremely detailed nature. The second step is that the clinician make the most thorough and detailed evaluation possible. "The point is that evaluations of this sort must be done with the highest level of professional skill possible; no other standard is possible when the purpose is deciding who shall live and who shall die."[10(p46)]

With regard to the issue of due process, the difficulty arises in jurisdictions in which statutes do not provide for challenge by the defendant in an adversarial process of the psychiatrist's opinion about his or her competency. Where that is the case, the authors "conclude that a finding of competence requires more certainty, clarity, and comprehensiveness than a finding of incompetence. . . . The burden of proof is on those who believe the prisoner is competent to die."[10(p48)]

More specific guidelines cannot be provided than the background information offered above. State statutes vary radically, and a clinician, should he or she actually make the choice to participate in such evaluations, must be familiar with the law in his or her own state. The authors reiterate that, in their opinion, psychiatrists ought not to participate in competency for execution evaluations if the death penalty is not first commuted to a life sentence.

REFERENCES

1. Reidinger P: Death penalty. *ABA J* 1987; 47–55.
2. Korn RR: Life followed by execution. *Crim Justice Behav* 1983; 10: 121–128.
3. Andersen K: An eye for an eye. *Time,* January 24, 1983, pp 28–39.
4. *Ford v Wainwright,* 752 F.2d 526, 530 (11th Cir. 1985) (Clark, J., dissenting), *rev'd,* 106 S. Ct. 2595 (1986).
5. Blackstone W: *Commentaries,* vol 4, §§395–396.
6. Coke E: *Third Institutes,* vol 6, ed 6, 1980.
7. Hawles J: *Remarks on Tryal of Charles Bateman,* in Howell T (ed): *Eleven State Trials,* 1816, §§ 474, 477.
8. Insanity of the condemned *Yale Law J* 1979; 88: 533–564.
9. *Gregg v Georgia,* 428 U.S. 153, 183 (1976).
10. Radelet ML, Barnard GW: Ethics and the psychiatric determination of competency to be executed. *Bull Am Acad Psychiatry Law* 1986; 14:39–40.
11. *McClesky v Kemp,* 55 U.S.L.W. 4537 (1987).
12. US Department of Justice, Bureau of Justice Statistics Bulletin: *Capital Punishment.* Washington, DC, Government Printing Office, 1985.
13. Bluestone H, McGahee CL: Reaction to extreme stress: Impending death by execution. *Am J Psychiatry* 1982; 11: 393–396.
14. Gallemore JL, Panton JH: Inmate response to lengthy death row confinement. *Am J Psychiatry* 1972; 129: 81–86.
15. Johnson R: *Condemned to Die: Under Sentence of Death.* New York, Elsevier North-Holland, 1981.
16. Davis C: *Waiting for It* 1980.
17. Gettinger S: *Sentenced to Die* 1979, p. 94.
18. *Ford v Wainwright,* 752 F.2d 256 (11th Cir. 1985).

19. Zonana H: *Ford v Wainwright:* Competency to be executed. *Am Acad Psychiatry Law Newsletter* 1986; 11: 8–10.
20. N.M. Stat. Ann. §§ 31–14–4 to 31–14–7 (1984).
21. *Solesbee v Balkcom,* 339 U.S. 9 (1950).
22. *Ford v Strickland,* 676 F.2d 471 (1984).
23. *Ford v Wainwright,* 4S1 So. 2d. 471 (1984); *Ford v Wainwright,* 752 F.2d 525 (1985).
24. *Caritativo v California,* 357 U.S. 549 (1958).
25. American Medical Association: *Principles of Medical Ethics with Annotations Especially Applicable to Psychiatry.* Washington, DC, American Medical Association, Sec. 1 No. 1, 1981 p 4.
26. Appelbaum PS: Competence to be executed: Another conundrum for mental health professionals. *Hosp Comm Psychiatry* 1986; 37: 682–684.
27. National Medical Association: *Position Statement on the Role of the Psychiatrist in Evaluation and Treating "Death Row" Inmates* (pp 1–5). Washington, DC, National Medical Association, undated.
28. Letter from Peter D. Ostreich, Chairperson, Florida State Hospital Human Rights Advocacy Committee, to Marchia Beach, Chairperson, Statewide Human Rights Advocacy Committee, Dec. 6, 1984.
29. Stone AA: Psychiatry and the death penalty. *The Psychiatric Times* III:9, September, 1986, p 1.
30. Radelet ML Barnard GW: Ethics and the psychiatric determination of competency to be executed (November 20, 1984, unpublished manuscript), cited in Ward BA: Competency for execution: Problems in law and psychiatry. *Fla St U Law Rev* 1986 14: 35, fn 59.
31. Sargent DA: Treating the condemned to death. *Hastings Center Report* 1986; 16:5–6.
32. Salguero RG: Medical ethics and competency to be executed. *Yale Law J* 1986; 96:167–186.
33. Curran WJ, McGarry AL, Shah SA: *Forensic Psychiatry and Psychology.* FA Davis Co, 1986 p 154.
34. Morse S: Crazy behavior, morals and science: An analysis of mental health law. *S Cal Law Rev* 1978; 51:527–654.
35. American Bar Association: *Proposed Criminal Justice Mental Health Standards.* Chicago, American Bar Association, 1985.
36. Group for the Advancement of Psychiatry: *Misuse of Psychiatry in the Criminal Courts: Competency to Stand Trial.* White Plains, NY, Committee on Psychiatry and the Law, vol 8, 1974.
37. Appelbaum PS, Roth LH: Clinical issues in the assessment of competency. *Am J Psychiatry* 1981; 138:1462–1467.
38. Appelbaum PS, Roth LH: Competency to consent to research. *Arch Gen Psychiatry* 1982; 39:951–958.
39. Owens H: When is a voluntary commitment really voluntary? *Am J Orthopsychiatry* 1977; 47:104–110.
40. Roth LH, Meisel A, Lidz CW: Tests of competency to consent to treatment. *Am J Psychiatry* 1977; 134:279–284.
41. Postel RI: Civil commitment: A functional analysis. *Brooklyn Law Rev* 1971; 38:1–94.

8

Stress as a Factor for Mental Health Professionals in Correctional Facilities

MICHAEL H. BELL

INTRODUCTION

There has been an increasing interest in the role of mental health professionals in correctional settings. Estimates of mentally ill inmates in prisons have ranged from as low as 5% to as high as 75% of the population.[1,2] Extrinsic factors, such as the deinstitutionalization of chronic mentally ill patients as well as the process of criminalization of the mentally ill, have contributed to this increasing interest as well as the growing numbers of mentally ill inmates in prisons. In this chapter, I will identify and discuss some of the factors that contribute to producing stress in mental health professionals who are working in correctional facilities. I will explore how stressful factors affect mental health professionals who venture into the locked doors of correctional settings in an attempt to offer treatment to a needy, often neglected population. In addition, I will attempt to discuss what, if anything, can be done to ameliorate the identified stressors. The observations in this chapter are based on my personal experience as a psychiatrist working in correctional settings as well as a review of representative literature on mental health professionals in correctional settings. My personal experience in the past includes working at the Correctional Facilities on Rikers Island in New

MICHAEL H. BELL • Department of Psychiatry and Mental Health Services, University of Medicine and Dentistry of New Jersey, Newark, NJ 07103.

York; doing consultation psychiatric evaluations at the Morris County Jail in Morristown, New Jersey; serving on the Bellevue Inpatient Forensic Unit in New York City; and performing psychiatric-legal evaluations at the Forensic Psychiatry Clinic in lower Manhattan. It is not my purpose in this chapter to either encourage or dissuade other mental health professionals from practicing in correctional settings. Rather, it is my hope that this chapter will be insightful for some, and that, for others, it will be sufficiently provocative to lead to further exploration and discussion of this subject.

It is not uncommon for mental health professionals who enter a correctional facility for the first time to have mixed feelings. For example, a psychiatrist visiting Rikers Island for the first time may feel awed by the process of getting to the mental health clinic. First, he must be cleared to cross over the bridge that leads to the island. Then he must pass through numerous checkpoints, barbed-wire fences, and jailbars. Correctional officers are seen everywhere, and the security is tight. There is a feeling of being isolated and segregated from the rest of society. The need for close security and the scrutiny of all who enter a prison remind the professional that he is entering a potentially dangerous setting. A new professional, who is not known to the correctional officers, is likely to be treated with caution by the officers on the gate and may even be subjected to a "patting down" (a bodily search) to insure that he is not bringing in any type of contraband. Thus, professionals may often find themselves experiencing mixed feelings of anxiety, fear, anger, or indignation when they enter into a corrections facility.

Even after the professional has come many times to a prison and becomes known to the correctional staff, he may still have confused feelings as a result of the nontraditional setting of his office within the prison. He may have difficulty with the punitive philosophy of prisons which is in contrast to the therapeutic, more humanistic settings that he has practiced in outside of prisons.[3] Prison security may often compromise the needs of the professional and the inmate to have an area where they can meet in privacy and maintain confidentiality. The professional must also be aware of the possibility of harm to himself. At any prison, the evidence of the potential for violence is everywhere. Inmates who suffer injuries that are caused by the actions of other inmates and from correctional officers can be a constant reminder to the professional that he, too, can be injured. At one jail, an inmate who was angry that a psychiatrist was not transferring him to a mental health facility chased the psychiatrist around the clinic before being subdued by the correctional officers. A week later, the inmate was back in the clinic where the corrections officers and nursing staff joked with him about his chasing the psychiatrist. The professional who is faced with the potential of physical harm to himself may overidentify with the correctional officers and seek to be punitive toward his patients, or he may foolishly deny his own fears and engage in provocative interactions with inmates, which may lead to his exposing himself to dangerous situations.[4]

As previously noted, inmates can also be a source of stress to the professional. In many prisons and jails, the inmate population may be overwhelmingly members of minority groups. For the professional working in such a setting, the possibility of stereotypic conceptualization, based on biased perceptions of ethnic groups by the professional, can become a problem. Professionals may find that the inmates, whom they are trying to help, are aloof, distancing, and suspicious of them. Other professionals have written of the difficulties of treating the antisocial person who has problems trusting and developing therapeutic alliances with therapists.[2,4] This phenomenon may be further exacerbated in the minority inmate who, based on his own experience of being a minority,[5,6] may feel an even more heightened distrust for the staff at the jail, whether they are correctional officers or mental health professionals. The professional who is white may feel overwhelmed by the racial countertransferential feelings arising in him as well as the negative transference feelings "assaulting him" from the inmates.

For the minority mental health professional, the situation can likewise be stress producing. His own sense of identity and racial pride may be affected by a situation in which the inmate population is predominantly minority. He may, on the one hand, overidentify with the punitive aspect of the prison in order to separate himself from those inmates whom he views as being bad and an affront to the efforts that he has made to improve the beliefs that his white colleagues have about minorities and, by extension, himself. On the other hand, he may overidentify with the minority inmates and attribute their plight to the racism in society and may therefore attempt to separate himself from the "system" and the prison administration by enabling the minority inmate to avoid following the rules and regulations of the prisons. Either course of overidentification can lead to further stress for the minority professional and impinge on his functioning.

The mental health professional who attempts to work with inmates is often confronted with the simple fact that inmates are often not nice people. Many of them have committed heinous crimes. One cannot help but have reaction feelings about the inmate who, before being incarcerated, brutally murdered, raped, or assaulted people. Often the lack of remorse in an inmate can stun the professional. Moreover, the professional may find himself with a hostile inmate who is intent on being intimidating with him; or, conversely, he may find himself with an inmate who attempts to impress him with a detailed and horrifying description of his "exploits" while at large. Often the inmates may dress and behave in a fashion that is adaptive for survival in the prison setting but that is maladaptive and frightening to the professional who is unaccustomed to correctional settings.

Of those inmates who are seriously mentally ill, some have been noncompliant with treatment in the past and continue to reject treatment when they are incarcerated. Some inmates do not have identifiable symptoms that can be treated and may have been brought involuntarily to the mental health professional by the correctional staff because they are disciplinary problems. When the professional attempts to conduct an examination, other problems can arise, such as the reliability of the information that is obtained. A reply by one psychiatrist may summarize the skeptical attitudes that can develop with this population: When asked "How do you know when an inmate is lying to you?," his simple answer was "Whenever his lips are moving!"

The professional who works in a prison has to be aware of the conflict of being manipulated either by the inmates or by the prison system. Manipulation of the professional by the inmates can be understood when one looks at the process of incarceration as well as the character pathology of many inmates. Incarceration imposes tremendous physical and emotional strains on many inmates. Prisons are brutal places in which many inmates will be victimized by other more brutal inmates, as well as being subjected to often rigid, unempathetic prison staff. Punishment plays a role in all prisons[7] and, in many cases, the source of stress to the inmates is the incarceration itself. The code of silence in prisons can leave an inmate with little recourse for help when he is being victimized by others. Prisoners who inform on other inmates place themselves at risk to increased stress, physical harm, and even death. An inmate who is being terrorized and victimized by other inmates may possibly turn to the professional for help. In such a situation, the professional may in fact do more harm if he rushes in blindly and reports on the other inmates. In seeking to protect the victimized inmate, he may actually expose him to further danger. This dilemma may be frustrating to people who are trained to be direct in their crisis interventions and who may ultimately find that they did more harm than good to their patients.

Although the mental health professional may be well suited to crisis intervention, he may at times be confronted with the malingering that some inmates resort to in order to be transferred from the general population to a prison mental observation unit or to a civil mental hospital. Obviously, the professional is not able to transfer everyone or he would disrupt the prison system. Consequently, the inmate may then "up the ante" and feign psychosis or make manipulative suicide gestures or self-mutilating acts in order to be transferred. If the psychiatrist transfers too many inmates, he may be overburdened with other inmates who will attempt to get out of prison in any way possible, and, in addition, he will strain his relationship with the correctional staff. But if the psychiatrist "holds the line," an inmate may progress to more self-destructive actions or may try to physically intimidate the professional. The professional who finds that he has been manipulated or seduced by an inmate may experience anger and begin to believe that all the inmates are feigning illness and are not to be believed. Also he may encounter further ostracism by the correctional staff who see him as soft and interfering with the discipline of the inmates. Thus, the mental health professional may find himself in a "can't-win" situation as he tries to balance his obligation to the prison system and to his patients, while, at the same time, trying to differentiate the malingerers from the seriously ill.

The problem of manipulation by the prison system and/or the inmates can be seen vividly in the case of inmates who are placed in solitary confinement or in disciplinary cells, where they may be confined for up to 23 hours or more each day. In some facilities, the only early way out of such confinement for an inmate is through the mental health route: if he is deemed too mentally ill to continue the punishment, he can be removed from the confinement. Then, too, the inmate in question may well have been a disciplinary problem who was sent to confinement for punishment. The professional must therefore balance the needs of the prison versus the needs of the inmates. The professional can be influenced by the correctional staff, since he is dependent on them for his own protection, and also by the fact that the jail is the correctional staff's "turf." The correctional staff may also bring a problem inmate to the professional and then may be disappointed if the psychiatrist properly declines to medicate the patient or to transfer him to a mental health facility.[8] The psychiatrist who may already feel isolated and unappreciated may incur further alienation and the risk of not being accepted as part of the "team."

PROBLEMS WITH THE THERAPEUTIC RELATIONSHIP

In prison settings, the problem of confidentiality and other ethical issues can cause stress for the professional.[1,9] As mentioned previously, there is frequently a dilemma that is the result of the duty of the doctor to the institution versus the duty of the doctor to the patient. The professional who is working in prisons is aware of this conflict, because he is obliged to report certain information to the corrections personnel, such as when an inmate is identified as being suicidal, homicidal, or posing a clear danger of injury to himself or to others; when an inmate is presenting a clear and immediate risk of escaping or creating a riot; when an inmate is in need of psychotropic medication or requires a transfer for mental health reasons.[10] Along with the problem of confidentiality, the problem of informed consent can arise when treating inmates. In this regard, the professional attempts to serve two clients, the prison and the inmate, and conflicts may result even though it is possible to serve the best interests of each. Nevertheless, ethical problems, which are discussed elsewhere,[1,9] can occur when information is obtained from a trusting inmate. The psychiatrist is then obligated to report these findings to the correctional staff, which disclosure may result in punitive consequences for the inmate. This situation, however, is not unique to prison psychiatrists. Other psychiatrists, in military settings and in the private sector, who are faced with child-abuse cases or with patients who threaten harm to others (as, e.g., in Tarasoff-like cases) may have to break confidentiality because it is required by statute or by case law.

Other factors may interrupt the therapeutic relationship. Because of his background, the inmate may have difficulty forming a therapeutic alliance and may distrust the therapist. He may also act in ways that cause both the therapist and the correctional staff to react in a punitive, rejecting manner toward him secondary, for example, to his use of splitting and projective identification.[3] For the professional, his own countertransference can be a source of intrusion into the therapeutic alliance and a source of stress to himself. The difference between what is punishment and what is treatment can become a thin line for the therapist who may be strained by the countertransference toward the inmate. The desire to see an inmate punished may persuade the professional to withold treatment as a form of punishment; he may develop either a laissez-faire or a survival-of-the-fittest attitude toward an inmate who is in distress, which may lead to an increase of guilt feelings within himself. Furthermore, he may think that the institution is the cause of all the problems therefore leading him to do battle with the administration in the mistaken belief that he is helping his patient, instead of realizing that he is responding only to his own stressful situation.

The logistics of functioning in a security-minded environment can also interrupt the treatment provided by a professional. The problems of supplying medication to inmates, the difficulties in getting inmates to be seen in a setting where there are rituals that are carried out in set, regimented ways by the correctional staff, in addition to inmate count checks, inmates who are sent out to court hearings or are transferred to other facilities without warning, all can interfere with treatment. The professional has either to adjust to his role in the greater scheme of the prison system or his stress will increase.

EFFECTS OF STRESS AND COPING WITH STRESS

The effects of stress are varied. The professional can find himself losing interest in his work and experiencing fatigue, anger, depression, and a decline in his physical and in his mental health. If he develops maladaptive coping mechanisms, he may suffer a loss of his skills as a psychiatrist, as, for example, in diagnosing and in treating mental illness. He may develop a disdain for all patients and attempt to protect himself from his own frustrations by believing that all mental illness is malingered. The process of overidentification with the correctional department (which has been discussed) may lead to a desire solely for punishment of inmates. Conversely, the professional may overidentify with the inmates and place himself in a confrontational, more stressful position with the prison administration. A professional in a position of leadership may shy away from making decisions and delegate to others the right to make decisions that he is better qualified and trained to make. The professional may suffer a feeling of burnout and may even decide to terminate his affiliation with the correctional facility. The overstressed mental health professional working in prisons, like anyone else operating under a great deal of stress, may also find his life outside of the prison impinged upon, as he unsuccessfully attempts to cope with a situation that is now out of control. It becomes important then for the level of stress not to reach the point that the professional is unable to function at the level he is capable of.

COPING WITH STRESS

What can a mental health professional do to cope with the stress that is inherent in working in correctional facilities? One of the first things that can be done is to adjust to the environment of being in a prison. Prisons can be deplorable in terms of the physical conditions of the facilities.[1,8,9,11] It is important, therefore, to adjust to and understand the milieu of a prison. The mental health professional must also learn his place in the society of prison life whether it be with correctional officers, inmates, or the administration. I have already discussed examples of stressful situations that may be encountered, such as dealing with the correctional staff. The professional should see himself in the role of working with, as well as educating, the correctional staff about mental health issues as they relate to inmates and to the stress that the correctional officers themselves face. The professional can serve as a role model in offering a more humane way of dealing with problematic and mentally ill inmates.[3] Likewise the correctional staff can educate the mental health professional on aspects of working with inmates, as well as providing valuable clinical information that would otherwise not be available. Cultivating a liaison with other services and groups in the prison can help the professional to end the feelings of isolation and depression that come from being alienated from co-workers in the other disciplines.

Being aware of the problems inherent in working with inmates is also important if the professional is to cope successfully with stress. It is important for the professional to accept his limitations, because it is not possible, for a variety of reasons, to help everyone. It is essential for the professional to carefully select the inmates that he becomes actively and closely engaged with in treatment. Some researchers have recommended the importance of treatment groups and a team approach to working with inmates and/or people with antisocial syndromes.[1,4,11] Besides aiding other professionals with their sharing of the burden of providing services for a needy population, it also allows the treatment issues to be split from the forensic issues. In correctional facilities, for example, the problem of confidentiality can arise when information is also needed for legal purposes, such as competency to stand trial. Thus, some members of the team can be concerned with treatment issues while others can focus on psychiatric-legal issues. This division of purpose might avoid somewhat the problem of the professional becoming a double agent.[1,11]

Countertransference,[3,9,12] which has been mentioned earlier, can lead to the problem of the professional who fears harm from the inmates, who experiences intense anger at inmates and/or other co-workers at the prison, or who denies his own feelings. An understanding in the professional that his countertransference can affect how he functions is essential when working in prisons. It is important that the mental health professional realize he can serve as a role model for inmates and correctional staff alike in dealing with stressful situations.[3] The professional must walk a narrow line between attempting to provide help toward alleviating the problems of his patients, and exacerbating the problems by encouraging the inmates to be rebellious and uncompromising in an environment that demands conformity and adaptation by all. Countertransference problems can also lead to negative feelings toward inmates. Thus, it is important that the professional avoid labels and stereotypic characterizations of inmates. The professional must be aware that some inmates will attempt to con and manipulate him. Yet he must not allow these experiences to prejudice him into becoming cynical and punitive toward all inmates. Skepticism is a necessary attitude when working with some inmates, however, the professional should still be inquisitive and thorough in his evaluation of an inmate.

The manipulative inmate should be treated with a team approach, which should include the correctional officers. In his zest to be seen as mentally ill, the manipulative inmate may break prison rules by such actions as smashing furniture in his cell, flooding the cell, starting fires, or mutilating himself. The difficult inmate necessitates cooperation among several disciplines in order to handle appropriately the problems he presents. The correctional staff must be educated in terms of what may be psychiatric problems and what may be disciplinary problems so that they are better able to handle each situation. Once the professional has established a better relationship with the department of corrections, the pathologic inmate will be less able to create a split between the professional and the correctional staffs. Again, the problems of countertransference can arise in these situations and must be monitored.

The stress of working in correctional facilities should make the professional wary of working full-time in a prison. Although the psychiatrist may be better able to avoid this pitfall, some workers in the other mental health disciplines may not. If possible, working in more traditional settings outside of the prison part-time would aid the professional in decreasing stress, cynicism, and the burnout that can result in working full-time in the "trenches" of a correctional facility. In addition, the professional who is involved in other career activities, such as professional groups, medical schools, conferences, and educational endeavors, can aid in promoting a more distinctive image for those who work in prisons and who can easily become isolated from their peers.

Despite an awareness of all that has been discussed, a mental health professional may find himself succumbing to the stress of working in a correctional facility. Should such a scenario develop, the professional should attempt to identify what is causing the problem and then try to alleviate the problem. Some professionals may decide that the solution is to lessen their participation or to terminate entirely their participation. Knowing when the time has come to leave is also an important consideration and should be explored with supervisors, therapists, and friends. Working in prisons can be stressful. For some, the experience can be an opportunity to provide needed services to an underserved population; for others, it can be a quagmire, rife with stress and conflicts, which can appear to have no obtainable solution.

REFERENCES

1. Goldstein N: Psychiatry in prisons. *Psychiatric Clinics of North America* 1983; 6:751–765.

2. Lamb HR, Grant RW: The mentally ill in an urban county jail. *Arch Gen Psychiatry* 1982; 39:17–22.
3. Alder G: Correctional (prison) psychiatry, in Kaplan HI, Sadock BJ (eds): *Comprehensive Textbook of Psychiatry,* ed 4. Baltimore, Williams & Wilkins, 1985, pp 1990–1997.
4. Reid WH, Dorr D, Walker JI, *et al.* (eds): *Unmasking the Psychopath: Antisocial Personality and Related Syndromes.* New York, WW Norton & Co 1986.
5. Mayo JA: The concept of masked anxiety in young adult black males, in Klein DF, Rabkin J (eds): *Anxiety—New Research and Changing Concepts.* New York, Raven Press, 1981.
6. Bell M, Ellison R: Issues in the psychiatric legal evaluation of the black elderly, in Rosner R, Schwartz HI (eds): *Geriatric Psychiatry and the Law.* New York, Plenum Press, 1987, pp 327–335.
7. Shively D, Petrich J: Correctional mental health. *Psychiatric Clinics of North America* 1985; 8:537–550.
8. Kaufman E: The violations of psychiatric standards of care in prisons. *Am J Psychiatry* 1980; 137:5, 566–570.
9. Smith R: The state of the prisons: Prison doctors: Ethics, invisibility and quality. *Br Med J* 1984; 288:781–783.
10. Board of Correction: *Mental Health Minimum Standards for New York City Correctional Facilities, part VII: Confidentiality.* New York, Board of Correction, 1984, pp 6–7.
11. Valdiserri E: Psychiatry behind bars. *Bull Am Acad Psychiatry Law* 1984; 12:93–99.
12. Reid WH (ed): *The Psychopath—A Comprehensive Study of Antisocial Disorders and Behaviors.* New York, Brunner/Mazel, 1978.

III

Inmates' Rights

9

The Inmate as Patient

An Inmate's Rights in the Context of Health Care Services

NANCY N. DUBLER AND MARGARET D. WISHART

Rapid and positive developments in the prison health care field during the past decade have tended to obscure the fact that, prior to 1976, inmates of the nation's prisons and jails had no right to health care, even though it was impossible for them to obtain it by their own efforts, and, in most cases, received only the most rudimentary or no medical attention. Indeed, for much of recorded history, the societal expectation for prisoners has been torture and execution, and the health care obligations of jailers have extended only to keeping their charges breathing long enough to undergo these harsh and sanctioned punishments. Few were the prisoners who emerged alive or well from their dungeons or cells.

The Enlightenment movement of the 18th century, with its rationalist and humanitarian philosophy, together with the practical need to accommodate growing numbers of convicted criminals, encouraged the development in the Western world of a new type of prison, the penitentiary.[1] The new philosophy proposed that torture and execution were inappropriate for those of God's creatures who had fallen from the paths of righteous behavior. The penitentiary, it was argued, would not only perform the necessary function of segregating criminal offenders

NANCY N. DUBLER • Department of Social Medicine, Montefiore Medical Center, Bronx, NY 10467. **MARGARET D. WISHART** • Montefiore Medical Center, Bronx, NY 10467; Rikers Island Health Services, East Elmhurst, NY 11370.

from society, but would also reform these unfortunates, thus permitting them at the end of their sentence to gain a place within the proper world of commerce and industry. On a more pragmatic level, the development of prisons and jails in the new correctional model was also spurred on by the closing of America to the transportation of minor criminals from England and by the inability of Australia to absorb all of the convicts sentenced by the English courts.[2]

Although an institution designed for reform and rehabilitation must, of necessity, keep its subjects alive to fulfill its goals, from the beginning there was little discussion or concern about the rights of penitentiary inmates. Once committed to the institution, an inmate was considered civilly dead and no longer entitled to the rights and privileges of the general citizenry. There is a distinction, however, between a loss of the common rights of citizenship, on the one hand, and subjection to inhumane or torturous treatment, on the other. As the history of correctional institutions over almost two centuries demonstrates only too clearly, policies developed in a climate of moral condemnation of criminal offenders quickly degenerate into callous and barbaric regulations, however benevolent their objectives. As an example, the first attempt to introduce a minimal level of health care for prisoners occurred in England in the Gloucestershire penitentiaries in the 1780s. It succeeded only when the criminal justice and the medical authorities alike were persuaded that a few basic hygienic measures such as baths, however necessary for the public health of the institution, could still serve a punitive function. In a report proposing the shaving of prisoners' heads to prevent the spread of vermin, Sir George Onesiphorous Paul, a magistrate responsible for supervising the penitentiaries, argued that:

> Because so far as shaving the head is a mortification to the offender, it becomes a punishment directed to the mind, and is (at least so I have conceived) an allowable alternative for inflicting corporal punishment intended to be excluded from this system.[1(p 101)]

This opprobrious attitude toward penitentiary inmates was further strengthened by the rigid class distinctions between them and their overseers, all of whom were members of the middle and upper classes. In contrast to many political prisoners of preceding centuries, those men and women committed to the penitentiaries were almost without exception drawn from the ranks of the poor. Thus, the pattern for the prison or jail as the instrument for the segregation and largely unmonitored "rehabilitation" of the most disadvantaged members of society was set and remained unchanged for almost two hundred years.

THE CONSTITUTIONAL RIGHT TO HEALTH CARE

In the 1960s, however, a number of forces combined to focus judicial and public attention on the deplorable conditions of the prisons and jails in the United States. Civil rights protestors, an uncommon middle-class prison population, found themselves incarcerated. These educated and often well-connected inmates were able to stimulate interest in their own plight and in the situation of their fellow inmates. Investigative reporting documented the indignities, dangers, and degradations of prison life. Legal Services, staffed for the first time in 1968 by attorneys supported by federal funds, found itself able to litigate on behalf of classes of the dispossessed and the vulnerable. By the 1970s a number of court cases, media exposés, and prominent coverage of prison riots had documented that many prison systems in the United States not only confined and punished but, in addition, abused, tortured, and murdered. A prisoner, especially a black prisoner in the South, often disappeared into a prison system to emerge in a coffin or to be found later as a corpse buried in the prison yard. Finally, in response to all of these stimuli, the courts began to reexamine their previously held position that the reviewability of prison and jail administrative structures and decisions was beyond their jurisdiction.

In 1973, in *Procunier v Martinez*,[3] the Supreme Court decreed the end of the "hands-off" doctrine. That doctrine had held that the problems of prison and jails were so complex and intractable and so ill-suited to resolutions by judicial decree that policies of support for administrative discretion were adequate and appropriate. In the face of prison uprisings, and in response to the societal pressures that had emerged in the sixties, prison administrators, said the courts, now had to justify deprivations or policies of punishment by demonstrating that the "regulation or practice in question furthers an important or substantial government interest." Once scrutiny had been judicially permitted, the courts quickly became the regular forum for the presentation of evidence demonstrating the callousness and sometimes brutality of prison administrators. Institutions that had been designed to confine and punish through the deprivation of liberty had evolved into settings characterized often by unrestrained violence and disregard for human suffering.

The issue of whether inmates had a "right" to medical care became an early focus of litigation for obvious reasons. Medical care, or the lack thereof, represents one of the single most important elements in an inmate's existence. The lack of medical care, or its denial, results in pain, suffering, and long-term health disabilities which, the cases would argue, were not decreed by the sentence. The early cases struggled to create a standard that could be used to judge the adequacy of care without flooding the federal courts with inappropriate litigation that did not raise constitutional issues, but rather claimed malpractice. Some of these early cases argued that the provision of some or any care would meet the constitutional standard. Other cases argued that only adequate care would suffice.

In 1976, in *Estelle v Gamble*,[4] the Supreme Court stated clearly that persons have a constitutionally protected right to medical care when incarcerated. The Court grounded its decision in interpretations of the Eighth Amendment. This amendment was proposed originally to prohibit the bizarre tortures and horrible punishments, which had been the prerogative of the English king. Over the decades, however, the Supreme Court had held that this amendment changes according to contemporary standards of decency and dignity. Therefore, the Court stated, it could now prohibit the medical deprivations that had been proved to exist in prisons. The court reasoned that to put persons in prison where they cannot secure their own medical care and not to provide that care results in precisely the pain, suffering, and torture which the Eighth Amendment was designed to prohibit. In its opinion, the Court stated that:

> Deliberate indifference to the serious medical needs of prisoners constitutes the unnecessary and wanton infliction of pain . . . proscribed by the Eighth Amendment. This is true whether the indifference is manifested by prison doctors and their response to the prisoner's needs or by prison guards in intentionally denying or delaying access to medical care or intentionally interfering with treatment once prescribed.[5]

The scope of this standard was immediately challenged in federal jurisdictions around the country. Two primary questions were placed before various federal courts:

1. Could systemic deficiencies provide the basis for injunctive relief when buttressed by demonstrations of individual denials of care?
2. Did the scope of the right to care extend from care for somatic illness to care for mental illness?

Both of these questions were answered in the affirmative. The courts held that injunctive relief would lie in prison cases and thus not only could an inmate's constitutional right be vindicated, and an individual wrong be remedied by an individual federal suit, but the prison or jail could be ordered to alter those aspects of its health care delivery system that had led to the deprivation in question. The affirmative answer to the second question meant that treatment for psychiatric illness would be held to the same constitutional standard as treatment for medical illness.

The right to mental health care stands on the same analytic base as the right to medical care. Additionally, it is supported by a separate line of cases that decreed, in the late fifties and early sixties, that the mentally ill confined in large state institutions had a "right to treatment." Those cases reasoned that confinement in a mental institution by the state was a deprivation of individual liberty that had to be legally justified by a compensating individual benefit.[6] These cases were decided, in large measure, after the development of psychotropic medications and new psychiatric interventions, which made it possible, for the first time, to treat large numbers of mentally ill cheaply, effectively, and outside of confined settings. This legal and treatment context became the background for the articulated right of prison and jail inmates to mental health care, that is, an inmate is entitled to a physiological or psychiatric treatment if the prisoner's symptoms evidence a serious disease or injury which is curable or may be substantially alleviated, and the delay or denial of care could produce possible serious harm.

EXERCISING THE RIGHT TO CARE IN THE CORRECTIONAL SETTING

Providing medical or mental health care services in a prison or jail presents problems unlike those encountered in any other setting. In correctional institutions, where security concerns are always paramount, health care services are subservient to the goals of correctional authorities and are often in conflict with them. The goals of correctional administrators are confinement, custody, and control; the goals of health care providers, whatever the setting, are diagnosis, treatment, comfort, and cure. The correctional staff at institutions are trained to distrust and distance the inmate population. The medical staff must be governed by an ethic of caring and concern.

Some distinctions are made, but, in the main, inmates tend to regard all staff in correctional settings as "the others." Differences between and among correctional and civilian staff are difficult to establish and hard to maintain. Inmate existence is organized along lines of power over other inmates and manipulation of the administrative system. These principles can extend to the health care system, even when that system is an independent one, and often lead, it is charged, to attempts to manipulate health care providers in support of real, exaggerated, or even imagined complaints. In contrast, it is easy to see that, in a setting in which all ties to the outside world are severed, and physical and mental energies have few appropriate outlets, an inmate will focus inward on even minor physical or emotional distress and discomforts. Confinement, regimentation, close supervision by correctional staff, and oppression by other inmates are all calculated to raise levels of anxiety in those who are not mentally ill and to exacerbate preexisting mental illness. Given these stresses, medical and mental health care providers must work according to carefully designed protocols that enable them to diagnose and treat within the context of regimentation and restriction.

Especially in the area of mental health care, diagnostic skill must differentiate between an inmate's response to the devaluing and dehumanizing structure of prison life, which is calculated to cause discontent and unhappiness, and true mental health problems whose origins are not site-specific. In most cases, generalized discontent or unhappiness is not a treatable mental illness. But anxiety may be related to inter-inmate power struggles or disagreements with the administration. It, too, need not be a mental health problem. Disabling anxiety, however, whatever its reality base, and true mental illness, as defined by the Diagnostic and Statistical Manual of Mental Disorders (3rd ed., revised), do provide the basis for an inmate's right to treatment.

ACCESS TO CARE

There are particular problems of access to care in any correctional setting. Prisons and jails are designed to prevent ease of movement by inmates both to the outside and within the institution. Therefore, in addition to systems that permit inmates to communicate with the health care unit without hindrance, constitutionally adequate access to care requires an ancillary system under which medical and mental health care providers can reach out to the inmates who may not be able to communicate their needs directly. Health care staff must assure access in various ways. First, they must establish ways of informing inmates of the specific services available to them. Second, they must establish a regular system for the daily physical observation of inmates in segregation areas from which they are not readily allowed egress. Third, they must work with the correctional authorities to develop flexible systems that enable inmates to communicate easily with the health care staff. Fourth, they must educate correctional officers and their supervisors about those signs and symptoms of possible health problems in inmates that should be communicated immediately to the health care service.

Sign-up sheets or sick call slips, which can be filled out daily and sent to the medical clinic or the mental health center, are vitally important. However, especially for the mentally ill, the ability to mobilize effectively and use existing systems may be severely hampered. In such cases, observation of inmates by specially trained correctional officers, supplemented by regular observation by health care personnel, is essential.

THE RIGHT TO CONFIDENTIALITY

It is particularly difficult to assure the confidentiality of doctor–patient communications in a correctional setting. Outside of prisons, confidentiality is taken to be a primary characteristic of the doctor–patient relationship. Beginning with the earliest professional oaths, physicians have pledged to guard the medical secrets of their patients. In addition, the courts early recognized the existence of special relationships that formed the basis for a doctrine of judicial privilege. Four sets of protected relationships were identified by the English courts and were later codified by statute in all states in the United States. These four relationships are those between husband and wife, priest and penitent, lawyer and client, and physician and patient. The courts reasoned that communication was so central and critical to these relationships that a later claim for testimony in court about the content of conversations between the parties could be defeated by the protected parties' raising the issue of privilege. Not surprisingly, because the exercise of this privilege almost certainly excludes otherwise relevant testimony from the consideration of the court, it has been interpreted narrowly by most courts.

This doctrine of privilege, and the ethical obligation of confidentiality incorporated in all states under the licensing codes, establishes the formal supports for the obligation of physicians to keep the communications of their patients secret and private. Arrayed against these protections for the confidentiality of patient communications are third-party-reimbursement arrangements, which require a patient to authorize physicians to share information on diagnosis and treatment, the computerization of medical information, which provides large numbers of individuals with largely unrestricted access to stable data bases, and the growing system of team care, in which medical charts are used as the basis for communication among health care providers. Certainly, in a hospital or clinic, where various providers care for one patient, the concept of strict confidentiality is largely a myth. If it applies at all, it applies to those formal reports of a patient's condition, other than to third-party and government reimbursers, for which a patient's explicit release is required. In a prison or jail, there is no way to truly protect the confidentiality of an inmate's statement to a health care provider once it has been written in the chart. In many prisons and jails, the health care providers are direct employees of the correctional system, and the health charts are maintained and filed by correctional officials. Whereas the American Public Health Association *Standards* clearly state that maintenance of medical records by correctional personnel is an inadequate procedure,[8] it remains the norm rather than the exception. By their very nature, prisons are hotbeds of information. It has been said that the only way not to have a secret spread in a prison is not to think it—once articulated, secrecy and sanctity can never be assured.

This volatility of information requires all health care providers, but especially mental health care providers, to exercise particular care in attempting to guard confidentiality. Certain information, such as intimate details about an inmate's life, which are not necessary for diagnosis or treatment, should not be committed to the chart. Much information, however, will be relevant to treatment and should be carefully guarded. Even more than medical information, mental health histories demand stringent control over records. Locked file systems and limited access by professionals only may be necessary to assure confidentiality.

To inmates, confidentiality means not only the protection of information in the chart but also a guarantee that secrets once shared will not be retold unnecessarily to others. At the first encounter, the mental health worker should provide this guarantee. Concurrently, the professional should explain that the only exception to the doctrine of confidentiality will be those normal legal and moral obligations to respond to a clear and present danger of grave injury to the inmate or others, and the single issue of escape. The dynamic and dangerous nature of correctional institutions means that information about the potential danger of riots or attack, in addition to the danger of suicide, must be shared with authorities. A correctional setting is always potentially explosive and the overriding ethical obligation to care for the mental health of the general population must consistently be a factor in a caregiver's determination regarding the protection of individual information.

There are formal requirements a mental health service can impose on itself in order to demonstrate to inmates the seriousness of its commitment to confidentiality. For example, it can and should refuse to have any of its mental health practitioners testify at parole or punishment hearings. The purpose of a mental health service is the treatment of inmates, not the facilitation of the penal or criminal justice system. It should refuse all requests for information from the institution that are not directly related to a situation that could be a danger to the inmate or to others. It should insist that the layout of the treatment areas is such that correctional officers assigned there for security purposes can have inmates in sight, but are not permitted to overhear conversations between patients and staff. The balancing of institutional and individual needs requires a finely tuned sensitivity to the rights of inmates and an awareness of the needs of the correctional community.

THE RIGHT TO REFUSE CARE

Outside of correctional institutions, adult patients who are of sound mind have a clear right to consent to or to refuse medical care, even if the result of the refusal may be death. This right is grounded firmly in the common law concept of self-determination, in notions of liberty, and in the constitutional right to privacy.[8] Outside of prisons, even patients who are alleged to be mentally ill may refuse treatment, unless they satisfy the standard for civil commitment "a danger to self or others," at which point they may be judicially restrained for a limited and specific period of time.[9] Even persons who have been involuntarily committed to mental institutions have the right to refuse treatment absent proof of an emergency and irreparable harm.[10] Within prisons, however, the right to refuse care can be limited by considerations of prison administration, which may override an inmate's desires and decisions.[11]

Central to the refusal of medical or mental health care is the voluntary decision of a decisionally capable patient who is adequately informed by providers about the alternative treatments available and the risks and benefits of each. A patient who is capable of making health care decisions is one who is able to understand the risks and benefits of the proposed intervention, to weigh that understanding against personal preference and a set of values, and to communicate the decisions to the health care providers.[12]

Patients who are mentally ill may have severely compromised abilities to process information. They may be unable to identify personal preference and to focus on their own best interest. The panoply of civil commitment statutes is designed to rescue these patients from their ineffective intellectual and emotional calculations, which might leave them at risk, not by choice, to the ravages of illness. Whether the civil commitment standard is "a danger to oneself or others," or "behavior which is a product of mental illness," society has recognized an overriding obligation, supported by the *parens patriae* doctrine and the police powers of the state, to protect the mentally ill from themselves and to protect others from them.

Were these measures not sufficiently complex, the courts have recently constructed a range of protections for those who may meet the standard for involuntary commitment, but who may choose, nonetheless, within their confinement, to refuse the administration of psychotropic medications. The exact degree to which this right applies within the correctional setting is unclear.[10,13]

Refusals of medical or mental health care should be met with caution in correctional settings. Given the varying quality of institutions and their health care services, it is often impossible to distinguish whether a refusal is an informed voluntary decision of a capable patient or is, in the alternative, a denial of care. Certainly, if the consequences to an inmate from refusing care are potentially serious, may have long lasting health effects, or may lead to death, extraordinary scrutiny must be applied to assure that the refusal is grounded in the decision of a capable inmate, knowledgeable about the consequences, and is not a reflection of the denial of officials, oppression by other inmates, or the inefficiency of the system. It is not unknown for correctional officers to deny an inmate access to the health care service for punitive reasons. Conversely, many inmates fail to keep appointments with the health care services for a variety of often legitimate reasons, which do not indicate a desire to refuse care. In large urban jails, where there are growing numbers of non-English speaking inmates, patients may understand imperfectly the information that is provided and the appropriate response. For these reasons, all refusals of care for health problems of any severity should be confirmed by a health care professional directly with the inmate, with the provision of translation services if necessary. Providers must not accept a correctional official's report that an inmate has refused care for all but the most minor problems.

Inmates therefore have the right to refuse mental health care unless there is the direct and immediate possibility of harm to self or others. However, this does not mean that inmates exercising this right must necessarily be housed in the general population. The obligation of mental health care providers to the public health of the institution may require that they segregate troublesome inmates in mental observation or protective custody units over protest, although they may not be able to force treatment.

THE RIGHT TO ADEQUATE CARE

Ever since the landmark Supreme Court decision in 1976, the courts have struggled in numerous cases to define with greater specificity the requirements for constitutionally adequate health care for inmates. A major resource in this undertaking has been the development of professional standards for the delivery of health care to incarcerated populations by national organizations, such as the American Public Health Association (APHA) and the American Medical Association (AMA). Although both groups developed their standards in accordance with their perceptions of inmate–patients' needs and the particular circumstances of prison life, their approaches have been somewhat divergent. From the publication of the first edition of its *Standards for Health Services in Correctional Institutions* in 1976, the APHA has consistently supported the principle that incarcerated persons are entitled to a level of care that meets contemporary national standards. The AMA, which first published its *Standards for Health Services in Jails* in 1981, focused more on developing minimal guidelines for the provision of health care equivalent to that available in the less well-defined "community."

In the second edition of its standards, published in 1986, the APHA ensured that the standards "[took] into account the growth in sophistication of state and local public health officials, institutional administrators and health care providers in correctional settings", as well as "reflect[ing] the specific developments of federal law."[14(p ii)]

In line with this approach, the second edition of the APHA standards spells out quite specifically what constitutes satisfactory compliance with each standard, citing cases in support of its requirements.

The APHA standard for the adequacy of a mental health program is in general agreement with that of the New York City Board of Correction, whose 1985 *Mental Health Minimum Standards for New York City Correctional Facilities* are considered to be among the most advanced in the nation. Both organizations require a correctional mental health program to provide:

1. Crisis intervention and management of acute episodes, including immediate hospitalization when appropriate
2. A program to prevent suicide
3. Relief of present illness and the prevention of further deterioration
4. Elective therapeutic and preventive treatment as resources permit.

Clearly, the implementation of a mental health program that can promptly, consistently, and effectively provide these discrete services to a sizeable prison or jail population will require adequate numbers of highly qualified professional and administrative staff, and it will be costly. Evolving constitutional requirements and professional accountability demand no less.

REFERENCES

1. Ignatieff M: *A Just Measure of Pain—The Penitentiary in the Industrial Revolution, 1750–1850.* New York, Columbia University Press, 1980.
2. Hughes R: *The Fatal Shore.* New York, Alfred A. Knopf Inc., 1987.
3. *Procunier v Martinez,* 416 U.S. 396, 416 (1973).
4. *Estelle v Gamble,* 429 U.S. 97, 97 S. Ct. 285 (1976).
5. *Id.* at 104–105.
6. *Wyatt v Stickney,* 325 F. Supp. 781 (M.D. Ala. N.D.) (1971); 334 F. Supp. (1971); 344 F. Supp. 373 (1972); 344 F. Supp. 387 (1972).
7. Dubler NN: *Standards for Health Services in Correctional Institutions,* ed 2. Washington, DC, American Public Health Association, 1986, p 111.
8. *Schloendorff v Society of New York Hospital,* 105 N.E. 92 (1914); *Roe v Wade,* 410 U.S. 113, 93 S. Ct. 705, 35 L. Ed. 2d 147 (1973); Miller L: Informed consent: I. *JAMA* 1980; 244:2100; Miller B: Autonomy and the refusal of lifesaving treatment. *The Hastings Center Report,* 22, August 1981; Brant J: Last rights: An analysis of refusal and withholding of treatment cases. *Mo Law Rev* 1981; 337.
9. New York State Mental Hygiene Law, §§ 9.27–9.33; *O'Conner v Donaldson,* 422 U.S. 563, 45 L. Ed. 2d 396, 95 S. Ct. 2486 (1975).
10. Rhoden N: The right to refuse psychotropic drugs. *Harvard Civil Rights, Civil Liberties Law Rev* 1980; 15:363.
11. *Commissioner of Corrections v Myers,* 399 N.E. 2d 452 (1979).
12. President's Commission for the Study of Ethical Problems in Medicine and Biomedical and Behavioral Research: *Making Health Care Decisions: The Ethical and Legal Implications of Informed Consent in the Patient–Practitioner Relationship.* Washington, DC, Government Printing Office, 1982.
13. Rhoden N: The limits of liberty: Deinstitutionalization, homelessness and libertarian theory. *Emory Law Rev* 1982; 31:375.
14. Dubler NN: *Standards for Health Services in Correctional Institutions,* ed 2. Washington, DC, American Public Health Association, 1986.

10

Psychiatry in the Service of the Criminal Punishment System

Some Conceptual and Ethical Issues

JAY E. KANTOR

I will keep them from harm and injustice.

Hippocratic Oath

Ethical dilemmas seem to emerge whenever the health care system touches the criminal justice system. Those conflicts most commonly occur when the physician's patient is also a prisoner. The most difficult dilemmas arise when a psychiatrist seems called on to fulfill multiple and inconsistent duties. On the one hand, the psychiatrist is sworn to do no harm to his patients and, more than that, is obliged to do good for his patients. On the other hand, the same psychiatrist is working for the criminal justice system that at least appears indifferent to the ultimate interests of those who are arrested or are on trial and, after sentencing, seems intent on doing harm to those convicted.

How can the psychiatrist reconcile the seemingly conflicting demands of those two roles? This problem of "dual agency" can arise at every stage of the criminal justice process. Consider the following examples of possible sources of conflict:

JAY E. KANTOR • Department of Philosophy, New York University, College of Art and Sciences, New York, NY 10003.

1. A psychiatrist may be asked to evaluate a detainee in order to determine whether he is competent to stand trial. He may believe that, if he finds the prisoner competent, the prisoner's risk of receiving punishment is enhanced. Should he, in order to keep the prisoner free from harm, evaluate him as not competent even if he believes him to be competent?*

2. The psychiatrist asked to treat the prisoner who has been determined to be incompetent to stand trial may believe that treatment will restore the prisoner's competency. He is then faced with a similar dilemma: Should he treat the defendant and increase the probability that he will be punished, or should he leave things alone and "keep his patient from harm?"

3. If an insanity defense or a diminished capacity defense is in the offing, the psychiatrist may face still another related dilemma. A psychotic prisoner compensated with the help of medication may have a harder time winning his insanity defense than he would if he appeared before the jury untreated and in a crazed condition. Should the psychiatrist deny his patient treatment for the sake of the defense? Should he accede to the request of a defense lawyer who asks that his client not be treated?

4. If the prisoner goes to trial and pleads not guilty by reason of insanity, should the psychiatrist, believing the defendant to have been responsible for his criminal act, lie and weight his testimony to attempt to keep the defendant out of prison and thus out of harm?

5. If the prisoner is found guilty, and diversion to a mental health treatment facility is a possibility, should the psychiatrist lie to a judge in order to keep the prisoner out of prison?

6. If the psychiatrist is working with a diverted convictee who is not compliant with treatment, should he report his patient to the parole officer?

7. On the other hand, if the psychiatrist is working within a prison and can get prisoners out of hard duty by claiming they are ill, should he do so?

8. A psychiatrist is asked to evaluate a convicted sex offender to determine if he is a suitable candidate for chemical or surgical castration. Does that raise an ethical conflict for him?

9. And, most dramatic of the dilemmas, if the psychiatrist is confronted with a prisoner facing execution who has been determined to be

*The most famous instance where this was reputed to have been done was with the poet Ezra Pound, who faced charges of treason. In order to save him from harm, a psychiatrist reputedly did evaluate Pound as incompetent to stand trial even though the psychiatrist's professional judgment was that Pound was competent.

incompetent to be executed, should he treat him in order to make him well enough to be executed?

Although these are often called dilemmas of "dual agency," they might better be called dilemmas of "multiple agency."

Persons have different layers of obligations. First, we all have obligations toward each other as persons qua persons. So, for example, we all are bound not to harm other persons. Concomitantly, all persons have a right that other persons not harm them. In that sense, the *primum non tocere* of medicine is redundant. These obligations of persons toward other persons could be called "general" obligations, and they are usually correlate with "general" rights that all persons possess.

There are also "special" obligations that persons may have toward others. These special obligations arise out of agreements made between persons and they correlate to "special" rights. So, for example, if I own land, I may contract with you to give you a right to walk through the land. In return, as part of the contract, you may be obliged to pay a fee to me.

The special obligations of a psychiatrist qua psychiatrist and the special obligations of an employee of the criminal justice system qua employee are contractual creations. These obligations are created when a person takes on the role of psychiatrist, or when a person takes on the role of employee of an institution. They are not obligations that are demanded of all persons at all times. For example, although laypersons may have some moral or limited legal obligation to do good for others,* a physician's obligation to be beneficient to his patients is more encompassing. His obligation of beneficence in the physician–patient relationship is derived from the defining characteristics of the profession of medicine and from the requirement of the laws that give him privilege to practice medicine. Similarly, contracts between employers and employees create special obligations and rights. An employee incurs certain obligations in return for rights to his salary and his other benefits. That may seem straightforward, after all, an employee's obligations may be neatly listed in his job description, and a psychiatrist's obligations may be neatly written out in licensing statutes and codes of ethics. Unfortunately, things are not that straightforward. First of all, a neatly written obligation may be ambiguous. For example, the American Psychiatric Association's amendments to the American Medical Association's Code of Ethics say that "a psychiatrist shall not take part in executions." Does that mean that psychiatrists should not evaluate condemned prisoners to see if they are competent to be executed? Second, there are profound questions about the nature of the obligations and rights that are created from

*For example, the requirements of "Good Samaritan" laws.

the contract between psychiatrist and patient, which we will now examine.

THE PSYCHIATRIST–PATIENT CONTRACT

Recent analysis and redefinition of the nature of the physician–patient relationship has left us with a number of questions about the obligations and rights created by the contract between the physician and his patient. The traditional view of the physician–patient relationship saw it as based on a paternalistic model. The primary* contractual obligation of the physician was to be beneficient to his patient in the same way that a parent should be beneficient to his small child. He was to make the proper treatment decisions for his patient, without having to take the patient into the decision-making process. Perhaps he was to tell fairy tales to his patients in order to make hard truths palatable, or to avoid the hard truths entirely.

This paternalistic model of the relationship is presently being abandoned.† The new model of the contract is based on a belief that the primary obligation of the physician is to recognize the patient's autonomy. In this model, the psychiatrist's obligation to be beneficent takes second place to his obligation to recognize the patient's right to self-determination. The increasing stress on informed consent, the right to refuse treatment, and truth-telling to patients are instances of this change. More and more, the physician is called on to do what his patient wishes even if the patient's wishes are in conflict with what the physician believes is good for the patient.

This new model of the contract is more congruent with the idea that "physician" and "patient" (and "employee") are really only roles. Underlying those contracted roles of "physician" or "patient" or "employee" are the basic being of the contractees as persons. Thus, the basic moral relationship between physician and patient is seen as person–person rather than simply as physician–patient. As persons, both the physician and patient have certain general rights and obligations that supercede and place limits on any special rights and obligations that may be created by a contract. These fundamental rights and obligations belong to all persons and ordinarily cannot be lost or bargained away by particular contractual agreements. For example, a patient does not lose his right to self-determination when he becomes a patient, and so retains his right to informed consent.‡

*After "Do no harm," of course.

†In theory, at least.

‡He may waive, however, the exercise of a general right at specific times.

This reevaluation of the physician–patient relationship is still in process, and we can see it reflected in the changing requirements for informed consent and, as well, in the increased recognition of the right to refuse both somatic and psychiatric treatment. In the interim, the change is presenting certain unresolved problems. For example, we are not certain about the extent of the physician's obligation to continue with a patient when the patient's wishes go contrary to the physician's judgment about the best course of treatment.

Similar problems exist for the employee–employer relationship. There are rights and obligations that cannot be bargained away when one becomes an employee. But which rights and obligations are retained by the employee? For example, does a physician lose his right to strike when he becomes employed by a hospital? Does he lose the right to select which patients he will treat? Must he treat patients who may pose some risk to his own health?

AUTONOMY AND THE PRISONER-PATIENT

The autonomy model presents us with special difficulties when we try to apply it to the physician–patient relationship as it exists in the criminal justice system. The ordinary patient is a person with rights first, and a patient second. However, a prisoner is neither an ordinary patient nor an ordinary person. Once he has been arrested, he has lost some of his rights.* If he has been convicted of a crime, he has forfeited even more of his rights. But how much and how many of his rights he loses along the way is another question subject to dispute. For example, does he retain the right to refuse treatment?† Does he, if convicted, as some of the public seem to believe, lose the right to the quality and amount of care they would afford to the innocent?‡

In sum, and thus far, that leaves us with the following sources of problems:

1. As an employee of the criminal justice system, the psychiatrist's

*He may also have gained rights; for example, the legal "care and custody" requirements of prisons may entitle him to treatment that he would not be entitled to as a free person on the streets.

†Thus, the court, in ruling that Mark Chapman, the killer of John Lennon, had no right to continue a hunger strike, cited the limitations of prisoner's rights as one rationale for forcibly feeding him.

‡In informal polls taken in many ethics classes, I have noted that health care providers of all types would prefer to deny convicted felons scarce medical resources in favor of persons innocent of such crimes.

obligations may be clearly defined but may conflict with his obligations as a psychiatrist.

2. As a psychiatrist, there is some dispute about the extent and nature of his obligations toward his patient. Are they first to be beneficent to his patient, or first to recognize his patient's self-determination? How much is he obliged to accede to his patient's wishes regarding treatment?
3. Does the prisoner-patient have the same rights as the ordinary patient in regard to his medical care?

Although the ethical issues that arise in pretrial, trial, and posttrial procedures are closely connected, I will concentrate here mainly on issues that come up posttrial and postsentencing.

PSYCHIATRY

Ethical problems are exacerbated for the psychiatrist and other mental health professionals who work in the criminal justice system. First, the criminal justice system and psychiatry sometimes seem to be working with mutually inconsistent theoretical assumptions. The law assumes that adult human beings are responsible for their actions. That is, it assumes that a person is in control of his behavior and, if he committed a criminal act, presumes that he had the ability to refrain from that action and hence is culpable for his act. In philosophical terms, the law assumes that persons have free will. Of course, the law allows for the possibility that a person was not responsible for his actions and thus is not culpable. Nevertheless, regardless of various jurisdictional differences in insanity defenses and defenses of diminished capacity, the legal burden to disprove responsibility effectively always lies with the defendant.

Contrary to the legal system's presumption that we have free will, psychological explanations of behavior traditionally have been pulled along by a deterministic undercurrent. For most of its history, psychology has attempted to grow up with the physical sciences. Classical physicalistic methods of explanation attempt to treat persons as they would treat any other objects in the universe—their behavior being totally a product of their innate states. This deterministic presumption is that a person's actions stem from causes outside of his control, be those causes inborn, physiological, social, psychodynamic, or conditioned. On the face of it, there appears to be no room for "free will" in that model of explanation.

Moral and legal principles of justice demand that we not hold a person culpable or morally responsible for behavior that he could not control. These basic principles of justice further demand that we punish only those who are responsible for their criminal actions. As we have said, the legal system implies that only *some* persons should not be punished, because those exceptional persons can be shown not to have been in control of their actions. However, the implication of the psychological deterministic tradition is that *no* persons ought to be punished for their behavior. In this view, we may try to change a person's undesirable behavior patterns by rehabilitating him, but it would be unjust to blame or punish him for his actions.

Along with that, the major traditions of psychotherapeutic treatment have other reasons for avoiding blaming patients. Expressing disapproval to a patient about his behavior is often considered counterproductive, if not deadly, to the therapeutic process. And although the criminal justice system may coldly try to bring a convictee's feelings of guilt to the surface so that he can stew and suffer over them, the therapeutic process more often tends to try more warmly to help the patient rid himself of feelings of guilt. This nonjudgmental aspect of treatment is also in accord with the belief that a therapist should possess a certain degree of empathy with his patient.

These factors may leave the psychiatrist with a conscious or unconscious theoretical bias against *any* system of punishment.

All in all, it is no wonder that psychiatrists often feel uncomfortable working in conjunction with the criminal justice system.

PRETRIAL EVALUATION ISSUES AND MULTIPLE AGENCY

There have been recent attempts within the mental health profession to deal with some of those dual agency issues that arise when the psychiatrist is serving as evaluator rather than as treating psychiatrist. These attempts range from suggestions that the psychiatrist warn the evaluee that he is not serving as a treating psychiatrist who is bound by obligations of confidentiality and the other obligations of treating psychiatrists, to suggestions that the evaluation and treatment processes be kept entirely separate, with separate case records, and with no psychiatrist serving both as evaluator and treater.

Although those attempts may help to dissolve some of the dilemmas of dual agency, there remain underlying problems not so easily solved. The psychiatrist who serves solely as evaluator is acting somewhat in the role of scientist. He is attempting to give a value-free professional judgment about certain facts in the world. The criteria used to determine competency may be shakier than (for example) the criteria used to determine the bacteria content of drinking water, but the facts are, presumably, the facts. However, we know that scientific facts always have implications that reach outside of science. The microbiologist's value-free and objective findings about bacteria content have implications for society's policies about water supplies, and the psychiatrist's value-free judgments about the competency of the evaluee have implications for society's treatment of that evaluee. The most striking example of the moral inadequacy of attempting to separate objective medical judgments from their eventual nonobjective use is that of the concentration camp physicians in Nazi Germany. Such physicians gave objective determinations about the fitness of inmates to work at slave labor or, by default, determined that the inmates were fit only to be exterminated. A plea on the part of those physicians that "I was only acting in my professional role, giving descriptive evaluations" would strike many people as being no more morally exculpatory than the plea "I was only following orders." Thus, the psychiatrist who feels moral satisfaction because he does not work with the same person as treater and evaluator, or the forensic service that has a policy of separating those roles, should not necessarily rest easy.

Like the patient, the psychiatrist is a person first, and a psychiatrist second. The total extent of his obligations cannot be solely defined by his "professional" role as a psychiatrist. He may have obligations as a person that are, or seem to be, in conflict with his role as psychiatrist and also may be in conflict with his role as employee of an institution. They may also be in conflict with the law. The present psychiatric code of ethics alludes to those obligations, stating "it is conceivable that an individual could violate a law without being guilty of professionally unethical behavior."[1] In context, the annotation clearly is intended to allude to "social protest" activities; nevertheless, one wonders what degrees and kinds of illegal activity performed for moral reasons would exempt a psychiatrist from professional censure. Thus, for example, the evaluating psychiatrist in the Ezra Pound case evidently felt that he had a moral obligation to break the law and to override his obligations as an employee of an institution. Should that clause in the code of ethics exclude him from criticism for his reputed actions?

Treatment

There are similar issues of "multiple agency" relating to psychiatric treatment. Like evaluation, treatment does not occur in a vacuum. It would be a mistake for the psychiatrist to suppose that treating a patient is an isolated phenomenon with no further ramifications for the patient or for society. That is particularly true when his patient is a prisoner facing trial or facing punishment.

Competency to be Executed

Dilemmas of multiple agency have drawn a great deal of attention since the Supreme Court ruled in *Ford v Wainwright*[2] that it is unjust to execute a prisoner who has been adjudged incompetent to be executed. I think that a discussion of this particular dilemma will be useful in clarifying, if not resolving, some of the other dilemmas I have written about above.

Those prison psychiatrists who were opposed to capital punishment may feel Ford's victory to be Pyrrhic, because they were then put into the position of being required to treat incompetent prisoners in order to make them well enough to be killed. Some psychiatrists have taken the position that, under those circumstances, the psychiatrist has an overriding moral duty to refuse to treat such prisoners.

There are various arguments that could be put forward against these psychiatrists. For example, to leave such prisoners severely psychotic may have the effect of denying them the ability to make last-minute appeals, or the ability to come forward with evidence that might free them. However, those psychiatrists who are opposed to taking part in treating such prisoners usually argue that these considerations do not outweigh the wrongness of taking part in the execution process.

For example, Dr. Douglas A. Sargent is a recent and typical example of those who are concerned with this dramatic problem.[3] He begins by speaking of the problem as an instance of the dilemma of dual agency; on the one horn, psychiatrists have an obligation to treat the prisoner. The obligation derives both from the general requirements of their profession and from the specific requirements of their employment contract with the prison. The other horn, claims Dr. Sargent, is the physician's obligation not to cause harm to his patient. Like many others, he believes that obligation requires that a physician not cause or be complicit in causing the death of his patient. To successfully treat the prisoner who is incompetent to be executed is, according to this argument, to help cause his death. Like many others, Sargent believes such treatment would be morally wrong, and he argues against those psychiatrists who are willing to treat such condemned prisoners. However, I think that those who take this position have misconstrued the issues.

First, we are in a time at which we can no longer say that "do no harm" always means "keep the patient alive as long as possible." We know that there are cases in which more harm may be done to a patient by keeping him alive instead of being an indirect (or, perhaps, even a direct) causal factor in his death. For example, a terminally-ill patient may be suffering needless pain because he is being treated aggressively.

Of course, condemned prisoners are usually not terminally-ill in the ordinary sense of the term; however, there may be an analogy. I think that Dr. Sargent is making the common mistake of assuming that all of the psychotic are in a state of blissful madness. Clearly, some psychotics are in a great deal of mental pain, perhaps to the extent that given the consequences of living with the denial of treatment versus the consequences of treatment and subsequent execution, they might themselves believe that they are better off dead. In those instances, it is not really clear that being "complicit" in the death of the prisoner by treating him necessarily constitutes "harm" to a patient.

There may be a way out for those who believe that making such prisoners competent to be executed is wrong. The prison psychiatrist or physician who is faced with a choice of leaving his patient in mental anguish or "treating him to death" might think of choosing another way of "keeping his patient from harm"—that of drugging the prisoner into a permanent blissful incompetence so that he cannot be executed. Yet, there seems to be something wrong with that option, even though it saves the prisoner from execution and also alleviates his mental suffering. Perhaps part of what is wrong with that option is that it would be inconsistent with some goals of psychiatric treatment; goals that are really quite consistent with some ideas about punishment.

The general acceptance of autonomy theory approaches in patient care has had effects on the concepts of medicine as well as having effects on the physician–patient relationship. Without going into detailed discussion here,[4] we can say that "mental health" is beginning to be thought of as either synonymous with "having internal autonomy," or thought of as inextricably tied to the possession of internal autonomy. This view replaces previous concepts that either tied mental health to conformity to specific sets of behavior patterns that society believes to be desirable, or saw mental health as necessarily descriptive of persons who are always happy or free from mental suffering. After all, to be autonomous means being an active participant in the world. That, in turn, may, as the existentialists point out, sometimes be more conducive to angst than to happiness. Conversely, a person is mentally ill to the degree that he lacks the mental ability to be a self-determined agent who is in control of and responsible for his actions. Implicit in this view of mental health is a rejection of any strict physicalistic determinist view of persons, and an acceptance of the concomitant belief that it makes sense to say that persons can be responsible for their actions. In fact, autonomy and responsibility are taken to be the essence of full and healthy personhood, and the role of the treating psychiatrist is to attempt to help his patient restore his internal autonomy. Thus, in this view, the primary obligation of a psychiatrist is not simply to make his patient happy, or not necessarily even to alleviate his suffering, or help his patient simply dispel feelings of guilt or remorse. For having the capacity to be unhappy, or suffer, or have feelings of guilt may be consistent with, and appropriate to, being a responsible being; and helping a person to get the capacity to have appropriate feelings of guilt or even have appropriate suffering may not conflict with the duty to "do no harm." In fact, in this view, the psychiatrist who alleviates a patient's suffering, at the expense of the patient's autonomy, has harmed the patient. Along with that, the psychiatrist who willfully fails to restore his patient's autonomy has violated his duty of beneficence. Being beneficent and acting in the patient's best interests can no longer be seen simply as providing happiness for the patient. Certainly, this sort of reasoning at least partially accounts for our intuition against drugging the candidate for execution, as well as our intuitions in general against those psychosurgical techniques that alleviate patient suffering at the cost of the patient's "spirit." That goal of psychiatry to restore autonomy may be quite consistent with helping to make a person competent to be executed.

This last point may become clearer if we examine some of the rationales given for the practice of punishing criminals.

PUNISHMENT

It is a commonplace that there are a few main rationales for the practice of punishment. These rationales may fit into three categories: (1) to express society's outrage and values, (2) to deter, and (3) to retribute. Present public attitudes toward capital punishment encompass all three reasons. For example, there is a widespread belief, justified or not, that capital punishment will deter others from committing similar crimes. Clearly, there is also a general belief (more easily justified) that capital punishment will deter the offender from a repetition of the crime. There is also a widespread belief that the capital offender "deserves" execution. And, of course, there is often general outrage in society about particular crimes and about the existence of crime in general. The outrage is accompanied with a hew and cry that the guilty be punished.

The belief in punishment as an expression of societal outrage is really parasitic on the rationale of punishment as retribution. That is, it is based on the belief that the person who committed the crime "owes" for what he did, and, therefore, must "pay" for what he did. This concept of punishment as debt is engrained in our legal heritage, and may be found among the natural law legal theorists as well as found among the legal positivists.

Thus, a contractualist such as Thomas Hobbes explains the function of punishment as a setting of a price on misconduct that would outweigh the possible and probable gains obtainable by the misconduct.[5] Any reasonable person, even one of "ill-will," can rationally weigh the risks and benefits of committing a crime and (on the assumption that punishment is probable), will decide that the risk of being punished, and the degree of suffering that punishment would include, outbalance his probability of benefitting from the crime.

Hobbes' theory combines deterrence and retribution. Any reasonable person will be deterred from criminal behavior by the thought of punishment. At the same time, any person who risks punishment by thinking he can "get away with it" is aware of what is at stake and is liable for paying the consequences if he gets caught. Such an account of punishment provides justification not only for the insanity defense, but also for the belief that those who are punished must know what is happening to them. In this view, someone who is insane is someone who is or was unable to understand or "keep' the contract. He is no more able to understand that "cost–benefit" analysis of crime and punishment than does a child or "wild beast."

Similarly, someone who is so "insane" at the time of punishment that he does not understand what is happening to him, and why it is happening to him, is not really being "punished." He is not really paying his debt. Presumably, punishment must contain an element of harm or suffering to the punished and must have a "fit" to the crime that the punished can understand. He must understand why he is getting a particular punishment as punishment. For an extreme example, how could we consider the imprisonment of a convictee who is in permanent coma to be "punishment?" An insane person may suffer from punishment, but if he is unaware of the connection between his responsibility for the crime and the punishment, it makes little sense to say that he is suffering *because* of his misdeed.

A strict retributionist such as Immanuel Kant would demand that those who are punished understand what is happening to them and why it is happening to them. Kant believed that those who are responsible for wrong actions ought to be punished as their just deserts. But here, too, the Kantian belief is that the person is to be punished *if* he is responsible. Punishment of a responsible person is a recognition of his responsibility for the crime and a recognition that he was and is capable of understanding the penalty attached to that crime. "Punishment" of one who does not realize what is being done to him cannot be conceived of as punishment, as "just deserts."

Thus, for example, Hegel, arguing along Kantian lines, claims that "punishment is regarded as containing the criminal's right and hence by being punished he is honoured as a rational [i.e., responsible] being."[6]

A retributive theory of punishment would require that the condemned be brought back to a condition in which he understands what is happening to him before he may be executed.*

Punishment as Deterrence

Whatever one may think of the efficacy of capital punishment as a general deterrent, it is clear that there is a widespread public belief that capital punishment does deter. Yet, with that, I think that public belief in capital punishment as a deterrent is only adjunct to a more fundamental communal belief in the retributive function of punishment. I think that even the most vociferous of those clamoring for more executions would not condone the execution of a truly innocent person, even if the execution served to deter many future crimes. Many people have a jaundiced view of the insanity defense. However, that may be more an indication of their distrust of its application, and their lack of knowledge about its complexities than an indication of their disagreement with the principle that only the truly responsible should be held guilty for criminal actions.† After all, the concepts of "responsibility" entailed in the defense are quite subtle and hard to grasp. The fact that juries do sometimes find for the defendants' pleading insanity is an indication that a public given enough facts and forced to think about those facts can come to accept that the physical act of committing a crime does not alone establish moral or legal culpability. I think that reflects a general belief that it is the responsible criminal who "deserves" punishment, and a belief that the primary justification for punishment is, in fact, that it is the criminal's "just deserts."

If we look at punishment in its function as a deterrent to future criminal behavior by the person punished (i.e., what is sometimes called "particular deterrence"), we naturally have to turn away from capital

*We can see this attitude poignantly displayed in the film "Paths of Glory" in which an unconscious condemned man is brought back to consciousness to face the firing squad. The directions about how to accomplish that are given by the army physician.

†I think that there is also a misconception about the frequency of insanity defenses. Again, by informal poll, I have found that even a majority of medical students and residents overestimate both the frequency and success of insanity defenses.

punishment cases. Although the executed criminal will not commit future crimes, the general rationale of particular deterrence really ties in to attempts to change the future behavior of the person punished. The assumption is that the punishment will cause enough suffering to the criminal to dissuade him from repeating his actions. Clearly, if this sort of deterrence is to work, the person punished must be aware of the reasons for his suffering. That is, the function of the punishment is to make the criminal averse to the sort of behavior for which he is guilty. If he is incapable of seeing the connection between the crime and his suffering, the punishment will not deter him.

Punishment as Justified Institutional Vengeance

Arguments have also been made to justify punishment as institutionally controlled forms of vengeance.[7] The claim here is that the desire for vengeance is a justified emotion, but that the public interest and public order require that it be satisfied through the law rather than through individual acts of revenge. Yet, here too, it is difficult to imagine that vengeful feelings could be any more satisfied by inflicting pain on one who does not understand the reason pain is being inflicted, than they could be satisfied by trying to vent the feelings by harming innocent persons or (Homer notwithstanding) by defiling the corpse of the criminal.

In general, one would think that anyone who strongly believes that those who are responsible for crimes ought to be punished would be bothered by the precedent set by punishing those who are not cognizant of the reason for their punishment. Such a practice would water down the tie that retributionists feel exists between responsibility and desert. A widespread acceptance of finding the insane guilty, and of punishing the insane, could probably only have the long-range effect of eroding the claim that the responsible are responsible and owe a debt.

Now it strikes me that, if a psychiatrist does believe that mental health is a state of internal autonomy, and further believes that the practice of punishing responsible criminals is justified, then his *prima facie* obligation as a psychiatrist is to treat his prisoner patients with the goal of restoring their internal autonomy. As I have said, that goal is not necessarily inconsistent with his duty not to harm his patient, or his duty to be beneficent to his patient. In fact, he may even be committed to the Kantian-Hegelian claim that to punish the responsible criminal is actually to show respect for his personhood. It is to say "you are a fully autonomous, responsible person and your actions are not simply products of determined causes that were outside of your control."

Castration and Autonomy

Stepping aside briefly from the issue of capital punishment, we can see how this analysis raises major problems about the practice of offering treatment to the prisoner as an alternative to punishment. "Treatment" in these cases may include chemical or surgical castration for sex offenders, psychosurgery for certain violent offenders, and rehabilitation programs for alcoholic offenders. Such practices seem to be inherently inconsistent. On the one hand, the alternative of punishment implies that the offender was totally responsible for his crimes. On the other hand, offering him the alternative of treatment implies the opposite explanation. It implies that there are psychological causes for the offender's criminal behavior and, thus, the offender is not totally responsible for his behavior.

The psychiatrist may reject the autonomy view of mental health and its assumption of free will. He may hold to a deterministic belief that persons are never morally responsible for their actions, and, hence, he may also believe that punishment is always inappropriate and unjust.

I am not sure that those bothered by the Ford case think that it is *always* inappropriate to punish persons, and, hence, always wrong for physicians to be a direct or indirect causal factor that leads to any punishment of persons. My suspicion is that they are really specifically bothered about the justness of *capital* punishment.

But that is a different issue for all of us, psychiatrists or not; it is an issue that cannot be argued by simply resorting to the claim that "Doctors are around to save lives, not to take lives." For as we have seen, on the face of it, there is no apparent logical inconsistency, no logically necessary dilemma of "multiple agency" existing for the psychiatrist who is a causal link on a chain that leads to justified punishment of his patient.

The dilemmas arise only if the psychiatrist believes that he is being asked to be complicit in causing the patient to undergo a type of punishment that, he himself believes, is unjust. What ought he to do? This is a question about the pragmatic application of ethical theory, and it is the sort of question that is most difficult to answer. It is usually far easier to talk about what is ethically correct than it is to do what is ethically correct. All we can do here is look at some options for action.

As we have said above, no special contract can require its contractees to perform duties that violate their general rights as persons. In that light, the psychiatrist who believes that capital punishment (or any other practice) is always an unjustifiable violation of a person's rights has an obligation to try to convince his professional organization to explicitly forbid its members from taking part in practices that violate person's rights. That, of course, may be easier said than done. He may also lobby for legislation similar to that now in place in Maryland.[8] There, a prisoner who has been declared incompetent to be executed has his sentence commuted to life imprisonment. That takes away some of the burden of treating psychiatrists who are against capital punishment. (Unfortunately, it may place another burden on their backs: Should they try to have all prisoners facing the death sentence declared incompetent to be executed?) He may also choose, at the outset, never to be directly involved with work that will put him in "moral danger." That is the route chosen by, for example, Dr Alan Stone, who refuses to do forensic cases. If the psychiatrist does stay involved with such work, and if his organization does not have an explicit statement, or his state does not give him a legislative remedy, then he is faced with a second, more difficult problem. What should he do if, as a prison psychiatrist, he is asked to take part in either an evaluation for competency to be executed or asked to treat a prisoner in order to make him competent to be executed? First, post-Nuremberg we can say that no one ought to be forced to do an action that he believes is immoral. One option then, is to refuse to take part in the process. He can do this by either refusing to work in the prison system at all, or by refusing to take part in those aspects of his employment that he finds morally repugnant. The last option presents certain difficulties. On the one hand, more and more institutions are becoming sensitive to the moral qualms of health care providers about issues such as abortion and "do not resuscitate" orders. Many hospitals explicitly allow providers to withdraw from such cases without prejudice to their employment. On the other hand, a health care provider has obligations toward his patients, who, in turn, have certain reasonable expectations about their rights to treatment when they enter a hospital. The provider also has obligations toward his peers who have certain reasonable expectations about their work loads, and how those work loads are to be shared. With that in mind, it would seem that, for example, a physician opposed to abortion simply should not be working in a hospital unit where abortions are routinely performed. Analogously, perhaps the prison psychiatrist who is opposed to capital punishment and who has to face these competency-to-be-executed cases should move his practice to another location.

Another option that may be open to the prison psychiatrist who is opposed to the death penalty is to remain in the system working as a "mole." That is, he may keep working trying to save as many condemned as possible from execution, doing anything from giving his evaluees the "benefit of the doubt" about their competence, to outrightly lying about his evaluations. Those who find this "option" abhorrent and "unprofessional" should ask themselves what they would think of a Nazi physician who stayed within the system but tried to save as many as he could from the gas chambers, lying, if necessary, about their physical condition. Do they believe that such a physician was acting "unprofessionally" and was morally culpable?

Clearly, there are many problems with that approach, problems that are theoretical, ethical, and pragmatic. We have spoken about the theoretical problem, namely, that it is not really apparent that psychiatric treatment is inconsistent with capital punishment. The ethical and pragmatic issues include considerations of the long-term consequences of such a "militant" approach. We know that a psychiatrist can get a reputation for the way he handles such cases. In the microcontext, such a psychiatrist may reach a point where his judgment is no longer trusted by the courts, and his services are no longer requested. Of course, a psychiatrist may be willing to risk that, believing that he, at least, has had the opportunity to save a few persons from what he believes to be injustice. However, there is the macrocontext to be considered, too. Once he is found out, he will be instrumental in breeding public distrust of psychiatry in general.

Of course, any prudent militant psychiatrist would have to be somewhat selective about the persons he attempts to save. After all, if he attempts to evaluate as incompetent every convictee who comes before him to plead incompetency, he will be out of the system in a very, very short time. That selectivity will raise another important ethical issue. What criteria will he use to decide who will be saved, and who will be killed? What right does he have to personally set *any* criteria for selection? Ezra Pound was saved from trial and possible execution because the evaluating psychiatrist believed that he was a great poet, and believed that great poets deserve special treatment. But what about those who are not great poets, those for whom the psychiatrist feels no empathy? Will the psychiatrist now playing God place *them* in a state of grace?

REFERENCES

1. American Psychiatric Association: *The Principles of Medical Ethics with Annotations Especially Applicable to Psychiatry*. Washington, DC, American Psychiatric Association, 1986, p 5.
2. *Ford v Wainwright,* 106 S. Ct. 2595 (1986).
3. Sargent DA: Treating the condemned to death. *Hastings Center Report* vol 16, no. 6, December, 1986, pp 5–6.
4. See, for example, Moore M: *Law and Psychiatry*. Cambridge, England, Cambridge University Press. 1984; also Culver CM, Gert B: *Philosophy in Medicine*. New York, Oxford University Press, 1982.

5. Hobbes T: *Leviathan,* part two, XXVII, XXVIII.
6. Hegel GWF: The Philosophy of Right, cited in Ezorsky G (ed.): *Philosophical Perspectives on Punishment.* Albany, SUNY Press, 1972.
7. Stephen JF: *A General View of the Criminal Law of England* ed 2. London, 1890, p 99. As discussed in Golding M: *Philosophy of Law.* Englewood Cliffs, NJ, Prentice-Hall, 1975.
8. Maryland S.B. 973 (May, 1987).

11

Forensic Evaluation and Treatment in the Same Institution

A Moral Dilemma

WILLIAM S. PACKARD

INTRODUCTION

When a physician is called upon to perform a forensic evaluation, there is often a presumption that no doctor–patient relationship exists, and that the physician is working for the court with the purpose of providing an opinion on a legal issue.[1] Although treatment recommendations may be offered, the forensic examination usually does not entail a subsequent implementation of a therapeutic regimen. However, in certain settings in psychiatric practice, psychiatrists are providing traditional clinical services while also performing court-ordered examinations. These settings include jails, prisons, and forensic psychiatric hospitals, where defendants receive treatment after a finding of not guilty by reason of mental illness, or of not competent to stand trial. The dilemmas and conflicts created by these two different tasks for psychiatrists working in correctional facilities will be the subject of this chapter.

Psychiatrists have long been providing clinical services in correctional facilities. In fact, the Supreme Court has recognized the constitutional requirement that the facilities attend to the medical needs of its inmates (*Estelle v Gamble*).[2] The extent of the psychiatric services provided may vary from a part-time consultant, who is present only one day

WILLIAM S. PACKARD • Mental Health Unit, Suffolk County Correctional Facility, Riverhead, NY 11901.

a week, to full-time or even around-the-clock coverage by a team of psychiatrists, psychologists, social workers, and alcohol and drug counselors. The clinical demands are often quite varied, and may include emergency evaluation of the disturbed behavior of a newly admitted psychotic inmate; crisis intervention with an inmate upset over his or her incarceration; the prescribing of medications; commitment to a psychiatric hospital; psychotherapy; and discharge planning. Inmates are referred for these services by correction officers, judges, members of their family, their mental health clinicians in the community, clergy, and probation or parole officers. The correctional psychiatric practice is usually quite busy, and combines elements of an emergency room, a clinic, and an inpatient unit.

While there has been some attention paid to the issue of psychiatric treatment in correctional facilities, [3–6] a review of the literature revealed no articles pertaining to the subject of performing forensic examinations while treating an inmate. While there is a recognition of the importance of the issues that arise, such as right to treatment and confidentiality,[7–8] little attention has been paid to this more difficult issue. Gutheil and Applebaum[9] do mention some problems inherent in the concept of mixed or divided agency, their term for treating and evaluating a patient for the court at the same time. However, they look at the issue from a more general perspective and make only brief reference to the issue in correctional settings.

CONFIDENTIALITY

When the demands of forensic evaluations are added to the already considerable problems met by the correctional psychiatrist, new ones arise. The first problem that presents itself is the issue of confidentiality. The court-ordered examination is one in which no confidentiality exists, because a report of the findings usually goes to the judge, the prosecution, the defense attorney, and, sometimes, the probation officer. In contrast, the psychiatric services provided in correctional facilities are protected by the traditional limits of confidentiality found in other settings. Concerns about danger to self and others are the only situations in which confidentiality can be breached. The American Bar Association recognizes the need for confidentiality in its *Criminal Justice Mental Health Standards* (sections 7–10),[10] although it extends its limits to include dangerousness to person and property as well.

The conflict over confidentiality occurs when an inmate has been seen for a forensic examination by the same psychiatrist. Often, the treating psychiatrist may obtain a history and observe behavior that the inmate might not want the forensic examiner to know. Because a court-ordered examination may be requested at a later point in the incarceration rather than when the inmate is first seen for treatment, it is difficult to avoid this situation. The psychiatrist could limit the data base for the court examination to just the information received at the time of the actual examination. However, this could lead to omissions that would not reflect the psychiatrist's true knowledge of the legal question being asked, and could cause problems if a hearing were held and the psychiatrist would have to testify.

As an example, an inmate who wants to be found competent to stand trial may choose to conceal a history of psychiatric treatment or psychotic symptoms, which may have been revealed earlier during a treatment session. Another example is the case of an inmate who, during a forensic evaluation, is trying to feign a mental illness in order to be found not competent to stand trial, who presented as having no major psychiatric illness during a previous contact. A third example is an inmate who is being examined for a presentence investigation who wants to conceal a history of antisocial behavior or drug and alcohol abuse.

THE THERAPEUTIC RELATIONSHIP

A second issue that can cause a dilemma is when the psychiatrist may feel that the duty to the inmate patient and the preservation of the therapeutic relationship are more important than meeting the needs of the court. Inmates are often concerned about whether the information they divulge to a mental health professional will be obtained by others. In order to gain the trust and confidence of an inmate that would lead to disclosure of material that reveals negative or unpleasant aspects of his or her character, there may need to be a guarantee of privacy. An intrusion into this privacy may irrevocably damage the relationship.

To illustrate this point, the following case is presented:

> A middle-aged woman was admitted to a local jail following her arrest for the murder of her husband. A call from a psychiatrist in the community, who had treated her in the past, revealed a long history of paranoid delusions focusing on her husband, about whom she had the belief that he had been replaced by an evil, alien being who was trying to drive her crazy and kill her. Acting on this belief, she killed him. While incarcerated, she maintained that she was not crazy and refused medications. She was in conflict with her lawyer over how to proceed because she saw her action as justifiable self-defense. The only person in whom she had any trust was her psychiatrist at the jail, who did not try to argue the validity of her delusions but maintained a sympathetic, supportive posture. After a peri-

od of time, she agreed to take neuroleptic medications which, unfortunately, did not alter the delusion about her husband, although she did become less suspicious and guarded. A competency examination was ordered, and the treating psychiatrist was one of the examiners for the court. Because she was still clearly delusional and could not assist her lawyer with a reasonable degree of rational understanding as required by the U.S. Supreme Court (*Dusky v United States*),[11] she was found not competent to proceed with her case. The effect of this decision on the therapeutic relationship was disastrous. She felt angry and betrayed by the psychiatrist, whom she had felt was the only person who listened to her. She stopped taking her medications, and whatever gains had been made in treating her were lost. Eventually, she was transferred to a forensic psychiatric hospital for treatment, but, on her return to the jail, she was not able to resume a therapeutic relationship with the psychiatrist. She saw him as an agent of the court and of the legal system that was harmful to her, not as a mental health professional who was trying to help her.

With regard to the issue of the therapeutic relationship, some psychiatrists take the position that it may not be relevant because the correctional institution imposes an environment that is not a free, open setting, so that a true therapeutic relationship does not exist. Inmates are present under coercion, and, therefore, the treatment that takes place occurs under artificial circumstances, with constraints imposed by outside forces, such as the court and the warden.

Many other psychiatrists feel that, although the setting does impose certain restraints, valid treatment can take place, so that the sanctity of the therapeutic relationship needs to be preserved. Even though there are impediments to performing treatment, the mental health professional must maintain the standards of his or her profession, and try to apply them despite the setting.[12]

THE FORENSIC EXAMINATION AS PART OF FORENSIC TREATMENT

The concerns about the therapeutic relationship in a correctional setting may seem overly scrupulous. To provide another point of view, one can compare the issue that arises in jails and prisons to the issue as it presents in forensic psychiatric hospitals. In most jurisdictions, court-ordered examinations can take place in psychiatric hospitals, where inmates are usually housed on a special unit. In addition, inmates who have been found not competent to stand trial, or not guilty by reason of mental illness, are usually committed by the court for inpatient psychiatric treatment in forensic psychiatric hospitals. These facilities are usually operated by the state, the county, or the local municipality. In both cases, the court is ordering the hospitalization, and the examinations are usually made for the court as part of the hospitalization. Frequently, the court will order a competency examination to take place inhospital because the inmate is so disturbed that he needs immediate inpatient psychiatric treatment. In addition, such an examination is ordered because the inmate refuses to cooperate with the examiners, or appears to be malingering a mental illness, and a period of daily observation in a hospital is needed to make an accurate assessment of competency. It is clear from the outset why the inmate is in the hospital: to satisfy the needs of the court. Although such treatment as psychotherapy and pharmacotherapy may occur, the evaluation for the court is the purpose for the hospitalization.

The same is true for the inmate who has been found not competent to proceed and is sent to the psychiatric hospital for the purpose of receiving treatment to become competent. The psychiatrist has an obligation to the court to provide the treatment and to examine the inmate in order to determine if competency has been restored. Once it has, the psychiatrist must report his findings to the court. Again, it is the court that has requested the treatment, and the psychiatrist is obligated to report back to the referral source.

The defendants who are found not guilty or not criminally responsible because of mental illness are also sent to psychiatric hospitals by the court for a specific purpose, which is to receive treatment with the ultimate goal of becoming not dangerous, and, if possible, of returning to the community. Because the court makes the decisions about any change in the restrictiveness of the environment which the patient needs, including transfer to another facility, retention at the same facility, passes, and release, the psychiatrist must again report to the court the results of examinations of the patient. From the outset, the psychiatrist has the role of being the court-appointed treater and examiner.

Turning to the case of court-ordered examinations done by treating psychiatrists in correctional facilities, the primary difference is that the treatment is not court-ordered. The inmate generally comes voluntarily for help, even when the referral is made by someone else, such as correctional staff, family, or previous therapists. In many cases, the inmate is self-referred. The psychiatric services provided are usually offered through the mental health department of the state, the county, or the local municipality, and not through the court or the department of corrections. Therefore, the treatment is rendered for the mental health needs of the community, not for a specific need of the court, and the court cannot require the transmission of mental health records or information obtained by the treatment services.

Even if the inmate does not voluntarily seek treatment within the institution, but behaves in such a way that treatment is necessary to prevent harm to himself or to others, the same standards of care and confidentiality must apply as if a similar situation were occurring in the community.

THE ETHICAL DILEMMA: WHOM AM I HELPING?

When the psychiatrist who treats inmates is asked to perform an examination for the state, the conflict between the psychiatrist's role as treater and as agent of the court arises. The court can gain access to information obtained by the treating psychiatrist when he becomes the examining psychiatrist for the court. Even though the evaluation may be more accurate because of the clinical information gathered during treatment, this is not the purpose for providing the treatment. If psychiatric treatment in correctional facilities were ever to be construed as having the purpose of providing information to the court, it would quickly lose its credibility, and it could also lead to a malpractice action against the practitioner or be seen as a violation of professional ethics.

As put forth by the American Psychiatric Association[13] in their *Principles of Medical Ethics* "a physician shall respect the rights of patients, of colleagues, and of other health professionals, and shall safeguard patient confidence within the constraints of the law" (section 4). Furthermore, it is stated that with regard to examinations for security purposes or to determine legal competence, "the psychiatrist must fully describe the nature and purpose and lack of confidentiality of the examination to the examinee at the beginning of the examination (sections 4–6). Also, the *Principles* acknowledge the right to withhold information "when ordered by the court to reveal the confidences entrusted to him/her by patients." If there is any doubt, "the right of the patient to confidentiality and by extension, to unimpaired treatment, should be given priority" (sections 4–9).

When asked to evaluate an inmate for a presentence investigation, or for a parole board hearing, the psychiatrist faces another dilemma, which is how to balance the best interests of society with the interests of the patient. If an inmate presents a hostile, arrogant way of relating, or gives a history of sociopathic behavior beyond what is known by the court, does the psychiatrist include all of this material in a report to the court, even though this information may have been conveyed to the psychiatrist prior to the order for the examination? As a physician the guideline to "do no harm" may not be very clear when an examination leads to a diagnosis of antisocial personality disorder. One may have to reinterpret that phrase in terms of the needs of society rather than the individual patient, although that may be contrary to the original intention of the concept.

Although there may be a positive therapeutic relationship, the psychiatrist may have an impression of the patient that would be seen as negative by the court, despite the psychodynamic understanding held by the psychiatrist. This may be difficult to transmit to the court, or the court may view the underlying psychodynamics as irrelevant to the disposition of the inmate. The compassion of a doctor for an inmate, whose upbringing may have been one of deprivation, can be difficult to transmit in a legal system where free will is seen as the underlying basis for human action, rather than psychic determinism.

Not every situation where this conflict arises is the same. A different way of approaching the problem might be to consider what was the original purpose of the encounter between psychiatrist and inmate. In some cases, a treatment relationship already exists with an inmate, and in the course of the treatment, a court-ordered examination is requested. In other cases, a physician performs a forensic examination, and subsequently begins to treat the inmate for psychiatric illness.

When a treatment relationship already exists, many would argue that the concerns of the patient come first, and the interests of the court should be dealt with secondarily, as if this were like any other treatment relationship occurring in psychiatric practice. If that were the accepted framework, then a psychiatrist would not reveal any information obtained from the patient without his express consent for such release, except for situations where confidentiality does not exist such as dangerousness to self or others, and child abuse. This should require doing a formal examination, and repeating the history taking and mental status examination after the customary warnings about the nature of the examination are given. In this way, no previously-acquired information would be given to the court without the patient's awareness that it was obtained during the actual examination for the court. If the patient inquires as to why the doctor is asking questions that have already been answered in previous treatment sessions, the response should certainly indicate a reflection of the doctor's concerns for confidentiality and an interest in separating the functions of treater and court-appointed examiner.

When discrepancies arise in the data that has been received in the past by the psychiatrist, and during the forensic examination, this should be pointed out to the patient to see what may be elicited. Sometimes alterations in details of the history may be done intentionally to suit a purpose, such as wanting to deny a history of psychiatric hospitalizations or to invent one that does not exist. Sometimes discrepancies may not be significant if they are suspected of arising out of poor recollection of dates and events. However, major changes in the details of a patient's life, or sudden changes in his behavior should be addressed during the examination, since having accepted the role of forensic examiner, the physician should do the best job possible, including identification of malingering.

In the second situation, where treatment is started after a forensic examination has taken place, many of the problems do not exist. Having seen the inmate for the court should not create any dilemmas regarding treatment unless there is a suspicion arising from the subsequent treatment sessions, that the inmate was malingering at the time of the examination. Should any information received after the examination be transmitted to the court, the psychiatrist could be accused of a breach of confidentiality. One solution might be for the psychiatrist to recommend to the court that another examination be requested, perhaps to be performed in a hospital to help determine if malingering is occurring.

Another potential problem may occur if the psychiatrist is asked to testify about the examination after a treatment relationship has started subsequent to the forensic examination. Having to discuss a patient's psychiatric condition and diagnosis in the presence of the patient may be harmful to the therapeutic relationship, regardless of the content. Such testimony might be especially difficult when issues of psychosis, dangerousness and sociopathy are brought up in front of the patient. It could certainly be harmful to a patient and to the therapeutic alliance to hear his psychiatrist say he has an antisocial personality disorder or schizophrenia. Certainly a more sensitive situation will occur when the psychiatrist has to testify if he has become aware, through the subsequent treatment that the patient was malingering during the forensic examination. Should this be conveyed to the court, risking a breach of confidentiality, or kept from the court, risking inaccuracy or perjury? Many psychiatrists would choose to reveal their true, current perceptions on the issue since the examination was performed to help the court, not to be therapeutic to the inmate.

SUMMARY

The task of the psychiatrist who performs forensic evaluations and treatment in the same institution is a complicated balance of different demands. As shown in the above examples, there can be competing interests that the psychiatrist will have to consider, and sometimes unexpected dilemmas will arise. It could be argued that the ideal solution would be to have different personnel performing the court-ordered examinations from those who provide treatment. In that way, there could be no obvious conflict. However, limitations in resources may limit the number of psychiatrists available in a given jurisdiction. Also, a case could be made for the professional who knows the inmate best to perform the examination for the court.

The psychiatrist who is in the position of treating inmates and evaluating them for the court should keep in mind these issues. Obviously, there is no clear solution to all the problems that can arise, but an awareness of the potential dilemmas will make one's work easier.

REFERENCES

1. Rosner R: A conceptual model for forensic psychiatry: a guide for the perplexed, in Rosner R (ed): *Critical Issues in American Psychiatry and the Law,* vol 1. Charles C Thomas, 1982, chap 1.
2. *Estelle v Gamble,* 429 U.S. 97 (1976).
3. James JF, Gregory D: Improving psychiatric care for prisoners. *Hosp Community Psychiatry* 1980; 31:671–673.
4. Valdiserri EV: Psychiatry behind bars. *Bull Am Acad Psychiatry Law* 1984; 12:93–99.
5. Petrich J: Rate of psychiatric mordity in a metropolitan county jail population. *Am J Psychiatry* 1976; 133:1439–1443.
6. Lamb HR, Grant RW: The mentally ill in an urban county jail. *Arch Gen Psychiatry* 1982; 39:17–22.
7. Kaufman E: The violation of psychiatric standards of care in prisons. *Am J Psychiatry* 1980; 137:566–570.
8. Tanay E: Psychiatry and the prison system. *J Forensic Sci* 1982; 27:385–392.
9. Gutheil TG, Applebaum PS: *Clinical Handbook of Psychiatry and the Law.* McGraw-Hill, 1982, chap 6.
10. American Bar Association Standards for Criminal Justice, 1984, sect 7–10.
11. *Dusky v United States* 362 U.S. 403 (1960).
12. Smith CE: Prison psychiatry and professional responsiblility. *J Forensic Sci* 1987; 32:717–724.
13. American Psychiatric Association: *The Principles of Medical Ethics with Annotations Especially Applicable to Psychiatry.* Washington, DC, American Psychiatric Association, 1981.

12

Patient Access to Medical Records in a Forensic Center

Patients' Rights to Information

ROBERT D. MILLER, BARBARA MORROW, MICHAEL KAYE, AND GARY J. MAIER

The past two decades have seen significant increases in the rights of mental patients. Persons facing involuntary commitment proceedings have won rights to adversarial hearings, representation by counsel, and (in some jurisdictions) the rights to remain silent and to refuse treatment. In addition, the presumption of generalized incompetency that previously attended involuntary commitment has disappeared, and most states have passed bills of rights for patients.

Another manifestation of increased recognition of individual rights as against the state is the provision of access to records held by various service providers, including medical providers. A number of states have passed laws or regulations, or have had court decisions, granting patients partial or full access to their records,[1–11] and several influential

Portions of this chapter were presented at the 38th Annual Meeting of the American Academy of Forensic Sciences, New Orleans, February 15, 1986.

ROBERT D. MILLER • Forensic Center, Mendota Mental Health Institute, Madison, WI 53704; Department of Psychiatry and School of Law, University of Wisconsin-Madison, Madison, WI 53706; Department of Psychiatry, Medical College of Wisconsin, Milwaukee, WI 53201. **BARBARA MORROW AND MICHAEL KAYE** • Forensic Center, Mendota Mental Health Institute, Madison, WI 53704. **GARY J. MAIER** • Forensic Center, Mendota Mental Health Institute, Madison, WI 53704; Department of Psychiatry, University of Wisconsin-Madison, Madison, WI 53706.

professional associations and task forces have recommended increased patient access to records.[12–14] Consumer advocates have challenged the traditional view that the medical record is the property of the treating clinician, arguing that the information in the records belongs to the patient who provided it, who should have the opportunity to discover what information is being used to determine his treatment and to correct errors.[11,15–17]

Another major development in individual patient's rights has been the extension of requirements for informed consent to treatment to psychiatric patients. In addition to the civil rights issues involved, proponents of informed consent argue that it will allow patients to become partners in their treatment rather than passive acceptors, with the result that compliance will go up and treatment will become more effective.[18–20] However, as Roth *et al.*[21] have pointed out, it makes little sense, clinically or legally, to ask patients to grant others access to their records when they themselves are ignorant of the contents of those records.

Although clinicians have led movements to provide many rights for patients, they have generally opposed efforts to permit patients access to their medical records. Many clinicians continue to feel that patients are not capable of understanding medical records and might be harmed by reading them. Psychiatrists have been particularly concerned that information in their records could be detrimental to their patients' treatment by presenting interpretive material prematurely or by allowing access to confidential information given to the clinicians by other persons.[22–31]

Other professionals have argued that at least limited access to records when interpreted by clinicians would provide information that could help patients understand their problems and need for treatment, help them to feel more a part of their treatment, and decrease paranoid fears of what was being written about them.[32–33] Lipsitt argued that many of the perceived problems may be realistic responses to physician behavior, such as being too secretive or authoritarian.[34] Kelm[35] not only advocated patient access to records but also the creation of a patient–clinician dialogue in the records themselves.

Most of these authors based their opinions on theoretical grounds or on their own clinical experience. There are, however, a few reports in the literature that have attempted to examine more systematically the effects of granting patients greater access to their records.

REVIEW OF THE RESEARCH LITERATURE

Most of the reported studies are nonblind, noncontrolled reports of the effects of granting patients access to their records. Golodetz *et al.*[36] examined the effect of giving 125 medical patients copies of their admission and discharge notes at the time of discharge. Nursing staff interpreted the notes and recorded their observations of the effect on the patients, and patients were sent a questionnaire two weeks after discharge. Forty percent of the questionnaires were returned. Eighy-four percent of respondents liked being informed, 50% asked for corrections, and 60% asked questions about their records. Discussions revealed that most staff felt that patient–staff relationships had improved as a result of the record sharing. Bouchard *et al.*[37] asked 100 medical patients to audit their own charts and then sent questionnaires to each patient after discharge. Almost all of the 93 respondents were strongly in favor of such access because of an increase in their understanding of their conditions. Eighty percent said they were more careful about following orders, 78% said they had changed their behavior as a result, and 97% said they worried less about their health.

Stein *et al.*[38] showed records to 88 psychiatric inpatients and then questioned patients and staff about their experience. Ninety-two percent of the patients were in favor of access, 86% felt they had better understanding of their problems, 85% felt they were more active in therapy, 71% said they were more self-confident, and 68% liked the opportunity to correct errors. Eighty-four percent said they were comfortable reading their charts, but 51% were upset by at least some parts of what they had read. Sixty-six percent felt that staff charting had become more accurate because of patient access to the records. After initial misgivings, 90% of staff were positive about patient access, and 79% wanted to continue the process. Seventy percent felt that open records improved therapy. Chart auditing revealed that erasures increased, as did recorded examples of disruptive behavior; the authors interpreted these findings to indicate that staff were more careful in their charting.

Three studies examined only patients who specifically requested to see their records. Roth *et al.*[21] interviewed 11 of the 12 psychiatric inpatients who asked and were allowed to see at least part of their records (4 were denied access) over an 18-month period in a university hospital. All but two, who were unhappy about some of the content (especially diagnoses), were positive about the access; those who were positive were pleasantly surprised at the accuracy of the records.

Seitz *et al.*[39] interviewed 11 of the 97 patients at St. Elizabeth's Hospital in Washington, DC, who asked to see their records over a 10-month period, out of approximately 5,000 admissions. All 11 said they were positive about the access; some were interested in using the information to secure their release (all patients interviewed were in the forensic division), but most were more interested in the content of staff charting, and said that they had not changed their attitudes about themselves or about staff after reading their records. Staff had feared that the patients wanted access in order to sue them; however, after the study, most staff indicated that they had become more precise and accurate in their charting.

In contrast to the generally positive findings of the previous studies, Altman *et al.*[26] monitored all medical patients requesting to see their records over a 6-month period in a large hospital with 5,000 admissions per year. They interviewed all 11 such patients and also looked retrospectively over a 3-year period at an additional 16 for whom psychiatric consultation had been sought, and who had also requested access to their records. All but one of the patients were diagnosed by the research team as having personality disorders, and all were rated by the researchers as being in conflict with medical staff at the time of the request to see the records. Ten patients were judged to be seeking evidence of ill will from staff, 9 were looking for evidence of staff skepticism of the validity of their symptoms, and 8 feared that they were actually sicker than they had been told. Nine of the group of 10 were angrier as a result of reading their charts, 2 of the second group were angry, but 2 were reassured after reading their charts, and all 8 patients in the last group were reassured by their charts. The authors concluded that patients with good therapeutic relationships with staff do not desire to see their records, and that those who see their records suffer as a result.

Altman's group has been severely criticized for methodological deficiencies and ideological biases in this study: critics have pointed out that the study sample was not representative of all patients; that the hospital policy discouraged all but the most assertive patients from seeking access to their records; that all the diagnoses were made retrospectively by researchers who were not blind to the fact that those patients had requested to see their records; and that the authors downplayed the positive results in accordance with their prestudy bias against patient access.[30,34,40,41]

There are two reports in the literature of more methodologically rigorous studies. Stevens *et al.*[42] compared 25 medical patients who were given free access to their records (and were told of the opportunity) with 25 patients matched for gender who had no access. Patients were screened for the study by passing a simple comprehension test of English. Staff were not blind to the identities of the 2 groups. Both patient groups were given pre- and posttests to measure their knowledge of their conditions and treatment, self-assessment rating scales of mood, and a rating scale of attitudes toward the health care system. Seven of the study patients asked to see their records, 17 passively accepted their records on ward rounds, and 1 refused to see her record. On completion of the study, there were no significant differences on any of the measures, although study patients scored slightly higher on the knowledge tests. Staff observation yielded the impression that, for most study patients, staff–patient communication was improved by access to the records.

McFarlane *et al.*[43] compared 44 acute psychiatric inpatients who were granted access to their records with 31 control patients who were not. At the end of 30 days, both groups were questioned about their knowledge of their diagnoses and the chart contents, and the charts were audited to investigate possible differences in medication refusal, unauthorized absences, discharges against medical advice, and PRN medications. The contents of staff notes were evaluated. Staff also rated both patient groups using the Nursing Observation Scale for Inpatient Evaluation (NOSIE) and Ward Atmosphere scales and a questionnaire concerning changes in patient behavior. Thirty-eight percent of the study group asked to see their records. There were no statistically significant differences revealed on the questionnaires except for the study patients' greater awareness of the staff chart notes, and there were also no significant differences on any of the rating scales. Twenty-three of the 24 staff questioned at the end of the study were favorable toward the patients' access.

Although the St. Elizabeth's study[39] did mention that forensic patients were disproportionately represented among those patients who requested to see their records (forensic patients made up 5% of the patient population but were responsible for 20% of the requests), there have been no previous systematic studies of granting a population of such patients access to their records. With the shift in characteristics of inpatient psychiatric populations toward more dangerous patients, who are more likely than in previous years to have criminal records[44] and to be litigious,[45] it is important to examine the results of granting such patients access to their records.

THE STUDY

The clinical administration at the 140-bed Forensic Center at Mendota Mental Health Institute in Madison, Wisconsin, determined on clinical and administrative grounds to permit increased access to medical records to their patient population. In order to investigate the effects of granting access to records to patients with histories of aggressive and antisocial behavior, we designed the following prospective study. We have previously reported preliminary results of this study.[46]

At the time of the study, the Forensic Center included four maximum, two medium, and two minimum security units, each with approximately 20 beds. Most of the patients, all of whom were male, had been committed for treatment after being found not competent to stand trial, not guilty by reason of mental disease or defect (the insanity defense), or having been convicted under the state's since-repealed Sex Crimes Law. Most of the patients found to be incompetent or insane were suffering from psychotic disorders, whereas the sex offenders were more likely to be diagnosed as having personality disorders and/or alcohol and drug abuse. The patients had been admitted initially to the maximum security division of the center, and had been transferred to less secure units as their conditions improved.

The Community Preparation Services Unit (CPS) was a 20-bed minimum security unit that was functionally a halfway house from which patients nearing release were able to go into the community to work or attend school. It was decided to pilot increased access to records on this unit, because the patients could be expected to be the most capable of understanding the information in the records and benefitting from the access, and least likely to become upset by anything they might read in their records.

Patients on the minimum security Forensic Services I Unit (FRS) and the medium security Crossroads Unit (XRDS), who would not gain increased access to their records during the initial pilot phase, were chosen as controls for the 4-month study period, in order to evaluate any effects of knowledge of the increased access by the CPS patients, with whom they had contact. Prior to the study, patients on all three units had been given written copies of their treatment plans every three months, plus monthly summaries of their progress notes, but no other access to their records until after discharge, at which time all patients had, by state law, the right to see their complete records. Although exact statistics were not kept, the institute medical records department reported that, in the year prior to the study, there were only three or four such requests out of 587 discharged patients.

Prior to the increased access, patients on all three units were informed of the proposed changes, and asked to fill out questionnaires concerning their attitudes about having increased access to their records. Staff on all three units also completed questionnaires concerning their attitudes toward increased patient access and their predictions of what would occur with the changes. All questionnaires were coded in a manner that permitted direct before or after comparisons of responses and ensured confidentiality.

Patients on CPS were then allowed to see all parts of their records upon request; a staff member was present to answer questions and to protect the record. Each patient's request to see a record was recorded in a log book. Because all the CPS patients had been on other forensic units prior to transfer to CPS, arrangements were made for them to talk with staff on other units if they had questions about previous charting.

After CPS patients had had access to their charts for two months, all study and control patients were interviewed. CPS patients were asked about their experience in reading their charts, and control patients were asked if their attitudes had changed in any way as a result of the changes on CPS. CPS patients were then permitted to write their own observations in a special section of their charts. They were instructed in appropriate charting methods, and all who wished to chart were required to sign consent forms indicating that they realized that their charting would be part of a legal document that could be subpoenaed by courts and transferred along with their full records upon a valid request.

After an additional two months, consenting patients on all three units were interviewed again to determine the final effects of both types of change on study and control patients. Staff on the three units were asked to complete a final attitude questionnaire.

Charts of all control and study patients were retrospectively audited by three of the investigators for three 1-month periods: six months prior to the study (before patients or staff were aware of the proposed changes) [Study Point A]; the second month during which CPS patients could read their charts [Study Point B]; and the final month of the study, when CPS patients could also write in their charts [Study Point C].

Raters were asked to record the following items for all charting concerning patients' mental status or behavior: number of entries, length of entries, profession of person charting, and the value judgment of the assessment (positive, negative, or neutral). At Study Points B and C, all study and control patients who were still at the institute were interviewed.

Patient Response to Increased Access

There were no significant demographic, clinical, or legal differences between study and control patients (Table I). On the initial questionnaire, many of the patients were unclear about what access to records they already had, even though all had been given copies of their treatment plans and given summaries of the daily progress notes on a monthly basis. Thirty of the 32 patients expressed a desire to see more of their charts. About half of these patients wanted to see the daily progress notes, whereas the rest wanted access to the whole chart. Reasons for wanting to see the charts included desires to see how the staff really saw them (13 responses, 41%), to check for accuracy and correct errors (6 responses, 19%), to increase communication and trust (4 responses, 13%), and to see how their treatment was going (3 responses, 9%). Some patients gave more than one reason. There were no statistically significant differences by diagnosis or legal status in patients' attitudes about their charts.

Twenty-four of the 32 patients indicated that they would like the

Table I. Patient Characteristics

	Study patients	Control patients
Age	35.8 ± 8.1	35.3 ± 9.3
Race		
Caucasian	15	18
Black	5	1
Native American	0	1
Marital status		
Single	13	10
Married	3	5
Divorced/Separated/Widowed	4	5
Type of commitment		
Sex offender	12	10
Insanity acquittee	8	9
Transfer from prison	0	1
Type of crime proved		
Rape	5	9
Child molestation	8	8
First-degree murder	3	2
Second-degree murder	2	0
Attempted murder	1	0
Arson	1	0
Burglary	0	1
Armed robbery	0	1
Diagnoses		
Mixed personality disorder	8	14
Antisocial personality	3	3
Other personality disorders	4	1
Schizophrenia	5	6
Alcohol/drug abuse	6	10
Pedophilia/Paraphilia	8	9
Sexual sadism	1	1
Borderline	1	0
Posttraumatic stress disorder	1	1

opportunity to make entries in their charts. Reasons given included a desire to be able to make corrections and increased feelings of control over their treatment (16 responses each, 67% of those expressing interest in writing in their charts); a desire to give their side of the story (9 responses, 38%); and a feeling that staff would be more careful of what they wrote if patients could respond in the chart itself (7 responses, 29%).

After the increased access was granted on CPS, neither CPS patients who chose not to read their charts nor control patients changed their opinions on the value of seeing their charts. The behavior of most study patients did not agree with their stated preferences: once access was granted, only eight study patients took advantage of the opportunity to read their charts, and only three read them more than once during the study period. Six of these patients had diagnoses of personality disorders and two were schizophrenic.

No patient requested to speak with staff on previous units to discuss past charting. There were no statistically significant differences between the characteristics of patients who looked at their charts and those who did not.

After the initial two months of access, only 11 of 17 (65%) study patients felt that access had been helpful; whereas at the conclusion of the 4-month study period, 13 of 15 (87%) felt it had been helpful. One patient was upset by some of the material he read; one felt he was breaking trust with staff on previous units by reading their charting; and one could not understand "all the big words" in the chart, despite staff assistance.

Most patients read only the daily progress notes (in addition to the treatment plans, which were already shown to all patients before the study). Desires to check on the accuracy of charting, to see staff opinions of them, and to correct inaccurate information (if it existed) predominated as reasons given for reading the charts after access was granted. Those patients who felt access had been useful stated that they were better informed about their treatment and about staff opinions of them. Most stated that any fears they had had about the charting were unfounded; and a number of patients who did not read their charts stated that they were reassured simply because they knew that they could read them.

When patients had the opportunity to write in the charts, none of them took advantage of it during the study period, although a few did so after the study ended. Half still thought it was a good idea, and several said that they planned to write in their charts, but "hadn't had time to write anything yet."

Staff Attitudes

Questionnaires before and after the study period were returned by 15 staff on the CPS (study) unit, and by 32 staff on the two control units (FRS I and XRDS). This represented 100% of staff who worked on those units during the entire study period. Prior to the increased access, the great majority of all staff favored some access to records and felt that at least some access would be helpful; but only half favored allowing access to the complete chart. A somewhat smaller majority favored allowing patients to write in their charts (Table II). Both before and after the study, the staff on the unit (CPS), which granted increased access, were

Table II. Staff Attitudes

Question	Study		Control	
	Before	After	Before	After
Patients should see some of their records	100%	100%	81%	88%
Patients should see all of their records	47%	67%	50%	34%
It is helpful for patients to see their records	100%	100%	81%	81%
Patients should be able to write in their records	80%	—	66%	—

more favorably disposed toward the changes than staff on control units. Differences in basic attitudes were not statistically significant by analysis of variance, but there were trends indicating that psychologists, social workers, and occupational therapists were more favorably disposed toward increased patient access to charts than were nursing staff (RNs, LPNs, and aides). There was also a nonsignificant trend for staff with the longest experience to be least favorable toward the changes.

Staff from both control and study units gave a number of reasons for their attitudes. Those who were favorable to access felt that it would help patients be better informed about their treatment and decrease suspiciousness (33 responses each, 70%) and improve staff record-keeping (22 responses, 47%); but there was also concern that patients might be upset by what they read (22 responses, 47%), that patient paranoia would increase (20 responses, 43%), that patients might read information harmful to other patients (14 responses, 30%), and that staff charting would become more guarded and less useful (7 responses, 15%).

On the prestudy questionnaires, those staff who felt that allowing patients to write in the charts was helpful argued that it would help patients participate directly in their therapy (32 responses), give them more of a feeling of control (30 responses), and would encourage staff to chart more carefully (19 responses). Those who opposed patient charting felt that patients would use it to harass staff (25 responses), and that it would divert too much patient energy away from therapy (18 responses). In meetings with staff prior to the study (but not on the written questionnaires), several staff complained that "the patients already have all the rights, while staff have none." Follow-up questionnaires yielded too few responses to these questions to permit statistical analysis.

Table III. Total Number of Entries

Unit	Period A	Period B	Average
Control 1	15.83	27.83	21.83
Control 2	11.78	11.78	11.78
Study	46.10	53.40	49.75

Staff Charting

To investigate possible changes in charting practices, Repeated Measures ANOVAs were performed with unit (CPS, FRS, XRDS) as the between-subject factor and study period as the within-subject factor. Data from the third study period were not included in the analysis due to reduced sample size. Four subjects from the experimental group were eliminated from analysis because they had been on a control unit during the prestudy audit period, making meaningful pre- or postcomparisons impossible. Dependent variables from the charting included the total number of entries, total number of lines of charting, average length of entry, and percentage and total amount of positive, negative, and neutral charting.

Initial between-unit differences ($P < .001$) were found in total number of entries, total number of lines, and average number of entries, but these differences remained constant throughout the study. Comparing the two study periods, there was a near-significant trend ($P < .09$) for more entries to be made in the second, and a significant ($P < .04$) increase in total lines of charting during the second time period on all three units (Tables III–V).

In addition to the initial between-unit differences in amount of charting, the types of judgments made also differed among the three units (Table VI). The percentage of neutral ($P < .01$), positive ($P < .06$) and negative ($P < .06$) entries differed among units in the prestudy period. These differences remained stable over the study period, and

Table IV. Total Lines of Charting

Unit	Period A	Period B	Average
Control 1	146.33	249.33	197.83
Control 2	87.67	79.78	83.72
Study	205.10	254.50	229.80
Averages between units		$F = 11.986$ $df = 2$	$P = .001$
Averages over study periods		$F = 4.749$ $df = 1$	$P = .038$

Table V. Length of Entries

Assessment	Control 1 A	Control 1 B	Control 2 A	Control 2 B	Study A	Study B
Negative	12.08	12.22	6.79	10.46	19.05	3.61
Positive	11.60	19.80	9.89	5.80	12.59	15.41
Neutral	5.85	5.95	3.73	3.71	3.35	3.73[a]

[a]$P = .044$.

did not change between study and control units. The total number of lines of neutral ($P < .001$) and negative ($P < .05$) charting varied significantly between units in the prestudy audit period, with percentage of positive charting ($P < .09$) nearing significance. These between-unit differences did not vary after study patients were given access to their charts.

Between the two study periods, there was an overall trend toward more lines of neutral charting ($P < .09$); total number of lines of positive and negative charting remained stable (Table VI). No change by treatment condition was found in the total lines of positive, negative, or neutral charting.

Only the average length of neutral entries varied initially between units. Over time, all units showed a near-significant ($P < .07$) tendency toward longer neutral entries. Staff on CPS showed a significant increase ($P < .05$) in length of neutral entries and a near-significant ($P < .08$) increase in the length of negative charting.

ADMINISTRATIVE RESPONSES TO INCREASED ACCESS

Initially, the hospital administration responded somewhat unfavorably to the plan to increase access to records. They held up the plan, in the Institute Research Committee, for nearly six months before approving it and objected specifically to permitting patients to write in

Table VI. Percentages of Entries

Assessment	Control 1 A	Control 1 B	Control 2 A	Control 2 B	Study A	Study B
Negative	25.5	12.5	8.3	17.7	2.1	2.1
Positive	24.3	34.8	24.9	24.5	10.5	7.8
Neutral	50.2	52.7	66.8	57.8	87.4	90.1

their charts and to permitting them access to information that we had received from other treatment facilities. Complaints from a few disaffected staff on forensic units that were not initially to grant their patients increased access through the hospital nursing office reinforced the administration's resistance. After the study results were available, the administration continued to be skeptical of extending access to other units and prohibited further access to outside material as well as the opportunity for patients to write in their official medical records.

EXTENSION OF PATIENT ACCESS

After the completion of the pilot study on CPS, patient access to records has been extended to the other medium security units in the Forensic Center. Because of the administrative ban, access was permitted only to materials in the records that originated at the Institute, and patients were not permitted to write in their charts. In addition, because of continuing objections (despite lack of problems) from staff on units from which patients had been treated previously, patients were allowed to see only the daily progress notes generated on the unit they were currently on. After transfer to another unit, the notes made by that unit's staff were removed from the active chart.

In the six-month period since increased access has been extended to other units, patient reaction has continued to be favorable. No formal studies have been done, but records kept on the units indicate that 28 of 54 (52%) of the patients have looked at their records at least once, 16 one time, and 12 more than once. One patient became sufficiently upset by something he read to require a brief period of seclusion; but otherwise, there have been no problems with the access. Ultimately, we plan to extend increased access to the entire Forensic Center.

DISCUSSION

Even though fewer than half the patients actually read any of their charts during the formal study period (in addition to the treatment plans that were already provided to all patients), it was clear from the interviews that the great majority of both study and control patients regarded the access to charts as positive. Many said that the very fact that they could see the charts obviated the need to do so and increased their trust in the staff. There was no evidence that any patients became worse from reading their charts during the formal study period. The only two patients who expressed strong negative feelings about their charts prior to the study did not take advantage of the opportunity to read them, so that access had no negative effects on their behavior or feelings toward staff.

Prior to the study, staff on all three units shared many of the same concerns about granting patients access to their records as have staff in other facilities: patients would not be able to understand their records; they might be harmed by premature disclosure of interpretations; patients' paranoid fears might be exacerbated; and staff time would be wasted in monitoring patients while they read their charts. But it was the criminal backgrounds of the patients that caused the most concern to our staff. They feared reprisals, especially with the sex offenders, the majority of whom were diagnosed as having personality disorders. Staff on units from which patients had been transferred to CPS were especially concerned, because they were no longer working with the patients and feared that reading past charting would reopen old wounds. These specific concerns had not been addressed in the previous literature, but were a major concern of our staff.

Prior to the commencement of the changes, the investigators met with staff on CPS and all the units from which patients were transferred to CPS, in order to explain the reasons for the changes and to reassure staff that previous experience with granting access at other facilities had not led to problems. A number of staff threatened to decrease their charting significantly, especially in the assessment section of the SOAP notes, because of the possibility that patients could read what they had written. Although the fact that all the patients had complete access to their charts after discharge did not seem to bother staff, the possibility of patients' seeing charts while they were still in hospital appeared to be more disturbing to some staff.

Despite staff fears, however, it is clear that few patients actually read their charts. The total time-study patients spent reading charts during the four-month study period was under 10 hours, and no time was spent in writing in the charts. Thus, staff fears that patients would devote too much energy (and waste too much staff time) reading their records were unfounded. In addition, threats that staff charting would deteriorate did not materialize, because no statistically significant differences in charting were found except for the greater length of entries with neutral assessments on CPS during the second study period. It must be noted, however, that several illiterate patients on CPS were reluctant to take up staff time in having their charts read to them.

It is also interesting that staff on the only unit in which patients actually saw their charts began with positive views about the increase, and that there was a nonsignificant trend for their views became more positive during the study, whereas staff on control units were originally less favorable and became even less favorable during the study. Staff resistance on the original control units has also diminished somewhat now that patients on their units have the same access, and with the protection that patients can no longer read charting from previous units.

The reaction of public hospital administrations and line staff to changes of any type has traditionally been negative.[47–49] Brown[50] has discussed the specific resistance of line staff to increases in patients' rights. We have pointed out elsewhere that one response to years of neglect and abuse of patients in public facilities has been to establish and protect patients' rights, while staff rights have tended to be ignored[51]. Others have demonstrated a continuum of attitudes toward an increase of patients' rights—the higher the eductional level of staff, the more positive about patients' rights.[52–55] Although the numbers were too small to achieve statistical significance, our experience with granting patients greater access to their records bears out these previous findings.

One conclusion is clear from our experience: it is imperative that staff feelings be taken into consideration before changes are made. As demonstrated by previous studies and confirmed by ours, there will be some staff who will remain opposed to any increase in patients' rights in spite of evidence that the changes are helpful (or at least not harmful.) While preparing staff for proposed changes in advance may not affect attitudes of some staff members, it may well prevent their attitudes from influencing other staff who are more open to change.

Acknowledgments

The authors wish to thank the staff and patients in the Mendota Forensic Center for their cooperation in this study.

REFERENCES

1. Privacy Act of 1974, Pub. L. No. 93–579.
2. Mass. Gen. Laws Ann. ch. 111, § 70 (West 1971).
3. N.Y. Rev. Stat. §§ 2A; 82–41–45 (1952).
4. Conn. Gen. Stat. Ann. § 4–104 (West 1969).
5. La. Rev. Stat. Ann. § 40:2014, 1 (West 1965).
6. Miss. Code Ann. § 41–9–65 (1972).
7. Mental Health Act 1975 Wis. Stat. ch. 51.30(4)(d).
8. North Carolina Department of Human Resources, Division of Mental Health, Mental Retardation, and Substance Abuse Services, Regulations, 10 NCAC Subchapter 18D, Sections .0100–.0414 (1980).
9. Shlensky R: Informed consent and confidentiality: Proposed new approaches in Illinois. *Am J. Psychiatry* 1977; 134:1416–1418.
10. *Pyramid Life Insurance Company v Masonic Hospital Association,* 191 F.Supp. 51,54 (1961).

11. Tucker G: Patient access to medical records. *Leg Aspects Med Pract,* October 1978, pp 45–51.
12. *Report of the Secretary's Commission on Medical Malpractice.* U.S. Dept of Health, Education, and Welfare, January 16, 1973, p 77.
13. *Personal Privacy in an Information Society.* U.S. Privacy Protection Study Commission, pp 1977, pp 293,298,299.
14. American Psychiatric Association: Model law on confidentiality of health and social service records. *Am J Psychiatry* 1979; 136:138–144.
15. Hinkle BJ: Living with the demands of confidentiality. *J Leg Med* 1977; 5:9–14.
16. Westin AF: Computers, health records, and citizen rights. Washington DC, National Bureau of Standards. (Quoted by Herrington BS: *Psychiatric News* 1977; 12:8.
17. Westin AF: Medical records: should patients have access? *Hastings Cent Rep* 1977; 7:23–28.
18. Katz J: Informed consent—a fairy tale? Law's vision. *U Pitt Law Rev* 1977; 39:137–174.
19. Simpson RE: Informed consent: From disclosure to patient participation in medical decision making. *NW U Law Rev* 1981; 76:172–207.
20. Meisel A: Making mental health care decisions: Informed consent and involuntary civil commitment. *Behav Sci Law* 1983; 1:73–88.
21. Roth LH, Wolford J, Meisel A: Patient access to records: Tonic or toxin? *Am J Psychiatry* 1980; 137:592–596.
22. Davidson HA: *Forensic Psychiatry,* ed. 2. New York, Ronald Press, 1965, pp 284–285.
23. Meissner WW: Threats to confidentiality. *Psych Ann* 1979; 9:94–105.
24. Halleck SL: *Law in the Practice of Psychiatry.* New York, Plenum Press, 1980, pp 182–183.
25. Grossman M: Confidentiality: The right to privacy versus the right to know, in Barton WE, Sanborn CJ (eds) *Law and the Mental Health Professions.* New York, International Universities Press, 1978, p 149.
26. Altman JH, Reich P, Kelly MJ, Rogers MP: Patients who read their hospital charts. *New Engl J Med* 1980; 302:169–171.
27. Steiner P: Patient access to the medical record: A study of physician attitudes. *Med Rec News* 1978; 49:77.
28. Tancredi LR, Lieb J, Slaby AE: *Legal Issues in Psychiatric Care.* Hagerstown, Md, Harper & Row, 1975, p 56.
29. Smith WH: Ethical, social, and professional issues in patients' access to psychological test reports. *Bull Menninger Clin* 1978; 42:150–155.
30. Bernstein RA, Andrews EM, Weaver LA: Physician attitudes toward patients' requests to read their hospital records. *Med Care* 1981; 19:118–121.
31. Fletcher JL: Patient right to acquisition of medical records. *IMJ* 1975; 147:31.
32. Shenkin BN, Warner DC: Giving the patient his medical record: a proposal to improve the system. *New Engl J Med* 1973; 289:688–692.
33. Bronson DL, Rubin AS, Tufo HM: Patient education through record sharing. *QRB* 1978; 4:2–4.
34. Lipsitt DR: The patient and the record. *New Engl J Med* 1980; 302:167–168.
35. Kelm M: The medical record—a dialogue? *JAMA* 1984; 252:1289.
36. Golodetz A, Ruess J, Milhous RL: The right to know: Giving the patient his medical record. *Arch Phys Med Rehabil* 1976; 57:78–81.
37. Bouchard RE, Tufo HM, van Buren HC, *et al.*: The patient and his problem-oriented record, in Walker HK, Hurst JW, Woody MF (eds) *Applying the Problem-Oriented System.* New York, Medcom Press, 1973.

38. Stein EJ, Furedy RL, Simonton MJ, Neuffer CH: Patient access to medical records on a psychiatric inpatient unit. *Am J Psychiatry* 1979; 136:327–329.
39. Seitz JF, Ward A, Dobbs WH: Granting patients access to records: The impact of the privacy act at a federal hospital. *Hosp Community Psychiatry* 1978; 29:288–289.
40. Shapiro M, Lehman A: Patients who read their hospital charts (letter). *New Engl J Med* 1980; 302:1482.
41. Annas GJ, Matthews D, Glante LH: Patients who read their hospital charts (letter). *New Engl J Med* 1980; 302:1483.
42. Stevens DP, Stagg R, MacKay IR: What happens when hospitalized patients see their own records? *Ann Intern Med* 1977; 86:474–477.
43. McFarlane WJG, Bowman RG, MacInnes M: Patient access to hospital records: A pilot project. *Can J Psychiatry* 1980; 25:497–502.
44. Steadman HF, Cocozza JJ, Melich ME: Explaining the increased arrest rate among mental patients: The changing clientele of state hospitals. *Am J Psychiatry* 1978; 135:816–820.
45. Miller RD, Maier GJ, Blancke FW, Doren DM: Litigiousness as a resistance to therapy. *J Psychiatry Law,* in press, 1986; 14:109–123.
46. Miller RD, Morrow B, Kaye M, Maier GJ: Patient access to medical records in a maximum security forensic center: A review of the literature and a controlled study. *Hosp Comm Psychiatry* 1987; 38:1081–1085.
47. Pearlin LI: Sources of resistance to change in a mental hospital. *AJS* 1962; 68:325–334.
48. Kaplan HM, Blain D: Organizational obstacles to change in a large mental hospital. *Am J Psychiatry* 1970; 126:1107–1114.
49. Fowlkes MR: Business as usual—At the state mental hospital. *Psychiatry* 1975; 38:55–64.
50. Brown P: State mental hospital staff attitudes toward patients' rights. *Int J Law Psychiatry* 1986; 8:423–441.
51. Miller RD, Maier GJ: Factors affecting the decision to prosecute mental patients for criminal behavior. *Hosp Community Psychiatry* 1987; 38:50–55.
52. Baker F, Schulberg, HC: The development of a community mental health ideology scale. *Community Ment Health J* 1967; 3:216–225.
53. Penn NE, Baker F, Schulberg HC: Community Mental Health Ideology Scale: Social work norms. *Community Ment Health J* 1976; 12:211–214.
54. Lindenthal JJ, Thomas CS: A comparative study of the handling of confidentiality. *J Nerv Ment Dis* 1980; 168:361–369.
55. Miller RD: Outpatient civil commitment of the mentally ill: An overview and an update. *Behav Sci and the Law* 1988; 6:99–118.

IV

Service Delivery Systems

13

The Prisoner as Patient

Assessing the Provision of Mental Health Care in the Correctional System

SARA L. KELLERMANN, MARJORIE A. ROCK, AND JANE A. BARKER

INTRODUCTION

Policy changes that have occurred at the interface of the mental health and the legal systems over the past 30 years have impacted significantly on individual clients as well as on the mental health and the correctional systems. A major consequence of these changes, debated in the literature, is the question of whether there has been an increase of mentally disabled individuals in the jails. Although some studies purport to document an increase in this population, other studies note that there does not appear to have been a highly significant increase of inmates who experience severe mental disorders.[1–6] What does appear to be clear, however, is that the general jail population is increasing at a rapid rate.[7,8] Therefore, even if the percentage of mentally disordered persons in the jails were to remain constant, the actual numbers of inmates with a need for mental health services would continue to increase.

Although the need for the provision of mental health services in the correctional system has been acknowledged, several problems persist in designing, implementing, and monitoring such services. A major problem, identified by Steadman *et al.*, is the "virtual absence of any em-

SARA L. KELLERMANN AND **MARJORIE A. ROCK** • New York City Department of Mental Health, Mental Retardation and Alcoholism Services, New York, NY 10013. **JANE A. BARKER** • Mental Health Services, Victim Services Agency, New York, NY 10007.

pirically grounded guidelines for establishing appropriate services for mentally disturbed inmates in jails and local correctional facilities."[9] Despite the absence of empirical guidelines, these authors note that professional associations have developed minimum standards for the administration, staffing, and provision of mental health services within the correctional setting. These standards serve to define criteria for providing at least a modicum of mental health services, usually including assessment, some form of treatment and/or referral, staff training, and a mandate for interorganizational communication between mental health and correctional staff, with provisions made to safeguard inmate confidentiality.

Given the paucity of empirical research concerning jail mental health programs, it is not surprising that there are few studies that discuss the evaluation and monitoring of such programs. One study in this area was done by Morrissey, Steadman, Kilburn, and Lindsey in which the authors evaluated two interorganizational variables in the provision of mental health service in the correctional setting—program auspice and program location—as predictors of the perceived effectiveness of jail mental health programs. The authors concluded that "there is no one best way" to organize jail mental health services; rather, a multitude of contingencies need to be considered in planning such services.[10]

The New York City Department of Mental Health, Mental Retardation and Alcoholism Services funds and monitors mental health services in the New York City correctional system. This chapter will therefore describe the structure of mental health services within the New York City correctional system. Then the role of the New York City Department of Mental Health, Mental Retardation and Alcoholism Services in the delivery of prison mental health services will be reviewed after which the department's evaluation protocol and site-evaluation findings will be discussed with regard to jail mental health services. Finally, implications for the provision and monitoring of jail mental health services will be discussed.

THE NEW YORK CITY MENTAL HEALTH AND CORRECTIONAL SYSTEMS

The New York City correctional system is the largest local correctional system in the United States. It is comprised of 13 institutions with a current inmate capacity (1988) of 13,651 and a projected capacity, by 1993, of 20,216 inmates. Mental health services are delivered in all 13 correctional facilities, with three separate and distinct levels of care provided. Levels of care consist of specialized mental observation units for those identified as needing initial assessment, intervention, and monitoring (433 beds), the Mental Health Center at Riker's Island (180 beds), for inmates needing more intensive care, and 136 inpatient prison beds in the municipal hospital system for those inmates requiring the most intensive level of acute inpatient care. In addition, all new inmates are assessed initially to determine whether there is a need for further services. Delivery of mental health services in such a large system is complex, requiring several municipal and voluntary agencies to work together to plan and implement services.

The New York City Department of Mental Health, Mental Retardation and Alcoholism Services, in its role under the City Charter and the New York State Mental Hygiene Law, is responsible for planning, funding, and monitoring all mental hygiene services in New York City, including services delivered in the correctional system. The local governmental unit was initially established in 1954 by New York State with the passage of the Community Mental Health Services Act—the first such act in the nation establishing a local mental hygiene authority.[11] The act established a system of state reimbursement to localities for the provision of community-based mental health services, based on a local planning process, and provided the mandate for localities to monitor community-based mental health programs. For more than 30 years, the department has administered the mental health network of New York City by planning for appropriate community mental hygiene services, developing and funding these services, and monitoring and evaluating the services provided to ensure that they meet quality assurance criteria. The evaluation and monitoring functions are accomplished by the department's Office of Program Review and Evaluation (OPRE), a centralized unit created for the purpose of carrying out on-going program monitoring of all contract agencies in order to assure that quality mental health services are provided.

PROGRAM REVIEW AND EVALUATION

Although the department's mandate has included the monitoring function since the inception of the department, the current structure of OPRE was established in 1978. At that time, a formalized evaluation protocol was developed for monitoring mental health agencies under contract to the department for the purpose of assuring compliance to contract specifications as well as to ensure generally acceptable standards of clinical care. Initially OPRE evaluated agencies on the following parameters: contract agency administration, chart review procedures, levels of service, admission, discharge, and referral policies, staffing patterns and credentials, appointment procedures, medical record procedures, environmental aspects of the agency, and consumer participation. The evaluation protocol incorporated regulations promulgated by the New York State Department of Mental Hygiene, the Joint Commission on the Accreditation of Hospitals (JCAH), Federal regulatory authorities, and generally acceptable clinical standards.

As has been noted, program evaluation traditionally involves three elements: structure, process, and outcome.[12] Because of the expense and methodological limitations of outcome studies, the department's primary focus has been to monitor the structural aspects of programs as well as the process of treatment. Recently, however, the New York State Office of Mental Health and the City Department have begun to address this aspect of program evaluation by the initiation of requirements that agencies develop internal measures of outcome, such as specific behavioral treatment goals and other measures of quality assurance.

OPRE's evaluation capabilities have paralleled the growth and diversity of the community mental health service sector, and, at this time, specialized protocols exist for the full range of services funded by the department.

Establishing a Database

The first formal evaluation of mental health services to inmates of the correctional system occured in 1979. This evaluation served two purposes: first, to establish a database on the services provided by Prison Mental Health Services on Riker's Island, that is, to describe the services, the patient flow, and the intersections with the correctional and medical system; and second, to provide the first qualitative assessment of service provision in the correctional system. It was noted that, of major importance, were the entry points into the correctional mental health system, which included state and local correctional settings, as well as the medical services and mental health services operated by a voluntary hospital and by the New York City Health Department.

The database provided by this first evaluation was comprehensive and descriptive, and provided, for each of the facilities, a review of program policies, staffing patterns, administrative procedures, patient flow, and environmental factors. Site-visit activities included administrative interviews, chart review, review of Department of Correction and Department of Health documents, and tours of the facilities. Each of the facilities that provided care was analyzed, utilizing criteria to evaluate intake and referral procedures, treatment modalities, suicide watch, staffing, environmental conditions, and chart review.

Mental Health Minimum Standards

This first systematic evaluation of the Riker's Island Prison Mental Health Services played a critical role in the development of the department's planning and policy approach toward the future provision of mental health services in the correction system. Two subsequent developments, which resulted in systems changes, were consequences of the evaluation report. In 1985, the Board of Correction issued the Mental Health Minimum Standards, a joint effort by the Department of Mental Health, Mental Retardation and Alcoholism Services, the Board of Correction, the Department of Health, and the Department of Correction, which were to have a major impact on the system; additionally, the delivery of prison mental health services was restructured. The development of the minimum standards represented an attempt by a municipality to codify program objectives and to develop a unified planning and delivery process for the provision of mental health services within the local correctional system. As noted by Steadman *et al.* the development of minimum standards for the delivery of jail mental health services by governmental units was slow to occur.[9] The promulgation of the New York City Mental Health Minimum Standards represents the first time a municipality has developed such standards.

One of the major findings noted in the recommendations of the first evaluation was that emphasis should be placed on triage and referral services, including effective screening and preliminary diagnosis, as opposed to attempting to deliver comprehensive, individual long-term care. In part, this emphasis was a response to the increasing rate of suicide in the jails. In 1978, there were six suicides, whereas by the end of April, 1979, four suicides had already occurred. Conceptually, from a policy perspective, this reflected a commitment to crisis intervention services—often a more effective method of utilizing limited mental health resources.

Subsequent Findings

The 1979 report noted the difficulty presented by the separate structures that operated the health and the mental health services on Riker's Island. At the time, the medical services were operated by Montefiore Medical Center, a voluntary teaching hospital, whereas mental health services were operated directly by a municipal agency, the Department of Health. The lack of coordination between the two agencies was reported in the evaluation and recommendations were made that a single administrative structure for the provision of both mental health and medical services be established.

A subsequent evaluation of the Prison Mental Health Services occurred in May of 1981. The key focus of this evaluation was on the assessment of interdepartmental and interagency linkages. The evaluation was carried out primarily through formal interviews with key staff in the Department of Correction, including administrative and line-level staff and the administrative staff of the prison mental health services. As a result of this evaluation, recommendations continued to stress the importance of communications among and between the systems.

A second focus of this site visit was on the quality of clinical documentation. This second evaluation employed a more sophisticated protocol for the review of the clinical records. The first protocol, in 1979, had assessed the presence or absence of the minimal components needed in a clinical workup, including a psychosocial history, treatment plan, suicide or homicide attempt, mental status exam, medical history, physical exam, and diagnosis. Finding deficiencies with only the presence or absence of those criteria, the 1979 report had recommended that mechanisms be developed to collect more extensive information. The 1981 evaluation assessed whether information was present or absent and what was the quality of the information. The ability of the department to monitor in this area paralleled the development of the chart-review protocols that were utilized by the department for the more traditional mental health system in the community.

In 1983, OPRE conducted the third site-visit evaluation of Prison Mental Health Services. Between 1981 and 1983, the inmate population in the New York City correctional system had shown a marked increase. This development was reflected in the 1983 evaluation report which noted the overcrowding of the correctional system and the concommitant decrease in availability of both correctional staff and mental health staff. As a consequence, mental health caseloads were high and support staff were insufficient. Despite these stresses on the system, the report acknowledged a number of improvements since 1981, including administrative improvement in Prison Mental Health, improvements in the Suicide Prevention Aide program, and environmental improvements at the Mental Health Center. Improvements were noted also in the quality of the clinical record. It became possible to distinguish between "short-stay" detainees and "long-stay" sentenced inmates, and two separate protocols were developed for these two groups. As noted previously, these improvements were primarily structural and process oriented: the major focus of the department's evaluations.

Recommendations in the 1983 report acknowledged that the Department of Health Prison Mental Health Services had instituted a sound framework for services despite the many stresses of the overcrowded system. Issues of coordination and linkages had begun to be addressed within this framework. The need for more formalized written policies was addressed, as was the need for more consistent clinical oversight of the system through the appointment of a Director of Psychiatry. In addition, recommendations included the development of a systemwide quality assurance mechanism, and the need for in-service training to improve clinical documentation.

In 1984, a restructuring of the health and mental health services on Riker's Island occurred. Montefiore Medical Center, a voluntary teaching hospital that had been providing medical services for the inmate population, was designated the provider of mental health services on the mental observation units, whereas the Department of Health became the sole provider of both health and mental health services in the Mental Health Center, the Riker's Island Hospital, and the Borough Houses of Detention. Essentially, Montefiore Medical Center assumed the role of the "outpatient" mental health services, and the Department of Health maintained responsibility for a more intensive level of care.

As a result of the major systematic changes that took place in 1984 and 1985, and with the promulgation of the mental health minimum standards by the Board of Correction, the Department of Mental Health delayed its biennial site visit until 1986. It should be noted that the minimum standards reflect, to a large extent, the concerns that had been raised by the department's evaluation process through the years. These minimum standards mandate clinical standards, services, and training for staff involved in the provision of mental health services. In addition, the standards formalize the role of the Department of Mental Health, Mental Retardation and Alcoholism Services in overseeing the planning, monitoring, and funding of mental health services in the correctional system.

Subsequent to the implementation of the standards, the department conducted a review of the mental health programs in the spring of 1986. Issues addressed in this site evaluation included the evaluation of the clinical program components and a further evaluation of the interface between the Department of Correction and the providers of prison mental health services. Findings from the evaluation illustrate the significant changes that had occurred in the system as well as the changes that had been made in the monitoring approach. Programmatic changes reflected the emphasis on crisis intervention and stabilization and indicated that these priorities were being met through prompt assessment, diagnosis, and treatment of inmates. In addition, written comprehensive policies and procedures had been developed; a Director of Psychiatry had been appointed and additional staff were being hired; and regular meetings were being held with the Department of Correction, Montefiore Medical Center, and the Department of Health to foster intersystem communications. In-service mental health training for correctional officers, a component that is frequently overlooked, had also been mandated on a systematic basis, utilizing a 28-hour mental health curriculum developed for this purpose.

Recommendations in the 1986 report also included issues related to the transfer of patients between Montefiore facilities and Department of Health and Health and Hospitals Corporation facilities. Collaboration was recommended between Montefiore, the Department of Health, and the Department of Mental Health with regard to developing aftercare resources for the discharged inmate.

In summary, the 1986 site-visit evaluation noted the major improvement in the communications and interface of all systems in this complex network. The process of developing the Mental Health Minimum Standards had tangible results in terms of improving the quality of care for the inmates and less obvious results, but no less important, of improving the working relationships between the many institutional parties involved in the oversight and provision of prison mental health services.

IMPLICATIONS

This chapter has presented the structure of the delivery of mental health services in the New York City correctional system and a review of the New York City Department of Mental Health, Mental Retardation and Alcoholism Services' role in the planning, funding, and monitoring of these services. It has also presented the Department's findings in regard to the evaluation process.

A review of the principles of the department with regard to assessing jail mental health services point to several underlying assumptions, namely, that there is a need for mental health services in the jail system. Inmates often enter the system with severe pathology and/or develop psychiatric symptomatology while in the system. Often the stress of entering the correctional system may precipitate or exacerbate a need for mental health services. Inmate mental health needs must be addressed from a humane point of view. In fact, legal precedents have been established that mandate "adequacy of," and "reasonable access to," mental health care in the correctional system.[13,14] Although underlying differences in function and mission between correction officials (safety and protection) and mental health officials (treatment and rehabilitation) may initially cause conflict in organizing mental health services, both agencies will need to develop priorities that are reasonable, humane, ethical, professional and cost effective.

Perhaps the most significant lesson to be learned is the need for the maintenance of ongoing communications between the systems. Open communication at all levels of the system represents the "glue" that makes programmatic success possible. Communication, in fact, may be more important than specific program auspice, as noted by Steadman *et al.*[9] This is no doubt true in a smaller system, but especially vital in a "megasystem" such as in New York City.

Furthermore, where both time and resources are limited, an emphasis on appropriate triage services, including screening, crisis intervention, and appropriate referral procedures, are an effective means of utilizing mental health funds, while providing necessary mental health services.

Mental health minimum standards provide the framework for the delivery of mental health programs and serve to develop a unified approach to planning, as well as for service delivery and evaluation. Mental health minimum standards, which are developed jointly by the correctional system and the mental health system, also provide a vehicle for developing communications, trust, and mutual understanding, as common goals are delineated among the two systems. The role of planning for future service needs in conjunction with both mental health and the correctional system is equally important. Without this kind of "exercise," mental health services would tend to be haphazard and reactive to particular crises. However, with an agreed upon framework and thoughtful joint planning, efforts can be devoted to providing and ensuring quality services through the evaluation and monitoring process.

An area that needs to be further developed with regard to mental health services in the jails is that of discharge planning and case management programs. This need was noted in the department's 1986 site evaluation of the program. This area is important in all systems, but especially so in large "megasystems" where released inmates with ongoing mental health needs can easily "fall through the cracks" upon discharge. As the case management system becomes an integral part of the mental health services spectrum, more thought should be given to integrating case management services for prison detainees with mental health needs in the larger mental health services system.

Finally, it should be noted that the systematic planning and monitoring of mental health services can have a positive effect on the structure of the relationship between the correctional system and the mental health system. As mutual understanding and positive relationships are fostered, the impact on the inmate/client will become more significant, and the inmate/client will be the recipient of more effective services.

REFERENCES

1. Abramson M: The criminalization of mentally disordered behavior: Possible side effects of a new mental health law. *Hosp Community Psychiatry* 1972; 23:101/105.
2. Zitrin A, Hardesty A, Burdock E: Crime and violence among mental patients. *Am J Psychiatry* 1976; 133:142–149.
3. Whitmer G: From hospitals to jails: The fate of California's deinstitutionalized mentally ill. *Am J Orthopsychiatry* 1980; 50:65–75.
4. Lamb HR, Grant R: The mentally ill in an urban county jail. *Arch Gen Psychiatry* 1982; 39:17–22.
5. Teplin L: The criminalization of the mentally ill: Speculation in search of data. *Psychol Bull* 1983; 94:54–67.
6. Monahan J, Steadman H: Crime and mental disorder: An epidemiological approach, in Morris N, and Towery M (eds): *Annual Review of Crime and Justice,* vol 4. Chicago, University of Chicago Press, 1982, pp 145–189.
7. Correction board moves to ease Riker's crowding. *The New York Times,* August 12, 1987, sect B, p 1, col 2.
8. Department of Correction, The Mayor's Management Report, New York City: *Citybooks,* January, 1987 p 25.
9. Steadman HJ, McCarty DW, Morrissey JP: *Developing Jail Mental Health Services: Practice and Principles.* Rockville, Md. National Institute of Mental Health, (ADM) 86–1458, 1986.
10. Morrissey JP, Steadman HJ, Kilburn H Jr, Lindsey ML: The effectiveness of jail mental health programs: An interorganizational assessment. *Crim Just Behav* 1984; 11:235–256.
11. Ozarin LD: Mental health in public health: The federal perspective, in Wagonfeld MO, Lemkau PV, Justice B (eds): *Public Mental Health: Perspectives and Prospects.* Beverly Hills, Sage Publications, 1982, p 34.
12. Donabedian A: *Explorations in Quality Assessment and Monitoring,* vol 2. Ann Arbor, Mich, Health Administration Press, 1982 p 90.
13. *Inmates v Pierce,* 489 F. Supp. 638 (1980).
14. *Estelle v Gamble,* 429 U.S. 97 (1976).

14

Policy Implications of Private Sector Involvement in Correctional Services and Programs

THOMAS A. JOHNSON

The purpose of this chapter is to stimulate research and encourage policy analysts to distinguish between what governments and the private sector can and cannot do with reference to our correctional programs. In short, we must begin to determine how well governmental policies that were designed to cope with correctional institutions and their programs actually work. Does the traditional approach of relying on government-sponsored correctional programs and institutions better meet our public interest goals than the slowly emerging privatization of these services? Levine *et al.* suggest that, if our concern is to determine the effectiveness of government policies in meeting public interest goals, we should pursue this analysis through a "policy impact approach."[1(p 63)]

A brief word of caution is needed before policy analysts begin to look at this problem; that is, we should stipulate that for many decades the governmental sector has imposed four specific policies, all different, and by and large incompatible, to guide their correctional philosophy. These policies that have been used to direct correctional institutions and

This chapter was originally read at the annual meeting of the American Academy of Forensic Sciences, Las Vegas, Nevada, February 10–16, 1985.

THOMAS A. JOHNSON • Criminal Justice Division, California State University, Sacramento, CA 95812.

their programs are: (1) rehabilitation, (2) deterrence, (3) retribution, and (4) incapacitation.

It is precisely this lack of similarity and compatibility that makes rational planning for the future in this field so difficult. In short, the political forces obstructing change are powerful and the reformers (not to mention the emerging field of private sector entrepreneurs) have no agreed upon program. On occasion, they may agree upon what is wrong, but they cannot agree upon what should be done to correct it.[1(pp 307–310)]

Regrettably, these diverse and incompatible policies, plus the absence of any real ability to focus on public interest goals with any degree of rational planning, are incredibly costly, not only in terms of public policy but also in terms of public funding:

> Nationwide, corrections is a multibillion dollar industry with most of the money going for institutional maintenance and salaries for prison employees. There are more than 200,000 employees working under federal, state and local jurisdictions, which process 2.5 million offenders annually. These operating costs would be extremely hard to eliminate or drastically change.[1(p 339)]

There are additional structural weaknesses that are attendant to assessing the policy implications of private sector involvement in our correctional field. These are specifically related to what Quade terms the unsatisfactory state of public policy-making. Quade notes that among the weaknesses is the difficulty the public decision maker confronts in the organizations and bureaucracies that he must work with (including his own and any that interact with it) in terms of the: (1) red tape, (2) poor communication, (3) low morale, (4) inadequate staffing, (5) inadequate records, and (6) the pressures from special interest groups with readymade solutions. Moreover, governmental organizations do not have the same reputation for attracting or making efficient use of individual skills and competence that is usually attributable to private industry.[2(p 20)]

The legislative process itself is not a model of great efficiency in terms of its contributions to a rational state of public policy-making. Another reason for failures within our traditional governmental correctional programs is the simple fact that despite the increasing complexity of problems now confronting them, the methods used by public authorities for their resolution have remained virtually unchanged since the beginning of government.[2(p 21)] In fact, Quade suggests that governmental programs rarely have an automatic regulator that indicates when an activity has ceased to be productive, or could be made more efficient, or should be replaced by another activity. In the private sector, businesses rely on profits and competition to furnish such needed incentives. The private sector has the discipline then to invoke the necessary decisions.

It is precisely these sets of facts that have encouraged the movement toward privatization of our correctional system. We have seen similar efforts in the fields of mental health, alcohol, and substance abuse, and within segments of our social welfare field. Policy analysts can engage in comparative research and perhaps extrapolate some of the strength and weaknesses in these fields and apply them to this emerging movement.

Because of their very nature as social problems, however, public policy problems within the correctional field tend to be more pluralistic and ill defined. Investigators in the fields of systems analysis and operations research (both precursors to the policy analysis field) addressed problems that related more to engineering and to other technology. They concerned themselves with public policy problems that were easier to formulate and to resolve using quantitative methods.[2(p 25)] Thus, the challenge to the private sector will be to avoid, if possible, some of the pitfalls that confront the public sector and that, we hypothesize, will not be avoidable due to the social problem nature of these issues. In other words, the private sector may be moving into this field with misplaced confidence in their engineering, their technology, and their decision-making process as related to their profit-making concept. It is safe to suggest that the motivating factor to the private sector is the multibillion dollar correctional industry and the possibility of tax advantages through lease-back financing arrangements. Obviously, the notion of profit through others' misfortunes will provide many philosophical challenges to the private sector, not the least of these will be the timely release of inmates despite the loss of daily fees once that inmate is released. Certainly today, with our incredible prison overcrowding and jail backlog, this should prove no immediate additional threat to the public. However, what about 5, 10, or 15 years from now?

Another aspect of the dimension of the social problem that the private sector will be confronting was best stated by Quade:

> It takes far more than the discovery of a solution on paper to eliminate any major public policy problem. There are additional tasks of communicating the proposed solution to all involved and convincing them that it is a valid solution. Also, problematic is the addressing of jurisdictional problems and boundaries, and the marshalling of the necessary resources. . . . In short, the problems of public policy are wicked problems in that they may have no definite formulation and no stopping rule to tell the problem solver when he has a solution. Moreover, a proposed solution is not true or false but good or bad. There may be neither an immediate nor even an ultimate test of a solution, as the set of potential solutions is not enumerable; every such problem is essentially unique and is a symptom of another problem.[2(p 25)]

Finally, and most importantly for the private sector, is the frequency with which public policy problems cut across established political and administrative boundaries, presenting jurisdictional issues to overcome, as for instance, when the indirect costs to the public from a project dwarf the direct costs and benefits. The difficulty with many of these problems is more in deciding what needs to be done rather than how to do it. The allocation of resources for efficiency may be secondary to the question of equity, that is, Who benefits? Who pays?[2(p 26)]

The private sector will also have an immense problem with the concept of vicarious liability litigation. Indeed, a rough estimate of Section 1983 liability reveals pending claims in excess of $20 billion, with judgments on the rise. In fact, over 40 states have major cases pending, and, in the past five years, we have experienced in excess of 1,700 court decisions in this important area. Of further concern to the private sector should be the ease with which these claims are litigated. In fact, most attorneys refer to this area as "boilerplate litigation."

Another area of legal vulnerability for the private sector is the First Amendment right of prisoners. We have no precedent established with reference to private operations as yet. Also, there is a question of bonding risk with reference to no-limit lawsuits. Although the corporate veil will protect investors, the corporation and its officers will still remain at risk and vulnerable.

Other areas of potential legal concern to the private sector, which should necessitate assessment of policy implications, reside in the many actions that fall under Section 1983. In all probability, these will be tort cases and insurance claims in the private sector. Therefore, the importance of insurance to private providers will be immense. Insurance companies are just beginning to recover from their industry's worst three years ever in the casualty area. Provided that full or partial coverage will be available for all areas, premiums promise to escalate substantially. Therefore, the concept of risk management and risk assessment will be paramount concerns confronting the private sector.

We have no empirical data that suggest that privatization within our correctional field is or could be as effective or more effective than our present public sector operations. This is not to say that we should not experiment with this concept. However, where we do experiment, let us provide the adequate research design to offer sound judgments as to its strengths and weaknesses.

REFERENCES

1. Levine JP, Muscheno MC, Palumbo DJ: *Criminal Justice: A Public Policy Approach.* New York, Harcourt Brace Jovanovich Inc, 1980.
2. Quade ES: Analysis for public decisions, in Nagel SS (ed): *Policy Studies: Review Annual.* Beverly Hills, Calif, Sage Publications, 1977.

15

Models of Mental Health Service Delivery to Correctional Institutions

GARY J. MAIER AND ROBERT D. MILLER

The provision of mental health service to convicted mentally disordered offenders is in crisis again.[1] This perennial problem has remained unsolved for a number of reasons. A principal reason underlying our lack of success (resolve?) is the basic conflict between the principles of the criminal justice system, punishment, retribution, deterrence, and rehabilitation,[2] and the basic premise underlying the therapist–patient relationship—trust.[3] The practice of punishment prevents the possibility of trust formation. In our opinion, this basic conflict in values underlies all the apparent levels of conflict. The perennial problem of the insanity defense, where law and psychiatry collide, and the deep difference between the roles of security and treatment staff in prisons are two obvious examples of this basic difference.

Furthermore, there are a number of reasons why this crisis is apparent at this time. First, our prisons are overcrowded. There was a 34% growth in population between 1978 and 1982, straining already scarce resources. Second, the movement to deinstitutionalize the chronic mentally ill in the 1960s and 1970s has not only created "the bag lady," but

GARY J. MAIER • Forensic Center, Mendota Mental Health Institute, Madison, WI 53704; Department of Psychiatry, University of Wisconsin-Madison, Madison, WI 53706. **ROBERT D. MILLER** • Forensic Center, Mendota Mental Health Institute, Madison, WI 53704; Department of Psychiatry and School of Law, University of Wisconsin-Madison, Madison, WI 53706.

also crowded jails, and then prisons, with patients who used to reside in hospitals. The criminalization of the mentally ill is well documented.[4,5] Third, the trend toward giving longer sentences has kept prison beds full. More important, however, in this swing to the right, is the growing trend to decrease the judge's authority at the time of sentence and to decrease the flexibility parole boards have in granting early release to selected inmates, especially those who have participated honorably in prison rehabilitation programs. Psychiatric/psychological treatment is losing credibility with the public and the parole board.

For these reasons and others, it is not surprising that recent surveys of psychopathology in prison populations continue to demonstrate that, at any given time, 20% to 25% of the inmate population experience significant, and in other circumstances, treatable symptoms of mental illness.[6–8] The fact that mental health services to the mentally disordered offender have been neglected for years; that most departments of corrections are understaffed compared to European staffing standards[9] in custodial and mental health professionals; that, in a recent survey of state correction facilities, 28 states had defined standards for mental health services for the convicted and that only 16% of these complied with their standards, it is understandable that the human suffering of the mentally ill has come to the attention of the courts. Although the *Wyatt v Stickney* case[10] in Alabama does not offer the promise that was first sought in the court's entrance into setting standards in a psychiatric hospital, Metzner[6] reported that 20 states are now under court order to provide mental health services. Overcrowding, environmental health conditions, the lack of medical and mental health care, and violence are the four major issues addressed by this litigation.

Given this pessimistic picture,[11] is there any reason to believe that the current effort to address this issue will have any success? Class action suits will bring some relief.[12] There is also a growing emphasis and body of knowledge in correctional mental health, as attested by the scope of the papers presented in Chicago at the Eighth National Conference on Correctional Health Care.[13] Of 40 major topic areas, 30 had a direct clinical focus. There were more than 100 separate papers presented in these topic areas. Interest and information are growing.

In the following discussion, we will review models of delivery of mental health services in prisons and discuss the advantages and disadvantages of each. We will not discuss mental health services to jails or to juveniles nor will we deal with important system issues or specific treatment approaches. We can say that there are no standards to judge the effectiveness of any of these models and that, in spite of all our efforts, recidivism rates remain unchanged.

The judgments that we make arise from personal experience and from a review of surveys of psychopathology found in prison settings.[6,8] The first model is explained in greater detail, as the basic issues of intention, administration, and separating the mentally disordered offender from other inmates are considered common to all models. Other models are then discussed in regard to their unique advantages. All other factors are held constant.

MODELS FOR THE DISPOSITION OF CONVICTED MENTALLY DISORDERED OFFENDERS

Wardlaw,[14] in an excellent article, identifies and discusses the advantages and disadvantages of five models of mental health service to convicted mentally disordered offenders. We have followed his lead in describing these models. A number of solutions have been attempted as a means of coping with the dispositional problems posed by mentally disordered prisoners. Although they are not entirely mutually exclusive, five major approaches may be broadly distinguished. These are: (1) a centralized psychiatric prison, (2) small psychiatric units attached to major prisons, (3) regional forensic psychiatric centers, (4) regional security units at psychiatric hospitals, and (5) a centralized psychiatric security hospital.

Regardless of the model, the central problem lies in the fact that neither the prison system nor the health system wants jurisdiction over the mentally disordered offender. Mentally disordered prisoners fall in a "no-man's land" and are not properly cared for by either prison or psychiatric hospitals. This situation arises principally from disagreements over what role each should play. On the whole, prisons view mentally disordered prisoners as inappropriately placed in their institutions, arguing that prisons are neither equipped nor staffed to deal with their problems. On the other hand, the mental health system generally is reluctant to deal with prisoners, particularly those who are labelled "dangerous."[7] Often psychiatric staff believe prisoners/patients to be merely trying to avoid the rigors of prison life and thus to be wasteful of resources and frequently to be disruptive to the ward routine. More seriously, they fear that the need to provide security for prisoners is diametrically opposed to the general movement toward open wards in psychiatric hospitals. Further, it is argued that a large proportion of mentally disordered offenders are, for practical purposes, untreatable, and there is thus no justification for their occupying scarce hospital beds. It is easy, therefore, to see the pressures and interests that exist in both systems to divest themselves of this problematic group.

Psychiatric Prison

A psychiatric prison seems an ideal solution to many. Hartz-Karp,[15] in her analysis of dispositional modes, argues that the three major reasons most frequently cited for constructing psychiatric prisons are administrative efficiency, humanitarian concern, and protection of the offender and the community. It is argued that it is important to separate the mentally disordered from the criminal so that the former are "treated" and the latter are "punished." In particular, it is felt that it is inappropriate to subject the mentally disordered to a regime officially labelled as punishment. It is then argued that only in a special purpose institution will those who are mentally disordered be afforded proper treatment and not be subjected to punishment. The psychiatric prison holds the hope of dealing appropriately with mentally disordered individuals by removing them from a punishment environment and placing them in a treatment one, thus satisfying humanitarian concerns. It provides security that alleviates community fears, and it removes what is said to be a particularly difficult and often violent group from normal systems, thereby removing considerable administrative difficulties for those systems.

Further, administrative difficulties are said to be caused in prisons by the presence of the mentally disordered, because facilities do not exist to segregate those who are violent, exhibit bizarre or unpredictable behavior, or are in other ways difficult (for example, refuse to work or obey orders). Proponents of a psychiatric prison accept that many of these problems have a psychological/psychiatric basis and that a treatment facility would be the most appropriate place to deal with them.

Separating the violent from the mentally disordered, who may also be violent, is another difficult issue. Often the tendency is to lump both groups together because they both cause management and administrative problems. When undifferentiated, the group with characterological pathology becomes a major problem to the treatment milieus whether in psychiatric prisons or mental hospitals. Accurate diagnosis in the prison is important.

The final argument advanced in favor of a psychiatric prison is that it would be an ideal protective device. Mentally disordered prisoners would be better protected from the depredations of other prisoners and the stresses of prison life (to which it is thought it is "unfair" to subject someone suffering under a mental disability) if housed in the "protective environment" of a treatment facility.[16] Further, such persons will also be protected in the sense that the treatment offered theoretically holds out real hope of a "cure," which will eliminate mental disorder or dangerousness or both. The community also benefits. It is protected because the dangerously mentally disordered offender is housed in secure conditions and is receiving treatment that will eliminate his or her dangerousness. Of course, the ultimate benefit derived from a psychiatric prison is claimed to be when the treatment staff themselves control release decisions and can release mentally disordered prisoners only when the staff considers them "cured."

Although all the above arguments stem from real concerns, the solution offered, a psychiatric prison, is based on, at best, unproven assumptions. The most important assumptions underlying psychiatric intervention are that persons whom the administration finds "difficult" (be they violent, noncommunicative, or not amenable to discipline) have psychiatric disorders and that psychiatrists are able to provide accurate diagnosis of and treatment for these disorders. The first assumption is widely challenged and the second and third are largely disproven by an increasing number of empirical studies that show that psychiatrists are extremely poor at arriving at reliable diagnoses in court,[17] and, even should they be able to do so, there is no specific treatment that can offer any realistic chance of success for the character disordered who would be so diagnosed.[18]

Much of the attraction to the idea of a psychiatric prison lies in the belief that psychiatry and psychology are powerful and accurate tools. The evidence suggests otherwise, however, and to be responsible we must carefully assess the claimed expertise and benefits. (Although it should be noted that the attraction of psychiatric prisons may simply be asylum, that is, getting the most disruptive inmates out of the general population, it may be considered by some prison administrators to be a sufficient rationale in and of itself, regardless of their beliefs about the power of psychiatry and psychology.) Further, as Ericson[19] argues, although psychiatry (and, by association, psychology) is not necessarily powerful as a treatment tool, it certainly may be powerful as a control. The great danger of assigning all the difficult prisoners to one institution and making treatment personnel primarily responsible for them is that the control function may become paramount. And as Ericson also notes, "Once set in motion, programs of this nature have a tendency to act to a maximum capacity, seeking and finding a perpetual supply of subjects to tinker with."[19(p 25)]

Apart from the question of whether or not we have the treatment tools to change significantly the behavior of seriously disturbed offenders, the concept of a centralized psychiatric facility within the prison system suffers from a number of other potential disadvantages. First, it is obvious that a psychiatric prison will not be capable of dealing with all the mentally disordered individuals within the prison system. But the mere existence of such a facility could well remove the pressure to provide adequate mental health facilities for all prisoners, because of the diversion of scarce and costly resources into the treatment of the most severely disturbed cases, and because the physical reality of the institution is visible "proof" that something is being done for the mentally disordered, thus diverting attention from the remaining problems. A second problem is that of the difficulty of involving the families or friends of the inmates in treatment as a result of the distance of a centralized facility from the areas in which many of the offenders and their families live. A decentralized system, on the other hand, at least allows the possibility of placing the offender in a facility within easy visiting distance of family and friends, where it is thought that this may be of assistance in recovery from mental disorder. Finally, experience with a number of psychiatric prisons has shown that, often, there is an inherent inflexibility in the regimes in such institutions that does not seem to be present to such a degree in smaller units. The emphasis on security, in particular, often seems to pervade the thought that goes into devising programs for all offenders in the institution rather than only for those who truly require it. There often seems more willingness to experiment with innovative programs in smaller units, with large psychiatric prisons being, frequently, more rigid in their attitudes to such innovations.

Small Psychiatric Units Attached to, or Part of, Major Prisons

An alternative to a psychiatric prison, which still accepts that the prison system must bear the major responsibility for convicted mentally disordered offenders, is to disperse psychiatric units through the major prisons. This concept involves having a psychiatric unit either attached to, or within, a number of prisons. Such a model is seen as countering the disadvantages of a psychiatric prison (such as an excessive concern for security, the holding together of large numbers of disordered and sometimes dangerous offenders, and the administrative and treatment conservativeness that seems to accompany larger institutions) as well as offering its own advantages. The first advantage is that such a system is able to cope with a greater number of individuals within the prison system because it is not geared primarily to the most severely disordered group. A unit, as well as being a secure facility for the treatment or containment of the severely disordered, should also serve the general population of its parent prison, providing day-care or outpatient-type services. Having a number of such units also allows for the development of specialist services so that, for example, different units may aim to provide special programs for different problem groups. In the United

States, New York State has developed a comprehensive system in this mold,[20] and North Carolina has also adopted this model, as the following mission statement indicates:

> The North Carolina Division of Prisons has the responsibility to deliver comprehensive mental health services which will provide for the care and treatment of mentally disordered inmates. Treatment programs will contain multi-disciplinary responses designed to prevent, contain, reduce, or eliminate those conditions which contribute to the patient's mental impairment. These services will include but are not necessarily limited to: (1) patient identification and diagnosis, (2) services for the acutely ill inpatient, (3) outpatient services, (4) special programs for selected diagnostic categories (e.g. passive inadequate, mentally retarded, etc.) and (5) preventative services. There will also be a program evaluation and a staff development component as a part of the mental health program.[22(p 26)]

A formal Memorandum of Understanding exists between the North Carolina Department of Human Resources (which is responsible for the state's mental health services) and the Department of Correction, which specifies that:

> The Department of Human Resources will be responsible for service delivery for the mentally ill, the mentally retarded, of the substance abuser prior to the time they are actually committed to a state prison. Once they enter the gate of a state correctional facility, the responsibility for their treatment shifts to the Department of Corrections. When they leave prison, either through parole or by "maxing out," the responsibility reverts to the Department of Human Resources. The Memorandum of Understanding further specifies that the two agencies cooperate in every way possible to provide an orderly flow of the patient into and out of the prison system to facilitate continuity of care.[21(p 24)]

The major advantage of this sort of formal agreement is that each department knows exactly where it stands and what its responsibilities are. The existence of such an agreement, together with the provision of adequate resources to enable the Department of Correction to fulfill its mandate, eliminates the disagreement between departments, which is characteristic of many jurisdictions. More important, it eliminates the ping-pong game that is played as many mentally disordered offenders are shunted back and forth between hospital and prison (what one cynic has called "bus therapy").

The major disadvantages appear to be those of cost. It could be argued that many services that could be provided by the civil mental health system are unnecessarily duplicated with resultant unnecessary cost to the community. However, it could equally be argued that such duplication as does exist is a small price to pay for the advantages that such a system offers.

Regional Forensic Psychiatric Centers

In Canada, one solution to the disposition problem has been the establishment of regional forensic psychiatric centers that have a mandate to cater exclusively to mentally disordered offenders.[22] In Canada, these centers are under the control of the federal prison authorities, but other models envisage control being vested in the mental health authorities on a joint service. There are a number of possible ways of organizing such centers. To set them apart from the psychiatric prison model, some examples would seek to offer a comprehensive forensic service to both convicted and unconvicted mentally disordered offenders. Thus, such a unit would provide long-term accommodation, short-term care for those on temporary transfer from a hospital or a prison, outpatient services for probationers/parolees and possible prisoners, and assessment and diagnostic services for the courts (including facilities to hold remandees for psychiatric observation and report).

The advantages seen in this model center on the presumed expertise that would be gained by having a large, comprehensive service–delivery agency capable of dealing with the problems of both prisons and mental hospitals. The disadvantages come from having to accommodate such a mixture of problem types and security levels. It is argued that, in the final analysis, the security needs of the dangerous, mentally disordered offenders could easily come to dominate, thus reducing many of the benefits that might otherwise flow from such a facility.

Regional Secure Units in Psychiatric Hospitals

The British solution to the problem of hospitals' being unwilling to accept certain groups of mentally disordered offenders, either from the courts or from prison, was to build a number of regional medium secure units within the confines of psychiatric hospitals. These units are designed to take only those offenders who, the medical staff considers, have a good chance of responding to treatment. They accept patients from the hospitals as well as from prisons, and thus such units are not exclusively for offenders but rather for those who need more control than is considered appropriate in a normal psychiatric setting. The criteria for admission to one such unit (The Wessex Interim Secure Unit) are as follows:

(a) An agreement between the relevant doctors and staff that the patient is both mentally disordered and should be treated in hospital.

(b) The patient's behavior is too difficult or dangerous for him (or her) to be managed in an ordinary psychiatric ward, but is not so difficult or dangerous that he/she requires the high security of a Special Hospital.

(c) The patient is either legally detained (e.g. by court order using the Mental Health Act) or is willing to stay as an "informal" patient, or as a condition of probation.[23(p 690)]

It is obvious that although the concept of such units, firmly in the civil mental health system, could have merit, it is only a very limited solution to the problem of where to locate the mentally disordered offender. Because of the limits on security and the criterion of treatability, such units exclude a large number of potential inmates (that is, the dangerous and the "untreatable").

A Centralized Psychiatric Security Hospital

The model of having a large, secure institution within the mental health system to cater for the dangerous mentally ill has been adopted all over the world, but has also been the subject of intense criticism over the last few years. Such institutions (e.g., the British Special Hospitals such as Broadmoor or maximum security hospitals such as Atascadero in California) usually cater for both civil and criminal patients. On the whole, they have been justly criticized for an overconcern with security, fostering institutionalization, and being conservative and inward looking.[24] They are frequently overcrowded and lack any real attempt at treatment. Security and control usually take precedence overall. Apart from the negative effects of the institutions themselves, the psychiatric security system, with its emphasis on security, is an inappropriate place to treat many sorts of mentally disordered offenders. But, if ordinary psychiatric hospitals are unwilling to take prison patients, many end up, inappropriately, in security hospitals—often with negative impacts on their chances of recovery or rehabilitation.[25] Thus, the presence of such a facility either means that it contains inappropriate patients or that these individuals may remain untreated in the prison system. Some complementary institution is still necessary.

DISCUSSION

We have been dealing with the relative strengths and weaknesses of each of these models. Recently, in Wisconsin, the Division of Corrections (DOC) and the Division of Care and Treatment Facilities (DCIF) collaborated to develop a hybrid institution called the Wisconsin Resource Center (WRC). Mentally disordered offenders from the DOC can be transferred to the specialized programming under DOC transfer statutes. The facility, however, is administered by the DCTF so that although it is not a mental hospital by statute, it has a progressive staffing pattern and mental health orientation. Further, even though contracting the services of mental health professionals to jails, correctional facilities, and prisons is more and more in vogue, such professionals tend not to develop allegiance to the secure facility or, with time, to feel that their services, while admittedly needed, are of any value. The WRC has been able to recruit a cadre of well-trained PhDs, MSWs, ATs and RNs who, because they have positional authority and mental health philosophy, feel that their needed services have impact. In addition, the collegial relationships that have formed over the last two to three years with forensic clinicians have made a difference to the morale of mental health professionals working in the rest of the DOC service facilities. They have also maintained an excellent relationship with the Mendota Forensic Center, the maximum security mental health facility to which they refer the mentally disordered offenders who meet commitment standards and refuse to cooperate with treatment. The WRC appears to be acting as the bridge institution from the small mental health units in each prison to the state's only maximum security hospital at Mendota Mental Health Institute. There is a belief that the WRC prevents deterioration in a number of inmates simply because the environment is more humane and less deprived than the security prisons. This hybrid facility, while youthful, bears watching as other states try to update mental health services to the mentally disordered offenders.

Finally, considering the models present, it is our opinion that small psychiatric units attached to major prisons with dual management have the most to offer. Prison and mental health expertise is required at the administrative level to ensure that security and treatment needs are met. Small units are less entrenched in excessive security, and offer a greater level of trust, better staff communication, and the possibility of specialization. Where morale is good, they even offer the potential of a rewarding career to the mental health professionals who would choose to work in this subspecialty.

REFERENCES

1. In Brief. Jails: *Intergovernmental Dimensions of a Local Problem.* Washington, DC Advisory Commission of Intergovernmental Relations, 1980.
2. Cavender G: Justice, sanctioning, and the justice model. *Criminology* 1984; 22:203–213.
3. Maier GJ: Therapy in prisons, in Madden DJ, Lion JR (eds): *Rage, Hate Assault and Other Forms of Violence.* New York, Spectrum Publications Inc, 1976.
4. Steadman HF, Cocozza JJ, Melich ME: Explaining the increased arrest rate among

mental patients: The changing clientele of state hospitals. *Am J Psychiatry* 1978; 135:816–820.

5. Sosowsky L: Explaining the increased arrest rate among mental patients: A cautionary note. *Am J Psychiatry* 1980; 137:1602–1605.
6. Metzner JL: Evaluation of a prison mental health system in litigation. Read before the Fifteenth Annual Meeting of the American Academy of Psychiatry and the Law, Paradise Island, Nassau, Bahamas, Oct. 27, 1984.
7. Gunn J, Robertson G, Dell S, Way C: *Psychiatric Aspects of Imprisonment.* New York, Academic Press, 1978.
8. McKay HB, Jayewardene CHS, Reedie PB: *The Effects of Long-Term Incarceration and a Proposed Strategy for Future Research.* Minister of Supply and Services, Ottawa, Canada, 1979.
9. Ward D: Inmate rights and prison reform in Sweden and Denmark. *Crim Law Criminology Police Sci* 1972; 63:240–255.
10. Stickney SB: Problems in implementing the right to treatment in Alabama. The *Wyatt vs Stickney* Case. *Hosp Community Psychiatry* 1974; 25:453–460.
11. Maier GJ: Relationship security: The dynamics of keepers and kept. *J Forensic Sci* 1986; 31:603–608.
12. Isele W: *Constitutional Issues of the Prisoners' Right to Health Care.* Chicago, American Medical Association, 1980.
13. *Program.* Eighth National Conference on Correctional Health Care, Chicago, 1984.
14. Wardlaw G: Models for the custody of mentally disordered offenders. *Int J Law Psychiatry* 1983; 6:159–176.
15. Hartz-Karp J: *The Mentally Ill within the Criminal Justice System.* Research and Information Series No. 19, Western Australian Department of Corrections, 1979.
16. Kittri N: *The Right to be Different: Deviance and Enforced Therapy.* New York, Penguin Books, 1971.
17. Bartholomew AA, Milte KL: The reliability and validity of psychiatric diagnoses in courts of law. *Australian Law J* 1976; 50:450–458.
18. West DJ (ed): *Psychopathic Offenders.* Papers presented to the Cropwood Round-Table Conference. (Cambridge, England, University of Cambridge, Institute of Criminology, 1968.
19. Ericson RV: Psychiatrists in prison: On admitting professional tinkers into a tinker's paradise. *Chitty's Law J* 1974; 22:29–33.
20. Wright JB: Mental health services in correctional settings, in *A Report to Governor Hugh L. Carey on the Insanity Defense in New York.* State of New York Department of Mental Hygiene. Feb. 17, 1978, pp 119–130.
21. Kiel RA: Mental health for the convicted offender: A model that works. *Corrections Today* 1981; 43:20–27.
22. Arboleda-Florez J: Forensic psychiatry services in Canada. Strengths and weaknesses. *Int J Law Psychiatry* 1981; 4:391–399.
23. Faulk M: Mentally disordered offenders in an interim regional secure unit. *Crim Law Rev* 1979; 17:686–695.
24. Gostin LO: *A Human Condition. The Law Relating to Mentally Abnormal Offenders: Observations, Analysis and Proposals for Reform* London, MIND (National Association for Mental Health), 1977.
25. Bluglass R: Advances in forensic psychiatry in England and Wales. *Int J Law Psychiatry* 1981; 4:199–212.

16

Reform by Decree

Litigation and the Provision of Mental Health Services in Jails

SUSAN O. REED

INTRODUCTION

Jails are different from prisons. This statement should be so obvious as to constitute a truism, but it is not. The majority of citizens use *jail* and *prison* as interchangeable terms, not understanding the difference in function of the two types of institutions and the consequent constraints imposed by those functions. Jails hold defendants prior to trial and offenders serving very short sentences. Prisons hold offenders serving longer sentences. Both institutions must house and care for some mentally ill inmates, but the numbers of these inmates, the criticality of their needs, and the resources available are different for each.

Until recently, the jail operation was the least visible part of a sheriff's duties. Few people knew or cared much about jails. That political invisibility has become less of a shield for jail administrators as attention has become focused in recent years on conditions of confinement in jails. For "attention," one may read "litigation," which has been the primary mechanism for organizational reform in state prisons and mental hospi-

The material in this chapter has appeared in Susan O. Reed: *Reform by Decree: The Provision of Mental Health Services in Jails and the Threat of Litigation,* dissertation. New York University Graduate School of Public Administration, New York, New York, 1987.

SUSAN O. REED • Department of Public Affairs, Criminal Justice Program, University of Wisconsin-Oshkosh, Oshkosh, WI 54901.

tals. Adequate medical and mental health services, basic hygiene issues, and acceptable methods of restraint and discipline have become more clearly defined through the process of litigation. Mental health services in jails, however, have not been sifted and illuminated so thoroughly by the litigation process.

One obvious reason is that until recently standards for mental health services to jail inmates have not been generated in sufficient detail to be of use to litigants. Standards first formulated by the American Bar Association, the American Medical Association, the American Correctional Association, and the American Public Health Association were framed in relatively general terms (i.e., the desirability of providing service).* This is in striking contrast to the specificity of standards relating to medical services, physical hygiene, access to legal counsel, and other conditions.

A second reason may be that our knowledge of what it is that jails do in response to the mentally ill offender is fairly primitive. This is certainly true with regard to small jails (62 inmates or less), which constitute over 75% of the total.[2(p27)] The gap in knowledge is exacerbated by the fact that we are not always clear on the difference between jails and lock-ups and thus cannot decide whether the pool of jails is 3,400 plus or 5,000 plus.† In other words, what should we be surveying?

> [Jails are] unbelievably bad for those who enter their gates either with incipient physical or mental health problems, or even for those who have no more than average resistance to physical or mental health problems, or even for those who have no more than average resistance to physical or mental stress.[3(p1)]

Jimmy Hoffa is not the most articulate critic of jails to be found. Yet his testimony, redundant as it is, states what others, more fluent and more impeccably credentialed than he, have said: jails make people worse. It has been noted often that jails are not pleasant places in which to work. Most are aging structures—noisy, dank, and lacking in areas where private interviews can be conducted. In short, the physical structure of jails is counterproductive to the delivery of mental health services.

Further, psychiatrists who work in correctional settings do not earn praise from their peers. The image of the "prison doctor" has been that

*As an example, admission screening to identify the mentally ill offender by "medical staff" with follow-up supervision by "trained personnel" is recommended. Further, "maximum cooperation" between "custody personnel and health care personnel" is deemed "essential."[1]

†A *lock-up* is usually a holding facility operated by police or other law enforcement agencies where arrestees are held while booking and other prearraignment processes are being completed. A *jail* is usually where postarraignment inmates are detained and is operated by the sheriff's office or the municipal correctional agency.

of the flawed or incompetent hack who has "sold out" to the brutal oppressiveness of the correctional administration. Rundle, a psychiatrist who serves as consultant to reform-minded outsiders to corrections systems decried in 1974, "psychiatrists, who work within the prison system, who have prostituted themselves personally and professionally."[4(p17)] Rundle may be correct about some of the stresses and some of the psychiatrists found in jails and prison, but not to the extreme he takes. It is true, however, dedicated mental health professionals are cut off from their peers because of the stereotype of their patients, their co-workers, and their own competence. They are paid significantly less than colleagues who work in noncorrectional settings. Good practitioners are hard to recruit, hard to retain, and hard to protect from burnout, the "dead above the neck" syndrome.*

The pyramidal authority structure in jails and prisons often has forced medical and mental health professionals to be accountable to custody staff. Goldsmith comments that this practice coupled with the lack of administrative leadership characteristic to part-time–staffed medical departments further weakens the position of medical (and mental health) staff. To maintain equilibrium, "some medical staff do become adjuncts of custodial personnel by using their talents to dispense tranquilizers in an effort to keep the prison quiet and to calm inmates."[5(p24)]

Another deterrent to good medical and mental health service delivery originates in characteristics of the patient population. Inmates often come to prison clinics to escape boredom, obtain drugs, and evade work assignments.[5(p22)] Doctors, by their treatment decisions, find themselves arbitrating disputes between inmates and custody staff regarding the degree of illness of inmates. If perceived as soft on inmates, doctors may find themselves working with the least competent and most uncooperative custody staff available. Other decisions can lead to enduring verbal abuse and intimidation from inmates.[5(p23)]

Much of the literature dealing with problems for the jail clinician follows the line developed above: psychiatrists may be asked by correctional administrators to medicate or otherwise treat inmates inappropriately in order to control unacceptable behavior. The correctional version of this conflict flows from the fact that many of the mentally ill in jails got there because they are assaultive and become more assaultive in jail. The legal rights of incarcerated mental patients have been a developing problem not only for mental hospitals in dealing with acting-out

*The researcher draws on her own experience in developing the medical/mental health programs at a state prison, at a juvenile institution, and in administering a forensic psychiatric service. The problem of recruitment in non-urban settings is so severe that one may begin to assume that candidates for employment are flawed, rather than the contrary.

patients but also increasingly for jails and prisons. According to Michaels, "there is general agreement that voluntary patients have an absolute right to refuse treatment."[6(p254)] But what about jail inmates? Does arrest and incarceration impact upon this right? The rights of inmates also include protection from harm from other inmates who may be dangerous because they are mentally ill but still legally competent to refuse medication.

It is this kind of patient/inmate that is the catalyst for much of the friction between correctional and mental health professionals. The high percentage of people in jails who present behavior management problems sometimes makes the right to refuse medication inexplicable to jail staff. The anger generated by the psychiatrist who refuses to medicate (because an inmate is competent to refuse), leaving the inmate to be controlled by jail staff, is long-lived and bitter.

Prior to 1978, it was difficult for jail inmates to sue their keepers for holding them in constitutionally inadequate conditions. Then a trio of Supreme Court decisions struck down the immunity from civil litigation that had protected county and municipal governments.[7(p160)] By 1980, inmates could litigate on violations of constitutional law as well as local law and regulations, be awarded punitive damages, and recover attorney fees in successful suits. This situation placed local detention administrators, usually sheriffs, in a perilous position. As the elected head of the county law enforcement agency, the sheriff had previously considered that the administration of the jail was a small portion of his responsibility. Certainly, it was the least understood and, to most constituents, the least visible component of the sheriff's duties. Sheriffs did not usually win elections by promises to improve (expensively) conditions for jail inmates. And few local voters understood the impact of court decisions that eliminated the sheriff's immunity from suit on wrongful conduct that could be brought by inmates.

In most states, the anticipated spate of inmate litigation did not materialize, nor did lawsuits from other categories of local service consumers. However, the trickle of litigation did produce great increases in premiums for liability insurance. Where it could be shown that a jail administrator was directly or indirectly responsible for a civil rights violation, punitive damages could be levied, and neither the city or county or the insurance provider would pay the damages.[8(pp71–72)] Small cities and local units of government seemed to face more litigation than larger units of government. Although figures are not available detailing the problem for county governments, a survey of small cities and townships found increases in insurance premiums ranging from 23% to 456%.[9(p2)]

As they faced new levels and kinds of liability risks sheriffs were hampered by their professional identification as law enforcement officials, not correctional administrators. They were likely to be members of police organizations and were not involved in the ongoing dialogue about judicial review that characterized the activities of professional correctional associations throughout the 1970s and 1980s.[10(p129)] In short, they were caught short and caught between the unwillingness of voters to pay for reforms and the demands of appellate courts to institute reforms.

The problems faced by jail administrators—aging physical plants, overcrowding, lack of minimal hygiene, and no programmatic resources—have been delineated often in other works. It suffices to state that jail administrators began to fear that they were ripe for successful suits by inmates, that they might be personally liable to pay damages, and that their constituents would not be willing to pay for jail reforms. The vigorous judicial oversight of jail operations from approximately 1970 to the present proved that they were right.[11]

It has been said that one function of jails may be as the temporary storage site for the chronically mentally ill citizen of the obtrusive, untidy, or dangerous variety. With the tightening of mental health commitment laws, many of these patients constitute a problem to themselves and others that (to citizenry demanding immediate solutions) can only be solved by the use of the authority of the criminal justice system. The segment of the mentally ill population thus selected to be admitted to jails seems to be most at risk for suicidal and self-injurious behavior, a problem which most jails had not been equipped to identify or treat. These tendencies may be exacerbated by the isolation, the shame of incarceration, the dank physical plants, and the abusive attitudes of jail employees who are neither selected for nor trained to have an ability to sensitively interact with emotionally fragile inmates.

These problems are compounded by conflicts within the mental health professions regarding the prediction and appropriate clinical response to the violent patient. The resultant confusion enhances the suspicion with which correctional workers regard mental health "interlopers." Mental health professionals find few incentives to attract them to correctional mental health beyond the rare (in any field of endeavor) dedication to serve the neediest. They are paid less, looked down on by colleagues, stereotyped as incompetent or worse, and work in relationships with correctional staff that are conflictual and detrimental to sound clinical practice.

Finally, the clients themselves discourage good mental health practice. Extremely discouraging people to work with, they are largely from the most disadvantaged socially and economically of the chronically mentally ill population. Other inmates demanding mental health service represent some of the most skilled and repellent malingerers to be encountered. Burnout for the dedicated mental health worker is common, quick, and widely reported. The prison doctor stereotype has been earned not only by the incompetent who *enters* the field of correctional mental health, but by the incompetent who *remains* in the field.

With this background in mind, one goal of this project was to examine the patterns of mental health service delivery in jails: what is it that jail administrators call "mental health service"? A second set of goals was to examine the relationships between incidents of suicide, self-injury, successful inmate litigation, and alterations in patterns of mental health service provision. One might hypothesize that suicides and self-injury generate litigation which generates reformation of mental health services in jails. This has been true of the processes that led to institutional reformation of state prisons and mental hospitals. Is there a similar path to the courts for jails with some characteristic organizational structure of services?

DESCRIPTION OF THE PROJECT

All jail administrators in Wisconsin, New Jersey, and New York were asked to complete a survey.* The survey instrument elicited data describing the jail (capacity, staffing patterns, budget, average daily population); the mental health services (schedules, type of professional employed, aegis of provider); and problems (incidents of suicide or self-injury, litigation).

Jail administrators whose responses indicated incidents of self-injury, suicide, and litigation by inmates were asked to participate in a structured interview. The interview focused on the jail administrator's decision criteria with regard to mental health services. Where major changes in the mental health package had been made in the recent past or were contemplated or desired for the near future, sheriffs and jail administrators were asked to detail the unacceptable service package (past or current) and the desired package (current or future). Data defining factors that made specific amendments to service attractive (type of service, type of provider, and costs) were sought.

New York State Local Detention

The summer of 1986 was an unfortunate period in which to poll New York detention administrators about mental health services in their

*The survey used for New York jail administrators did not contain all the items contained in the instrument used in New Jersey and Wisconsin.

jails. The insurance industry in the state had responded to the rise in litigation against public agencies by greatly increasing premiums. As a result, many local officials (sheriffs) were either not personally covered against judgments resulting from inmate litigation or feared that county officials would not insure them should they be named in future litigation. Consequently, the New York State Sheriffs' Association had just adopted a policy of not participating in any research that would focus on programs and services for jail inmates.

Recent research would seem to indicate that the New York Sheriffs were assessing their situation accurately. A survey of the lawsuits brought under Section 1983 of the Civil Rights Act of 1871 between 1977 and 1983 showed New York, Illinois, and Pennsylvania as having higher numbers of suits brought against them than other states. The average number of suits for all states but these three was 22. In contrast, New York had 248; Pennsylvania had 200; Illinois had 146.[7(p163)]

As a consequence, the polling process in New Jersey and Wisconsin was more successful because sheriffs and jail administrators were urged to participate in the survey by the leaders of their professional organizations. In New York, the survey was done by calling individual sheriffs and jail administrators and requesting that they both participate in the survey and agree to be interviewed. Some of those who agreed to be interviewed were helpful in obtaining the cooperation of a few of their peers. A general mailing of a vastly shortened survey instrument was then used in an effort to achieve a wider response. Even so, the resulting response was only 20 (34%).

Major gaps in information could be filled with the assistance of the New York State Office of Mental Health (OM), Bureau of Forensic Services, and the New York Commission on Correction (COC). The latter is the agency that develops standards on conditions of confinement in state and local correctional institutions and has the statutory authority with which to secure compliance. The Commission reviews all inmate deaths and requires a report on all inmate injuries and self-injuries. COC was the source of data on incidents of self-injury, suicide, jail capacity, and average daily population (ADP). The OMH was the source of information on some referrals of jail inmates to psychiatric hospitals.

At the time of the survey, many of the New York sheriffs interviewed were expressing their sense of isolation and beleaguerment. They perceived themselves at risk because of the insurance crisis and the indifference to or ignorance of the liability problem on the part of their local elected officials. Many expressed the opinion that the responsibility for remedying inadequate mental health programming for inmates properly rested with local mental health agencies. Leaders of these agencies were generally seen as unresponsive to the needs of jail inmates.* Often, when mental health services were not offered by county mental health providers, services were offered by contracts with external providers rather than by salaried jail employees.

Without exception, New York sheriffs and jail administrators indicated that self-injury and suicide were major worries for them, because of the liability risks these presented and because of humanitarian concerns. The COC and the OMH were beginning a joint program to offer training for suicide/self-injury prevention and were in the process of developing full mental health services by region, but most sheriffs interviewed were not aware that relief was on the horizon.

New Jersey Local Detention

Sheriffs in New Jersey were no strangers to the threat of inmate litigation. The wave of court orders and consent degrees defining conditions of confinement had hit many New Jersey county jails several years earlier. Consequently, the concern about liability was tempered by considerable sophistication and the presence of adequate (by standards recognized by most of the relevant judiciary) mental health programs in several jails. Several of the counties bounded by the Hudson River were in the process of or had finished program augmentation to satisfy court decrees. The New Jersey County Jail Wardens' Association has furnished leadership in this area.

New Jersey is more urban than New York and Wisconsin with all the attendant criminal justice demographics. The majority of New Jersey jails are large, with capacities of 100 or more. The larger jails offer mental health services by a variety of arrangements ranging from using jail employees to contracting with private sector, for-profit providers. Jail administrators in New Jersey do not *wait* for county mental health agencies to offer services to inmates. Given the history of litigation in the state, they know they cannot afford to be without at least minimal coverage.

New Jersey sheriffs and jail administrators interviewed did not speak much of a state mental health role in the definition and provision of adequate mental health services. Unlike New York sheriffs who speak resentfully of the monitoring role of the Commission on Correction, New Jersey local detention officials seem to feel that the shape of mental health services is theirs to define. References to state mental health

*The time frame and scope of the project did not allow for the interviewing of local mental health officials. Thus, information is not available to rebut or confirm this impression.

providers arose when they were discussing the need for psychiatric hospitalization on an intermediate or long-term basis.

According to those interviewed, the inspection and monitoring of conditions of confinement in local institutions are performed by the state correctional agency, which has the power to close down a jail for noncompliance. However, the state's enforcement powers did not seem to loom large. Most New Jersey county jails are boarding New Jersey State inmates because of overcrowding in the state system. As a consequence, drastic action on the part of the state compliance-monitoring unit is perceived as unlikely by respondents in the interviews.

Wisconsin Local Detention

Both mental health services and correctional services are provided by the same mega-agency, the Department of Health and Social Services. Technically, all mental health services to jail inmates are overseen by the Division of Community Services of the Office of Mental Health. Regulations exist that define the mandate of county mental health agencies to provide service to jail inmates. However, unlike New Jersey and New York, Wisconsin does not have standards that concisely define the scope and level of effort of these services. Hence, there is substantial variability in services from county to county:

> If an individual in jail *is willing to accept treatment on a voluntary basis,* it then is the responsibility of the county community services board . . . to provide that treatment. Some counties do have a system to provide . . . mental health services to jail inmates; others do not. (Italics added)[12(p51)]

Jail administrators, because the county mental health agency is the provider (by state regulation), do not generally use other providers. Because there are no guidelines for mandated service, the mental health providers respond on an "as-needed" basis. Costs for these services are not available to the jail administrators and frequently not to the mental health administrators. Services to jail inmates in most counties were not broken out in the agency budget as such. Thus data describing costs, hours of service by mental health practitioners, and types of service were unavailable. This is not to say that the services were not offered, but rather that the level of effort could not be documented.

Wisconsin sheriffs and jail administrators are as sensitive to liability issues as their peers in New Jersey and New York. But, given the lack of litigation on conditions of confinement in Wisconsin, they are not as fearful. This happy state is probably due in part to the leadership of the Division of Community Services, Forensic Services, and the Badger Sheriffs' Association. The latter group constitutes a powerful and sophisticated lobby and source of education for its members and works with the Forensic Services unit on mental health problems. It is unlikely that Wisconsin Sheriffs are caught napping as new liability issues develop.

PRESENTATION OF FINDINGS

Several factors are cited frequently by correctional professionals as causally linked to suicides and self-injury by jail inmates. These include: (1) the size of the institution (with larger institutions perceived as generating more stress on inmates); (2) the ratio of mental health practitioner hours to inmate; (3) the ratio of jail deputies and correction officers (COs) to inmates; (4) the occupancy rate or degree of overcrowding; (5) the ease of commitment to a psychiatric hospital or "turnaround rate" on hospital referrals by jail administrators; (6) The "turnover rate" of inmates as an indicator of stress on personnel making admissions' decisions about inmate mental health needs; (7) the screening at admission for mental health problems; (8) the provision of suicide watch; (9) the routine presence of mental health staff (especially during evenings and weekends when most suicides occur); (10) the availability of and speed with which emergency services can be obtained; and (11) the availability of alcohol and drug detoxification services (given the high incidence of substance abuse by suicides).

Descriptive Data*

Most jails in the sample were not crowded. Of the 78 jails for whom occupancy was computed, 34% were at 80% of total capacity; only 15% were over 100% of capacity. There were some differences between states. In Wisconsin, 70% of the jails were under 80% occupancy. New York and New Jersey had 16% and 18%, respectively, under 80% capacity. New Jersey had the most overcrowded jails with 82% at 100% capacity or more. This was in contrast to New York and Wisconsin at 21% and 5%, respectively, with more than 100% capacity. For the most part, the overcrowded New Jersey jails are those in the group that have been involved in major litigation with regard to conditions of confinement, in the Hudson River counties abutting or near New York City.

*Unless there were significant differences between states on the incidence of specific variables, data by state will not be presented. There were 79 jails in the survey sample; however, the number of cases will vary because not all respondents answered all questions. Therefore, pairwise treatment of variables will drop some cases from the analysis.

Table I. Rate of Turnover by Size of Jail

	Rate of turnover[a]				
Jail size	0–18	19–23	24–32	32 +	Row total
0–49	1(3)	13(34)	11(29)	13(34)	38(52)
50–99	6(38)	2(13)	5(31)	3(19)	16(22)
100–199	3(43)	3(43)	0(0)	1(14)	7(10)
200 +	8(67)	1(8)	2(17)	1(8)	12(16)
N(%)	18(25)	19(26)	18(25)	18(25)	73(100)

[a]Number of inmates per bed per year.

The jails differed in average size by state. New Jersey, a densely populated state, builds large jails; 81% are 100-bed capacity or larger. In contrast, 35% of New York jails and 30% of Wisconsin jails are 50 beds or smaller. Wisconsin and New Jersey each have only 5% of their jails with more than 100-bed capacity. It should be noted that New York and Wisconsin jails with regard to size, occupancy rates, and types of crime are more representative of most jails than New Jersey.

In all three states, the smaller jails had higher turnover rates.* Of those with capacity or 49 or less, 34% had a turnover rate of 32 or more inmates per bed per year. In contrast, most jails with a capacity of 100 or more had turnover rates of 18 or less (Table I).

Range of Mental Health Services

The three states differ in the provision of the eleven services measured in this study. New York, where sheriffs reported minimal (even hostile) relations with local mental health providers, is consistently below sample norms for service provision. Wisconsin, where the state mental health agency must provide services to jail inmates, offers the highest frequencies of services except for neuroleptic medications prescribed by a psychiatrist. New Jersey, where responsibility for service is unclear but with extensive experience with successful inmate litigation, closely follows Wisconsin in provision of services (Table II).

Most jails had routine arrangements for offering drug and alcohol counseling (usually volunteers), response to psychiatric emergencies (usually a referral out to a hospital), and drug and alcohol detoxification

*Data on average length of stay by legal status often is not maintained consistently by small jail administrators. So the turnover ratio was used (yearly admissions/average daily population).

Table II. Range of Mental Health Services by State

	Wisconsin		New York		New Jersey		Total	
Service	No	Yes	No	Yes	No	Yes	No	Yes
Emergency	6 (14)	37 (86)	16 (80)	4 (20)	2 (15)	11 (85)	24 (32)	52 (68)
Psychiatrist medicating	11 (26)	32 (74)	17 (85)	3 (15)	2 (15)	11 (85)	30 (39)	46 (61)
Routine MH presence	16 (37)	27 (63)	16 (80)	4 (20)	4 (31)	9 (69)	36 (47)	40 (53)
Admission screening	10 (23)	33 (77)	16 (80)	4 (20)	5 (38)	8 (62)	31 (41)	45 (59)
MH acute care unit	15 (35)	28 (63)	17 (85)	3 (15)	8 (62)	5 (38)	40 (53)	36 (47)
Drug detox	6 (14)	37 (86)	17 (85)	3 (15)	3 (23)	10 (77)	26 (34)	50 (66)
Alcohol detox	5 (12)	3 (88)	17 (85)	3 (15)	3 (23)	10 (77)	25 (33)	51 (67)
Drug/alcohol counselling	5 (12)	38 (88)	16 (80)	4 (20)	2 (15)	11 (85)	23 (30)	53 (70)
On-going counselling	9 (21)	32 (79)	16 (80)	4 (20)	3 (23)	10 (77)	28 (37)	48 (63)
DD/MR screening	17 (40)	26 (60)	17 (85)	3 (15)	7 (54)	6 (46)	43 (57)	33 (43)
Suicide watch	8 (19)	35 (81)	16 (80)	4 (20)	3 (23)	10 (77)	27 (36)	49 (64)
N(%)	43(100)		20(100)		13(100)		76(100)	

and suicide watch. What is interesting is *who* is providing these services (Table III). Jail deputies were the most frequent providers for emergency services (40%), suicide watch (64%), admission screening (58%), and screening for developmental disabilities (35%).

Suicide

There are no major differences between states in percentages of jails reporting suicides. In Wisconsin, each of five jails (12%) had one suicide; two New York jails (10%) reported one suicide; and two New Jersey jails (15%) each had one suicide.

With only 9 suicides reported by 79 jails, no conclusions can be drawn. Some data are interesting, however. Five of the nine suicides were in jails with 90% or lower occupancy rate (65% of the sample). No jail that had admission screening by mental health staff had suicides. Suicide watch was available in the jail for seven of the suicides; anecdotal

Table III. Mental Health Services Offered by Jail Deputies and Mental Health Workers[a]

Service	MH workers	Jail deputies	No service[c]
Emergency	23(29)[b]	31(40)	24(31)
Medication	33(42)	15(19)	30(38)
MH sick call	22(29)	20(26)	36(46)
MH screening	2(3)	45(58)	31(40)
Acute care	28(36)	10(13)	40(51)
Drug detox	34(44)	18(23)	26(33)
Alcohol detox	36(46)	17(22)	25(32)
D/A treatment	41(53)	14(18)	23(29)
MH treatment	41(53)	9(12)	28(36)
MR screening	8(10)	27(35)	43(55)
Suicide watch	1(1)	50(64)	27(35)

[a]$N = 78$.
[b]N(%).
[c]There were 60 jails with at least one service; 19 jails had no routine services.

data indicate that many of the victims were or had been on suicide watch. Eight jails with no weekend coverage had eight of the nine suicides reported in the survey. CO or inmate ratios did not seem to matter; seven of the victims were in jails with intermediate ranges of COs to inmates. Three of the suicides occurred in jails reporting no self-injuries. Eight of the suicides occurred in jails with from none to three incidents. The ninth suicide occurred at an intermediate size jail reporting four incidents of self-injury.

Self-Injury

Because of the difference in state policies for the monitoring of self-injury (the definition of self-injury and presence or absence of a requirement to report such incidents) self-injury rates by state cannot be compared.

Occupancy Rates, Jail Size, and Population Turnover

Of the 336 incidents of self-injury, 44% occurred in jails with occupancy rates of 100% or greater (23% of the sample). Jails with under 50-bed capacity (57% of the sample) represented 57% of the jails with incidents of self-injury; jails with under 100 beds had 72% of the incidents. Jails with 90% or less occupancy (65% of the sample) had 66% of the incidents (Table IV).

The data do not support the argument that large jails generate

Table IV. Rate of Self-Injury by Occupancy Rate

Occupancy rate	Self-injury rate[a] Low	Medium	High	Row total
0–80%	1(4)	12(48)	12(48)	25(50)
81–90%	2(25)	2(25)	4(50)	8(16)
91–100%	1(13)	3(38)	4(50)	8(16)
+ 100%	2(22)	3(33)	4(44)	9(8)
N(%)	16(23)	5(7)	48(70)	69(100)

[a]Low: 0–.087; medium: .088–.291; high: .292–7.5 per 100 yearly admissions.

more self-injury than small jails. Self-injury computed in a ratio to yearly total admissions seems equally distributed throughout a range of jail size.

It has been suggested that high inmate turnover stresses the ability of corrections staff to know and appropriately react to the needs of inmates. The data seems equally distributed throughout a range of jail size (Table V). Jails with low turnover (a rate of 0–23 inmates per bed per year or less) represented only 30 of those with high rates of self-injury; there was a slight overrepresentation of jails with high turnover rates and high rates of self-injury. Jails with high self-injury rates (59% of the sample) were 62 percent of those with high turnover rates (Table VI). Crudely put, perhaps getting out of jail quickly prevents more self-injury than remaining in jail so that correctional staff can be able to identify the potential self-injurer.

Inmate/Staff Ratio and Self-Injury

Jail administrators hold that staff/inmate ratios are a key factor in controlling inmate self-injury. The results of this survey do not appear to confirm or reject this opinion (Table VII). It is true that 50% of the

Table V. Rate of Self-Injury to Average Daily Population

Self-injury rate[a]	Jail size 0–49	50–99	100–199	200 +	Total jails
Low	6(38)	3(60)	12(32)	2(20)	23(33)
Medium	3(19)	2(40)	15(39)	3(30)	23(33)
High	7(44)	0	11(29)	5(50)	23(33)
N(%)	16(23)	5(7)	38(55)	10(14)	69(100)

[a]Low: 0 to .087 per 100; medium: .088 to .291 per 100; high: .292 to 7.5 per 100 yearly admissions.

Table VI. Rate of Self-Injury[a] and Rate of Turnover[b]

Turnover rate	Self-injury rate: Low	Medium	High	Row total
Low	1(4)	11(44)	13(21)	25(41)
High	5(14)	10(20)	21(50)	36(59)
N(%)	6(10)	21(34)	34(56)	61(100)

[a]Low: 0 to .087 per 100; medium: .088 to .291 per 100; high: .292 to 7.5 per 100 yearly admissions.
[b]Low: 0–23 inmates per bed per year; high: 24–32 + inmates per bed per year.

jails with the high CO/inmate ratio had the highest rate of self-injury. It is also true that 46% of the jails with the low CO/inmate ratio had the highest rate of self-injury.*

Mental Health Costs, Hours of Service, and Self-Injury

There were no significant differences by state. Of the 28 jails that offered a routine presence of mental health practitioners, 54% reported 12 minutes or less per inmate.

Smaller jails generally spent less per inmate on mental health service. However, costs for mental health service did not seem to be related to the incidence of self-injury. Of the 32 jails reporting incidents of self-injury as well as cost data, 47% spent nothing on mental health service.† Jails spending $50 per inmate per year or less represented 67% of jails reporting incidents (which were 60% of the respondents). Data describing numbers of incidents by cost of service per inmate are similar; 74% of the incidents occurred in jails with a per annum mental health budget of $50 per inmate or less (60% of the respondents).

Perhaps dollars per inmate is not a useful measure of service. However, when mental health hours per inmate is used, there still appears to be no relationship between level of mental health services and inmate self-injury. Jails with the lowest levels of mental health services (0–12 minutes per inmate per week) report 48% of the incidents and comprise 54% of jails reporting any incidents.

*This ratio was created by using average daily correctional staff employed and average daily population. It is an inflated figure because not all correctional staff are responsible for inmate supervision, and it does not take into account that average staff totals are deployed among three shifts.

†As discussed above, zero costs reported by jail administrators often mean that the costs for mental health services are not found in the jail budget. Information obtained from the 21 interviews suggests that where the local mental health agency *routinely* offers services to jail inmates rather than on an "as-needed" basis, the jail administrator has access to cost data and did report costs in the survey response. So "zero costs" may mean either no services or no routine service.

Table VII. Relationship of CO/Inmate Ratio to Rate of Self-Injury[a]

CO/inmate ratio[b]	Rate of self-injury Low	Medium	High	Row total
Low	3(12)	11(42)	12(46)	26(52)
High	3(13)	9(38)	12(50)	24(48)
N(%)	6(12)	20(40)	24(48)	50(100)

[a]Low: 0 to .087 per 100; medium: .088 to .291 per 100; high: .292 to 7.5 per 100 yearly admissions.
[b]Low: 0–2.5; high: 2.6–3.14 +.

Admission Screening, Weekend Coverage, Suicide Watch, and Psychiatric Hospitalization

There were major differences by state in the provision of a suicide-watch function. In Wisconsin jails, 81% reported the availability of suicide watch as compared to New York and New Jersey with 20% and 77%, respectively. Overall, 49% of all respondents offered this service.

Most jails did not provide weekend mental health coverage; 71 (91%) did not have mental health professionals routinely available on weekends. There were no significant differences by state.

Admission screening was offered by 44 (56%) of the 79 respondents. There were significant differences between the states surveyed. Of the Wisconsin respondents, 66% offered screening at admission for mental health problems; 7% of the New York respondents and 23% of the New Jersey respondents offered this service.

Jail administrators were asked to estimate the number of inmates who received treatment in a psychiatric hospital unit for more than 72 hours and those that they believed should receive hospitalization for longer than 72 hours. No major differences by state were observed. Most respondents (51%) agreed with the outcome of their referrals to psychiatric hospitals. However, a substantial number (38%) believed that too many inmates were kept for treatment (usually necessitating overtime costs for outposted correctional guarding). Only 11% felt that too few inmates were being admitted for treatment.

Admission screening does not seem to impact much on self-injury. There were 39 jails (51% of the total) with admission screening who reported 200 incidents (58% of the 345 total). It may be that screening is more useful in identifying the potential suicide, not the potential self-mutilator.

Weekend coverage by mental health staff may be linked to self-injury. Of the 52 respondents reporting on self-injury and weekend coverage, 90% (47 jails) did not provide this service. Forty-nine percent of these jails had high rates of self-injury, in contrast to 20% of the jails with weekend coverage.

The impact of suicide watch on self-injury is similarly unclear. The 29 (41%) jails without suicide watch had 117 (51%) of the 231 incidents. Eight jails had no incidents and no suicide watch; eleven jails had no incidents with suicide watch.

Jailers speak anecdotally of the inmate who "cuts up" or "hangs up" because the psychiatric hospital or psychiatric service refused to accept him over the jailer's better assessment of risk. The data here do not support this view. In fact, the converse appears to be true. Forty-six percent of the respondent who described self-injury and hospital referals reported that hospitals kept inmates *against* the jailer's assessment of no need for hospitalization. Of these jails, 53% had high rates of self-injury. This is in contrast to jails who had assessments that were consonant with that of the hospital (with regard to the need for hospitalization) or who reported the turnaround phenomenon (only 8%). These groups respectively contained 35% and 33% of jails with high rates of self-injury. Thus, it appears that not only does the turnaround phenomenon not occur, but that jailers may be critically underestimating the need for inmates to be hospitalized (Table VIII).

These results make sense if one assumes that the potential for suicide is a portion of the luggage the inmate brings to the jail, while the tendency toward repetitive self-injury is "jail behavior," not "street behavior." It seems that we are relatively skilled at identifying at admission the inmate who will attempt suicide. We know that suicide is a phenomenon that occurs soon after admission. It is not necessarily so with self-injury. Further, it has been suggested that jail conditions exacerbate or even generate psychological disturbance. The attitudes and behavior

Table VIII. Hospital Referrals and Rates of Self-Injury

	Self-injury rate[a]			
Referral outcome	Low	Medium	High	Row total
Held against jail assessment	1(6)	7(41)	9(53)	17(46)
Consonant assessments	2(12)	9(53)	6(35)	17(46)
Turnaround by hospital	1(33)	1(33)	1(33)	3(8)
Number of jails (%)	4(11)	17(46)	16(43)	37(100)

[a]Low: 0 to .087 per 100; medium: .088 to .291 per 100; high: .292 to 7.5 per 100 yearly admissions.

of correctional staff (not mental health staff) are powerful shapers of the jail ecology that affects inmates.[13(p153)] So the presence of mental health personnel for a brief period of time at admission (whether admission during the week or weekend) or the availability of psychiatric hospital services do little to prevent self-injury, if self-injury occurs because of conditions *in the jail.*

LITIGATION

Jail Size, Overcrowding, CO/Inmate Ratios, and Inmate Turnover

It can be said that litigation is a major tool for improving mental health services. It cannot necessarily be said that poor mental health services are a catalyst for litigation. Nor does it appear that overcrowding is associated with litigation in most jails. Of the 15 jails reporting litigation involving medical/mental health services and occupancy rates, six (40%) were over 100% occupancy. One other litigant was in the 90% to 100% occupancy range (Table IX).

Big jails get sued. Eleven jails with a 100-bed or more capacity constituted 73% of the litigants, though jails of this size were only 25% of the sample. *Big* overcrowded jails get sued more than *small* overcrowded jails.

Of the 15 (21% of the total) jails for which CO/inmate ratios were computed that were also involved in litigation, 8 (53%) had the lowest CO/inmate ratios. The intermediate and highest ratios had 4 (27%) and 7 (47%) cases, respectively. Thus, there may be some connection between incidence of litigation and CO/inmate ratios (Table X).

High inmate turnover does not seem to generate lawsuits. To the contrary, jails with the lowest rate (18 inmates per bed per year or less) had 40% (6) of the legal action, while jails with the highest rate of turnover (32 per bed per year) had 27% of the lawsuits reported (Table XI).

Table IX. Jail Occupancy Rates and Incidence of Litigation

Occupancy rate	Litigation: No	Litigation: Yes	Row total
0–80%	29(52)	5(33)	34(48)
81–90%	9(16)	3(20)	12(17)
91–100%	9(16)	1(7)	10(14)
+ 100%	9(16)	6(40)	15(21)
Number of jails (%)	56(79)	15(21)	71(100)

Table X. CO/Inmate Ratios and Litigation

CO/inmate ratio[a]	Litigation: No	Litigation: Yes	Total
Low	31(84)	6(16)	37(51)
High	26(74)	9(26)	35(49)
Number of jails (%)	57(79)	15(21)	72(100)

[a]Low: 0–2.5; high: 2.6–3.14 +.

Scope, Level of Effort, and Aegis of Mental Health Services

Nine jails had complete data for mental health costs and litigation; litigation was evenly distributed among the range of spending ($0–$181 or more per year per inmate). Mental health provider hours per inmate by incident of litigation (n = 6) were also uninstructive. No litigation was reported by jails without routine mental health coverage; the six cases were distributed evenly among jails with a range of mental health hours per inmate.

Twelve of the 44 jails in the sample that offer admission screening, report 70% of the litigation. Jails that offer suicide watch have similar patterns of litigation. Of the 17 jails reporting litigation, 12 had suicide watch. Perhaps suicide watch and admission screening are more a *post hoc* response to litigation than to inmate behavior or needs.

The presence of mental health staff on weekends may be a response rather than a deterrent to litigation. The 71 (91%) jails in the sample with no weekend coverage reported 14 (82%) cases of litigation.

Table XI. Inmate Turnover Rate by Incidents of Litigation

Turnover rate[a]	Litigation: No	Litigation: Yes	Total
−18	12(21)	6(40)	18(25)
+18 −23	17(29)	2(13)	19(26)
+23 −32	15(26)	3(20)	18(25)
+32	14(24)	4(27)	18(25)
Number of jails (%)	57(79.5)	15(20.5)	73(100)

[a]Number of inmates per bed per year.

Suicide, Self-Injury, and Litigation

It seems certain that the high incidence of suicide experienced in the late 1970s in large urban jails was a catalyst for the first wave of litigation against jail administrators. We have read of the suicides in the Tombs in New York, Allegheny County Jail in Pittsburgh, and in Harris County Jail in Houston. But that was then. The development of suicide watch and admission screening programs and the awareness of liability that followed these cases seem to have been effective in reducing the incidence of jail inmate suicides.

The minimal data on suicides obtained by this survey, data describing the circumstances of suicides reported in the surveys obtained from interviews (not reported here) and anecdotal material from the 21 sheriffs and jail administrators interviewed seem to indicate that litigation is not generated now by suicides for two reasons. First, we do not have shocking numbers of suicides. Second, self-injury, to those interviewed, seemed more shocking and related to the quality of jail services and management. Correctional and mental health professionals may be expressing the opinion of the public as well as their own in stating that suicide is somehow more understandable than self-injury because it is not entirely preventable (Table XII).

Of the 17 jails in the sample that were successfully sued by inmates, 13 furnished data describing incidence of self-injury among inmates. Jails with two or more incidents of self-injury are overrepresented among the 13 jails reporting litigation. This represents 92% of the litigation cases, but only 49% of the group with two or more incidents. One third of the jails with litigation had between two and five incidents of self-injury.

Table XII. Rate of Self-Injury and Litigation

	Litigation		
Rate of self-injury[a]	No	Yes	Row total
Low	4(10)	3(25)	7(13)
Medium	17(43)	4(33)	21(40)
High	19(48)	5(42)	24(46)
Number of jails (%)	40(77)	12(23)	52(100)

[a]Low: 0 to .087 per 100; medium: .088 to .291 per 100; high: .292 to 7.5 per 100 yearly admissions.

Table XIII. Aegis of Mental Health Provider and Incidence of Litigation

Mental health service	Aegis of provider	Litigation: No	Litigation: Yes	Row total
Emergency	None	24(39)	0	24(31)
	Jail staff	20(32)	11(69)	31(40)
	MH worker	18(29)	5(31)	23(29)
Routine mental health service	None	33(53)	3(19)	36(46)
	Jail staff	15(24)	5(31)	20(27)
	MH worker	14(23)	8(50)	22(28)
Mental health admission screening	None	30(48)	1(6)	31(40)
	Jail staff	31(50)	14(88)	45(58)
	MH worker	1(2)	1(6)	2(3)
Acute care	None	36(58)	4(25)	40(50)
	Jail staff	2(3)	8(50)	10(13)
	MH worker	24(39)	4(25)	28(36)
Drug detoxification	None	25(40)	1(6)	26(33)
	Jail staff	10(16)	8(50)	18(23)
	MH worker	27(44)	7(44)	34(44)
Alcohol detoxification	None	23(37)	2(13)	25(32)
	Jail staff	9(15)	8(50)	17(22)
	MH worker	30(48)	6(37)	36(46)
Number of jails (%)		62(79)	16(21)	78(100)

Aegis of Provider and Litigation

Jails that provide service via jailers seem to be involved disproportionately in litigation. For example, emergency mental health services were provided by jailers in 40% of the sample; this group had 69% of the cases of litigation. Jailers offered the admissions screening function in 58% of the sample; this subgroup had 88% of the litigation. This imbalance is also found with regard to jails where jailers offer the routine "mental health sick call," acute care, and drug and alcohol detoxification (Table XIII).

Summary of Findings

Jail size and staff to inmate ratios seem to have little relationship to the incidence of self-injury. There is some basis to believe that shorter lengths of incarceration generate fewer incidents of self-injury. Data for the relationship between occupancy rates, size, and self-injury suggest that very large, overcrowded jails and very small, underused jails may have higher rates of inmate self-injury. Given what we know about conditions in the largest jails and the picture of small jails partially delineated by this study, it would be *very small* and *very large* jails that would create the climate most likely to produce or exacerbate emotional instability among fragile inmates.

This study evaluates the impact of mental health professionals on inmate mental health morbidity rates, using crude ratios of service hours to number of inmates. One cannot assume that the maximum levels of service found in this study are adequate, nor can the assumption be made that the configuration of professional affiliation and the deployment of mental health staff are appropriate to the task. An additional caveat is that the number of jails giving reliable information detailing service hours is small (20), and there is considerable confusion raised by the "no service" or "no routine service (service as-needed)" issue.

Having hedged conclusions thoroughly, one may state that there is no reason to believe that mental health presence as indicated in total hours per inmate is associated with frequency of self-injury in the jails surveyed here. This may be due to the fact that the amount of mental health services per inmate are too minimal to impact on the problem. In specifics, however, there is reason to believe that weekend mental health coverage is a strategy for preventing self-injury. Of 52 jails reporting self-injury and coverage schedule data, 23 (96%) of those in the high-injury group were without weekend coverage.

With regard to the impact of external psychiatric hospital units, the "turnaround" factor is not associated with high self-injury rates. The converse of this appears to be a factor, however. The jails in which hospitals retained inmates whom correctional assessments would have returned comprise 56% of those reporting high-injury rates and hospitalization data. In other words, jailers, not psychiatric hospitals, may more probably underestimate the risk inmates present to themselves.

It is suggested, therefore, that the jail at risk for high levels of inmate self-injury comes in two versions: the small, underused jail with longer lengths of incarceration and no weekend mental health coverage; and the large, overpopulated jail with longer lengths of incarceration and no weekend coverage. Both of these jails may have policies that aim at avoiding the hospitalization of mentally ill inmates.

The jail at risk to be successfully sued, as delineated by this study, does not seem to be at variance with original expectations with the exception of the hypothesis that high incidence of self-injury would be associated with incidence of litigation. Self-injury itself does not seem to be associated positively with inmate litigation. Jails with high-injury rates were not more likely to end up in court than jails with low self-injury.

It is true that the study comes *after* the litigation for many of the respondents, who then altered the mental health service program. Jails, however, cannot alter their admissions/discharge ratios and usually not correctional staff/inmate ratios very much or very rapidly. These factors did not appear to generate high inmate self-injury rates as expected. However, many of these factors are associated positively with the incidence of litigation. Large, overpopulated jails are sued more frequently than small jails. Jails with high inmate/staff ratios get sued more often. This is not true for low turnover that, contrary to correctional lore, seems more likely to generate self-injury rates.

As mentioned above, it is difficult to know whether some types of mental health services are provided as a response to litigation or are generative of litigation. Anecdotal information obtained in interviews suggests that jail administrators of smaller jails have been unable to obtain mental health services from grudging local political leaders until the threat of litigation becomes vividly imminent. Thus, we suggest that association found here between admission screening, suicide watch, and weekend coverage (a slight overrepresentation among jails with litigation) and litigation occurs as a function of the postlitigation response. The lack of these services may have been a catalyst for litigation, and the provision of the services was part of the court-ordered compliance package.

There appears to be little ambiguity with regard to aegis of provider of mental health services and litigation. Jails that use jail deputies to provide mental health services get sued. Jails that offer service via mental health professionals get sued less. This situation helps to explain why sheriffs and jail administrators are so insistent that training in mental health issues and skills be part of any new mental health service package, but are sometimes loathe to receive training without augmented service by mental health professionals. Enhanced ability to recognize inmates with mental health emergencies means increased responsibility to get appropriate service to that inmate. Put another way, does one get sued quicker when totally ignorant about the mental health service needs of inmates, or more informed but with major gaps in the ability to provide service?

Some of the data appear to suggest that jails with no mental health service get sued least frequently. That may be explained by the common practice of "as-needed" coverage being reported as "no service" by survey respondents. This is most common in Wisconsin which is 56% of the sample, and the state that statutorily requires county mental health agencies to serve jail inmates. Thus, the incidence of an erroneous "no-service" response is most likely to occur in 56% of the responses, in jails that may be offering fuller coverage than jails that report routine service.

It is very clear that data from the survey and obtained in the interviews support the hypothesis that litigation is the catalyst for amendment of mental health services in jails. All jail administrators interviewed cited fear of litigation as the primary motivation for change and a belief that increased mental health service hours were necessary.

CONCLUSIONS

Jails face problems that prisons do not. They are the holding place for mentally ill/incompetent and medically at-risk defendants who will be diverted out of the criminal justice system. Small jails have problems that large jails do not. Local political leaders are loathe to fund programs for special inmates in jails so little used that they may at times be empty. Thus, small jails may suffer from political and fiscal invisibility.

This survey has attempted to document the lack of mental health services in jails, most of which have 50 beds or less. These holes in services to jail inmates will not be filled by jail deputies, even if the sheriffs could obtain training in mental health issues for them. Sheriffs who operate smaller jails report that a serious traffic accident in their counties can pull all jail deputies into the patrol function on the Friday, Saturday, and Sunday evenings that mental health and correctional people dread. These law enforcement emergencies are viewed as superseding the needs of jail inmates.

The data here suggest that attention should be focused not only on the huge jails of our great cities, but also on the smallest jails for which an adequate correctional officer complement and services for inmates are not "cost effective." Given certain conditions of confinement, the self-injurious inmate seems to be a constant percentage of inmate population. Incident by incident in the smaller jails, inmates are injuring themselves, but not in numbers great enough to trigger local concern and program improvement. Local officials cannot be expected to respond to the small number of incidents of suicide and self-injury that occur in small jails, even though the total comprises the majority of incidents nationwide.

Most of the larger jails in this sample are moving toward minimally acceptable service for the mentally ill offender. Their administrators and county officials know that to reject this road is to incur expensive judgments in court. They can pay now in expanded services or pay later in court costs. (Some have paid in both circumstances.) In many less populous counties, elected officials and county mental health administrators may not be receptive (if they are not actively hostile) to the idea of offering routine mental health service to jail inmates.

Sheriffs responsible for smaller jails report that local elected leaders considered jail inmates unworthy recipients of services, especially given the small numbers that require mental health programs. Local officials were perceived by jail administrators as unaware of the liability risk underservice poses. Many sheriffs interviewed described the "shoot-the-messenger" response to their attempts to educate county commissioners in this area. They feared that local elected officials would be angered by being forced to understand that substandard inmate services put the county at risk to successful inmate litigation. Thus, sheriffs wanted local leaders to become more sophisticated about the liability risks they faced, but they did not want to be the bearers of the bad news.

The lack of services documented here may not comfortably be attributed to indifference, deliberate or otherwise, on the part of local detention administrators. In less populous counties, many sheriffs lack the training, the clout, and the jargon necessary to obtain mental health service improvement unaided. Indeed, it appears that the inability to fluently speak mental health argot may be as great an obstacle as any other encountered. Most sheriffs come to their positions with substantial preparation in law enforcement. Consequently, they should feel at ease with most aspects of their role. Their preparation for the job, however, has generally not included mental health issues. Some are unfamiliar with mental health statutes. Thus, they may be forced to rely on unsympathetic local mental health providers for definition of what is minimal service to jail inmates. It is in this situation that the lack of "mental health speak" becomes problematic. For all that they fulminate about the lack of sensitivity of local mental health professionals to the plight of the inmate, some sheriffs feel at a disadvantage when disagreeing with mental health professionals in public forums. Thus, they are loathe to fight for broader mental health coverage for inmates.

The author has worked for many years at the juncture of the correctional and mental health systems. For her, the carefully maintained stereotypes of the overly idealistic mental health worker and the cloddish jail deputy are not amusing cartoons but serious impediments to reform. Several jails in the sample with more extensive programming were administered by sheriffs with prior and ongoing experience in mental health services. Their confidence in their knowledge of the field and the close working relationships they developed with local mental health leaders as a result of that confidence are clearly the foundation of the programs they develop and maintain in a nonsupportive political arena. This happy state may be considered serendipitous, however. It is unreasonable to await the election of law enforcement officials who are also mental health administrators as the solution to inadequate jail programs for the mentally ill.

Adequate services also were found in smaller jails when both sheriff and local mental health professionals had actively lobbied as a team rather than as combatants. Here the sheriff who wished to focus on law enforcement issues did not have to acquire knowledge of mental health issues as a weapon. Mental health officials accepted responsibility for treatment of the mentally ill inmate.

It may be that the existence of local mental health administrators who are eager to treat jail inmates is equally serendipitous. As has been stated earlier, the nature of many of these inmates is a hindrance to cooperation between jail and mental health workers. A substantial portion of jail inmates who require services are well known to mental health providers as some of the most difficult to treat and unattractive patients they see. That mental health workers strive to view them as correctional *inmates* rather than as *patients* is understandable though not acceptable. Correctional workers describe these inmates as "mental health problems"; mental health workers define them as "behavior management problems." Over the years, these few exasperating clients have generated enough friction to create and maintain the negative stereotypes described above.

This study was begun with a naïve hope that patterns of service could be revealed that are effective in preventing the exacerbation of jail inmates' emotional fragility and the resultants of suicide and self-injury. The data, depending on one's outlook, are either encouraging or downcasting. The good news is that (within the limits of the data) it appears that admission screening for emotional problems and suicide potential is efficacious. The routine presence of mental health professionals, especially on weekends is useful.

The bad news is that relationships with external mental health service providers—hospitals—does not seem connected to the incidence of self-injury. For the most part, referrals out to hospitals are accepted readily. Indeed, mental health facilities are more willing to keep and treat inmates than correctional professionals think is appropriate. So lack of treatment in external sites may not be the failing that causes the high incidence of suicide and self-injury in jails. We must look to what conditions exist in the jail to find the better way. This is not an avenue that will be welcomed by either correctional or mental health workers, neither of which want increased mental health presence in the jail.

This means that mental health care providers must *work in the jail* and that jailers must *keep their problems in the jail.** Thus, the most favored

*Not addressed is the obvious solution of diversion of the mentally ill from the criminal

strategy of moving the mentally ill inmate to another site and another agency's budget is not useful. And if one assumes that mental health workers and not jailers should be offering mental health services, this means that counties must fund new services and new positions. The interplay between the standard-setting, standard compliance-monitoring, and local service-provision agencies determines the pace and outcome of the process at the local level.

The three states studied serve as examples of various phases of this process. New Jersey detention administrators, with the sophistication gained in federal courts, do not speak much of state promulgated standards for service, though they have been developed. In New Jersey, the courts have developed standards for many counties and have affixed accountability for service without regard for the county's ability to pay. Sheriffs in New Jersey have learned from their colleagues that staying out of court means providing services. They do not have to convince local political leaders and mental health administrators; the courts have done so.

New York State is in the last stages of developing standards for mental health services to jail inmates. This work is the result of a collaboration between the state mental health agency and a free-standing agency with the single mission of monitoring and enforcing standards for institutional correctional services, state and local. What is not clear in New York is the responsibility at the local level for service delivery. Who is supposed to treat the inmate? Litigation or the fear of litigation is uppermost in the minds of New York sheriffs, but the state has not had New Jersey's history of litigation. Local political leaders still need to be convinced that lack of service is a liability risk, and sheriffs feel unable to educate them. Sheriffs are focusing on protection of themselves and personnel from liability in future or pending litigation, not on service reform. They are unable, as most have stated, to obtain the resources necessary to improve services.

Wisconsin has a tradition of providing excellent mental health services. There has been little litigation on conditions in local detention. Accountability for service delivery to jail inmates is statutorily assigned to local mental health agencies. However, no standards exist to define what that service should be. Hence, sheriffs faced with perilously inadequate mental health services find it difficult to obtain resources. They

---

justice system. Because the social climate currently supports the notion of incarceration no matter what the cost, I assume we will be dealing with increasing numbers of mentally ill in local detention for the perceivable future.

are told by local mental health leaders that service will be provided "as needed." Indeed, almost a third of Wisconsin jails surveyed had no services on a routine basis. Those that routinely offered programs did so via a quilt of multiple providers.

Adequate services do not come into being without the development of standards for those services. Standards are not implemented without accountability for monitoring that is affixed to an agency with sufficient resources to monitor. Such an agency cannot monitor unless the delegation of responsibility for local service provision is unambiguous. And, where local leadership is resistive to providing the service, litigation on the absence of the service is the igniter of reform.

Litigation, like most weapons, is most powerful when threatened but not used. And like most weapons, litigation may win a war but may also destroy much of the resources that were the object of the conflict. It also seems clear that to simply threaten sheriffs only serves to increase resistance to reform. A more creative brandishment of litigation would target sheriffs and mental health leaders as *partners* at risk. Thus, standards, programs initiated, and responsibility for monitoring would become a jointly designed outcome that could be sensitive to both local norms and resource capacity as well as to national standards. All the players necessary to craft the solution would be involved and invested in the process.

REFERENCES

1. American Correctional Association: *Standards for Adult Local Detention Facilities.* (Rockville, Md, American Correctional Assoc, 1985, pp 73–75.
2. Kerle KE, Rord FR: *The State of Our Nation's Jails.* Washington, DC, 1982.
3. Hoffa JR: The shame of our prisons: Forgotten americans—decaying health. [*sic*] Read before the 100th Annual Meeting of the American Public Health Association Atlantic City, NJ, Nov 13, 1972.
4. Rundle, F: Prisons: The crime of no treatment. *Psychiatric Opinion* 1974; 11.
5. Goldsmith SB: *Prison Health: Travesty of Justice.* New York, Prodist, 1975.
6. Michaels R: The right to refuse treatment: Ethical issues. *Hosp Community Psychiatry* 1981; 2.
7. Lee YS: Civil liability of state and local governments. *Public Administration Rev* 1987; 47.
8. Embert PS: Correctional law and jails: Evolution and implications for jail and lockup administrators and supervisors, in Kalinich DB, Klofas J (eds): *Sneaking Inmates Down the Alley.* Springfield, Ill, Charles C Thomas Publisher, 1986.
9. Liability costs rise in small towns. *Public Administration Times* 10.
10. Schafer NE: Jails and judicial review: Special problems for local facilities, in Kalinich DB, Klotas J (eds): *Sneaking Inmates Down the Alley.* Springfield, Ill, Charles C Thomas Publisher, 1986.

11. *Hamilton v Schiro,* 338 F. Supp. 1016 (E.D. La. 1970) (as an arbitrarily selected beginning of the litigation on conditions of confinement in jails).
12. Department of Health and Human Services: *Chapter 51: Wisconsin Mental Health Law.* Madison, Wi, Department of Health and Human Services, 1986.
13. Gibbs JJ: When donkeys fly: A Zen perspective on dealing with the problem of the mentally disturbed inmate, in Kalinich DB, Klofas J (eds): *Sneaking Inmates Down the Alley.*

Appendix: Mental Health Minimum Standards for New York City Correctional Facilities

The following mental health minimum standards are intended to improve the quality of mental health services delivered to inmates in New York City correctional facilities. These minimum standards shall apply to mental health services for all inmates in the care and custody of the New York City Department of Correction, except mental health services provided to inmates in the municipal hospital prison wards.

MENTAL HEALTH MINIMUM STANDARDS FOR NEW YORK CITY CORRECTIONAL FACILITIES

Part I - SERVICE GOALS

Section 1.1 *Service Goals*

Services for the detection, diagnosis and treatment of mental illness shall be provided to those persons in the care and custody of the New York City Department of Correction. The New York City Department of Health or a contracted service provider,* and the Department of Correction, with the approval of the Department of Mental Health, Mental Retardation and Alcoholism Services shall design and implement a mental health program to provide:

(a) crisis intervention and the management of acute psychiatric episodes;

(b) suicide prevention;

(c) stabilization of mental illness and the alleviation of psychological deterioration in the prison setting; and

(d) elective therapy services and preventive treatment where resources permit.

Part II - IDENTIFICATION AND DETECTION

Section
- 2.1 Policy
- 2.2 Receiving Screening
- 2.3 Training of Staff
- 2.4 Observation Aides

*Hereinafter referred to as the Department of Health

BOARD OF CORRECTION, CITY OF NEW YORK. Board Members: Peter Tufo, *Chair;* John R. Horan, *Vice-Chair;* Angelo Giordani; Wilbert Kirby; David Lenefsky, Esq.; Barbara Margolis; David A. Schulte; Rose M. Singer. Richard T. Wolf, *Executive Director.* John Rakis, *Deputy Executive Director.* Barbara E. Dunkel, *Counsel.* Elizabeth Armao, *Correctional Standards Review Specialist.* Joyce West, *Office Associate.*

Section 2.1 *Policy*

Procedures shall be developed and implemented which promote the timely identification of inmates requiring mental health evaluation.

Section 2.2 *Receiving Screening*

(a) Screening for mental and emotional disorders is to be performed on all inmates before they are placed in general population. This initial screening shall take place within twenty-four hours after an inmate's arrival at the correctional facility.

(b) Screening shall be performed by mental health services personnel or by appropriately trained medical personnel. Screening may be incorporated within the medical intake procedure.

(c) The Department of Health, with the approval of the Department of Mental Health, Mental Retardation and Alcoholism Services shall develop written procedures setting the topics to be reviewed in receiving screening. The review shall include, but need not be limited to: psychiatric history, including neuropsychiatric hospitalizations, contacts with mental health professionals, suicidal and violent behavior, history or presence of delusions or hallucinations, and an assessment based on behavioral observations of mood, orientation, impaired consciousness, indications of gross mental retardation and significant presenting complaints.

(d) The professionals conducting intake screening shall record their findings in a standard, written mental health intake form which the Department of Health shall develop with the approval of the Department of Mental Health, Mental Retardation and Alcoholism Services for use in all facilities.

(e) Receiving screening shall include a description of available mental health services and the procedures for access to those services:

(i) inmates shall receive a written communication in English and Spanish describing available mental health services, the confidentiality of those services and the procedures for gaining access to them;

(ii) the Department of Correction shall make provisions to assist in assuring that the procedures for gaining access to mental health services are verbally explained to illiterate inmates, and that inmates whose native language is other than English or Spanish are given prompt access to translation services for the explanation of these procedures.

Section 2.3 *Training of Staff*

(a) All correction officers and medical services personnel are to receive training and continuing education in programs approved by the Departments of Correction, Health and Mental Health, Mental Retardation and Alcoholism Services regarding the recognition of mental and emotional disorders. This training shall incorporate, but need not be limited to, the following areas:

(i) the recognition of signs and symptoms of mental and emotional disorders most frequently found in the inmate population;

(ii) the recognition of signs of chemical dependence and the symptoms of narcotic and alcohol withdrawal;

(iii) the recognition of adverse reactions to psychotropic medication;

(iv) the recognition of signs of developmental disability, particularly mental retardation;

(v) types of potential mental health emergencies, and how to approach inmates to intervene in these crises;

(vi) identification and referral of medical problems of mental health inmates;

(vii) suicide prevention; and

(viii) the appropriate channels for the immediate referral of an inmate to mental health services for further evaluation, and the procedures governing such referrals.

(b) No later than nine months from the effective date of these standards, there shall be at least one officer in every housing area on every tour trained in the application of basic first aid, including life support cardio-pulmonary resuscitation.

(c) Mental health services staff shall receive explicit orientation as well as continuing education and training appropriate to their activities:

(i) there shall be a written plan developed by the Department of Health and approved by the Department of Mental Health, Mental Retardation and Alcoholism Services for the orientation, continuing education and training of all mental health services staff;

(ii) in-service training shall include regular individual supervision of not less than one hour per week and not less than one hour per week of continuing education to be prorated for part-time staff.

Section 2.4 *Observation Aides*

(a) There is to be an organized program of observation aides trained to monitor those inmates identified as potential suicide risks as well as to recognize in those inmates not previously identified the warning signals of suicidal behavior. Inmates, including those housed in mental observation areas, may be employed as observation aides and shall be paid for their services.

(b) Written procedures shall be developed by the Departments of Correction and Health, to be approved by the Department of Mental Health, Mental Retardation and Alcoholism Services, defining the selection criteria for observation aides, the training they shall receive, the procedures they shall follow and the criteria for the evaluation of their performance as well as for terminating their employment where necessary:

(i) in developing a program of observation aides the Department of Correction shall consult with the Department of Health in order to provide for coordination of effort between the two agencies;

(ii) observation aides shall be trained to promptly inform correction or mental health services staff when they believe an inmate poses a suicide risk, presents an immediate danger of suicide or is engaging in bizarre behavior. This information shall be recorded in a systematic manner.

(c) Observation aides shall operate in all correctional facilities in the following housing areas: mental observation, punitive segregation, administrative segregation and new admission. They shall be employed in other areas as required.

Part III - DIAGNOSIS AND REFERRAL

Section 3.1 *Policy*

The Departments of Correction and Health, with the approval of the Department of Mental Health, Mental Retardation and Alcoholism Services, shall develop procedures to provide for the prompt evaluation and appropriate referral of inmates whose behavior suggests that they are suffering from a mental or emotional disorder, as well as the immediate evaluation and treatment of those in need of emergency psychiatric care.

Section 3.2 *Access*

(a) There is to be non-emergency access to mental health services. Inmates may refer themselves for preliminary evaluation, and they shall be seen by a member of mental health services staff as soon as possible but in no instance later than three working days after receipt of referral by mental health services staff. The Department of Correction shall ensure that notice of the request is received by mental health services staff within twenty-four hours.

(b) Inmates shall have twenty-four hour access to mental health services personnel for emergency psychiatric care and the management of acute psychiatric episodes:

(i) all inmates who report having been sexually assaulted shall be referred for emergency assessment;

(ii) inmates awaiting emergency evaluation are to be housed in a specially designated area with close staff supervision and sufficient security to protect inmates and staff;

(iii) the Departments of Correction and Health shall develop a written form for emergency evaluation referrals.

(c) Correction staff and medical services personnel are required to refer to mental health services those inmates in the general population who exhibit signs of mental or emotional disorders. A standard written procedure to include a description of the behavior upon which the referral is based shall be developed by the Departments of Health and Correction.

(d) The Department of Correction shall provide sufficient escort officers to ensure delivery of service in a manner that promotes the maximum efficiency of mental health services staff. The Department of Correction shall develop and implement procedures to provide that inmates requested for evaluation or follow-up be escorted to mental health services staff, or accounted for, the same day. In all cases where the inmate is still in custody, he or she shall be brought to mental health services staff within twenty-four hours.

Part IV - TREATMENT

Section 4.1 *Policy*

Adequate mental health care is to be provided to inmates in an environment which facilitates care and treatment, provides for maximum observation, reduces the risk of suicide, and is minimally stressful. Inmates under the care of mental health services, if in all other respects qualified and eligible shall be entitled to the same rights and privileges as every other inmate.

Section 4.2 *Criteria of Adequacy*

(a) The Department of Health shall develop written criteria to be approved by the Department of Mental Health, Mental Retardation and Alcoholism Services defining in accordance with current professional standards the mental health staff, supplies and equipment necessary to provide adequate mental health care.

(b) The Departments of Health and Correction shall develop written criteria to be approved by the Department of Mental Health, Mental Retardation and Alcoholism Services defining in accordance with current professional standards the space necessary to provide adequate and appropriate housing and treatment of inmates under the care of mental health services.

(c) No later than ninety days from the effective date of these standards, the written criteria shall be submitted to the Board of Correction for promulgation as an amendment to these standards.

Section 4.3 *Programs*

(a) Special housing shall be provided to those inmates in need of close supervision due to mental or emotional disorders, and to those inmates in the process of being evaluated for such disorders:

(i) twenty-four hour observation aides shall be assigned to special housing areas;

(ii) correction officers who have received not less than thirty-five hours of special training within the first year of their assignment shall be assigned to steady posts within these areas. These officers shall receive annual training enhancement. The Departments of Health and Correction shall develop a written curriculum to be approved by the Department of Mental Health, Mental Retardation and Alcoholism Services specifying the components and hours of the training programs;

(iii) inmates placed in special housing areas shall be seen and interviewed by mental health services staff at least once per week;

(iv) an individual member of mental health services staff shall be directly responsible for mental health services in each special housing area;

(v) the Department of Correction shall make provision for the allocation of dormitory space as special housing for the observation of potentially suicidal inmates.

(b) The Departments of Correction and Health shall develop specific written criteria and procedures for the admission to and the discharge from special housing areas for mental observation:

(i) it shall be the prerogative of mental health services to admit and discharge inmates from special housing areas for mental observation;

(ii) the placement of an inmate in special housing shall be reviewed by mental health services at least once per week.

(c) An individualized written treatment plan based upon the evaluation of the treatment team shall be developed for each inmate placed in special housing for mental observation and for all inmates to whom medication for mental or emotional disorders is prescribed:

(i) the treatment team must include a psychiatrist who shall personally examine each inmate evaluated by the treament team;

(ii) those members of the treatment team who are providing care to an inmate shall prepare a treatment plan, which shall be signed by the psychiatrist;

(iii) the Chief of Service or his or her designee shall approve all treatment plans;

(iv) the Department of Health shall develop written criteria to be approved by the Department of Mental Health, Mental Retardation and Alcoholism Services defining the nature and the specificity of the treatment plan;

(v) there shall be documented evidence of initial treatment planning within three days of the inmate being placed in special housing, and a treatment plan shall be prepared no later than one week after placement;

(vi) treatment plans shall be reviewed and assessed for effectiveness by professional mental health services staff at least every two weeks. Both the review and the inmate's progress shall be recorded in the medical chart;

(vii) a range of treatment modalities other than the provision of medication shall be made available.

(d) There shall be facilities appropriate for the observation, evaluation and treatment of acute psychiatric episodes.

(e) Where required, an inmate shall be transferred to a municipal hospital prison ward in accordance with New York State Correction Law Sections 402 and 508.

(f) Inmates identified as developmentally disabled shall be evaluated within seventy-two hours and mental health services staff shall make a recommendation to the Department of Correction as to whether such developmental disability makes it necessary for the inmate to be placed in special housing or otherwise separated from the general inmate population:

(i) inmates who suffer from developmental disabilities shall be housed in areas sufficient to ensure their safety;

(ii) if it is determined by mental health services that an inmate's developmental disability makes it clinically contraindicated that the inmate be housed in a correctional facility, then the Department of Correction shall immediately notify the court and a written notice shall be filed in the inmate's court papers.

(g) The Departments of Health and Correction shall use mechanisms approved by the Department of Mental Health, Mental Retardation and Alcoholism Services to identify inmates who are suffering from drug addiction or the disease of alcoholism. Inmates so identified shall be referred to available programs approved by the Departments of Correction and Health. Detoxification shall take place in a setting appropriate to the level of care required.

Section 4.4 *Informed Consent*

Except as otherwise provided herein, mental health treatment may be administered only upon the informed consent of the inmate after a disclosure of the risks and benefits of the proposed treatment in accordance with good clinical practice. The Departments of Health and Mental Health, Mental Retardation and Alcoholism Services shall develop procedures for the implementation of this section, which shall include the use of a written form to document the informed consent of the inmate.

Section 4.5 *Right to Refuse Treatment*

The city may not require treatment of an inmate without the inmate's consent unless, in an emergency, that person, by reason of mental disability or mental illness, poses a clear and present danger of serious physical injury to self or others. Then and only then may an inmate by examined, treated or medicated against the inmate's will, subject to the following conditions:

(a) the attending physician shall use only those measures which in his or her best professional judgment are deemed appropriate in response to the emergency;

(b) these measures may be used only with a written medical order;

(c) these measures may be used only with adequate explanation in the inmate's chart by the physician responsible detailing the length of the period of observation, the inmate's condition, the threat the inmate poses and the specific reasons for the specific intervention proposed;

(d) no order to treat an inmate against the inmate's will shall be valid for longer than twenty-four hours, without review and renewal and appropriate notation in the inmate's medical records;

(e) the Departments of Correction and Health shall develop procedures to be approved by the Department of Mental Health, Mental Retardation and Alcoholism Services for the implementation of this section, including the use of a written form to document an inmate's refusal to consent to a particular examination, procedure or medication.

Part V - MEDICATION

Section
5.1 Policy
5.2 Procedures
5.3 Pharmacy
5.4 Research

Section 5.1 *Policy*

Medication shall not be used solely as a method of restraint or means of control, but only as one facet of a treatment plan (as defined in Section 4.3(c)).

Section 5.2 *Procedures*

(a) The Department of Health, with the approval of the Department of Mental Health, Mental Retardation and Alcoholism Services shall develop and implement procedures governing the prescription, dispensing, administration and review of medication:

(i) medication for mental and emotional disorders is to be prescribed only by a psychiatrist, except in an emergency when a physician other than a psychiatrist may prescribe medication for mental and emotional disorders. Such a prescription must be reviewed by a psychiatrist within twenty-four hours;

(ii) except in an emergency, medication for mental and emotional disorders may not be prescribed to an inmate unless that inmate has had a physical examination including a detailed clinical history within the previous six months; in all cases the prescribing physician must first review the medical chart and all other medicine the inmate is receiving;

(iii) medication is to be administered only by appropriately trained medical or health services personnel.

(b) Psychotropic medication shall be dispensed only when clinically indicated, consistent with the treatment plan:

(i) all prescriptions for psychotropic medication must include a stop order; no prescription for psychotropic medication shall be valid for longer than two weeks;

(ii) every inmate receiving psychotropic medication shall be seen and evaluated by the prescribing psychiatrist, or, in cases of emergency when a physician other than a psychiatrist prescribes medication under Section 5.2 (a)(i), by the reviewing psychiatrist, at least once a week until stabilized and thereafter at least every two weeks by medical personnel;

(iii) female inmates who are prescribed psychotropic medication shall be informed of the potential risk of taking such drugs while pregnant and shall be given the opportunity to be tested for pregnancy.

Section 5.3 *Pharmacy*

(a) When stock medications are maintained within a correctional facility, the agency providing medical services shall develop and maintain a formulary of medications stored in that facility.

(b) The Departments of Health and Correction shall develop and implement a written policy to provide for the maximum security storage and weekly inventory of all controlled substances, syringes, needles and surgical instruments:

(i) "controlled substances" are defined as those so listed by the Drug Enforcement Administration of the United States Department of Justice;

(ii) written notice of this policy shall be given to all staff with potential access to any controlled substances or items under maximum security storage.

Section 5.4 *Research*

Biomedical or behavioral research involving any inmate in the custody of the New York City Department of Correction is prohibited, except insofar as it meets the requirements for approval of research which is subject to the Department of Health and Human Services' regulations, and in addition, has the approval of the Department of Mental Health, Mental Retardation and Alcoholism Services.

Part VI - RESTRAINTS AND SECLUSION

Section
6.1 Policy
6.2 Definitions
6.3 Procedures

Section 6.1 *Policy*

The Departments of Correction and Health shall develop and implement procedures subject to the review of the Department of Mental Health, Mental Retardation and Alcoholism Services governing the physical restraint and seclusion of inmates being observed or treated for mental or emotional disorders.

Consistent with the New York State Mental Hygiene Law restraints or seclusion shall not be used as punishment, for the convenience of staff, or as a substitute for treatment programs.

Section 6.2 *Definitions*

(a) Seclusion is the placing of inmates in their cells, or a seclusion room from which they cannot leave at will, during a normal lock-out period when other inmates in the housing area are given the option to lock out of their cells:

(i) seclusion shall be used only if the cells or seclusion rooms available allow adequate observation of the inmate by staff;

(ii) nothing in this Part shall restrict the ability of the Department of Correction to limit the lock-out rights of inmates for disciplinary purposes (punitive segregation).

(b) Physical restraint is the deliberate use of a device to interfere with the free movement of an inmate's arms and/or legs, or which totally immobilizes the inmate, and which the inmate is unable to remove without assistance:

(i) the Departments of Health and Mental Health, Mental Retardation and Alcoholism Services shall develop procedures defining permissible forms of physical restraints;

(ii) in no instance shall metal handcuffs be used to restrain an inmate; however, this proscription shall not preclude the application of appropriate security precautions during the transportation of inmates;

(iii) in an emergency, when an inmate presents a clear and present danger to himself or others, the inmate may be restrained, including with metal handcuffs, pending the arrival of a psychiatrist. Correction personnel shall immediately notify the mental health staff for response. The psychiatrist shall respond immediately, but in no event more than one hour after notification. When there is no institutional psychiatrist on duty, correction personnel shall immediately transport the inmate to a facility where a psychiatrist is present.

Section 6.3 *Procedures*

(a) The use of physical restraint or seclusion of inmates being observed or treated for mental or emotional disorders shall be permitted only where there is on-duty psychiatric coverage.

(b) Physical restraint or seclusion may be used only upon the direct written order of a psychiatrist which includes the reasons for taking such action.

(c) Physical restraint or seclusion shall be used only when the psychiatrist has examined the inmate and determined in light of all available mental health data that:

(i) the inmate presents an immediate danger of injury to self or others;

(ii) this potential for violence is the result of a mental health disorder for which the inmate is receiving treatment;

(iii) these measures are absolutely necessary to avert the danger and will be therapeutically beneficial; and

(iv) all other available alternatives are ineffective in preventing injury.

(d) An inmate put in restraints or seclusion shall be kept under constant observation and the need for continued restrictive measures shall be assessed by nursing or mental health staff:

(i) use of restraints shall be assessed every fifteen minutes and seclusion shall be reviewed every thirty minutes;

(ii) written findings of such reviews shall be noted on the inmate's medical chart;

(iii) vital signs (temperature, pulse, blood pressure and respiration) shall be recorded every hour.

(e) An inmate subjected to restraints or seclusion shall be released every two hours and given the opportunity to go to the toilet.

(f) A psychiatrist shall evaluate an inmate in restraints or seclusion at least once every two hours to determine whether continued restrictive measures are warranted.

(g) No order to place an inmate in restraints or seclusion shall be valid longer than two hours, and such an order shall be renewable only once, by a psychiatrist after evaluation of the inmate's condition.

(h) After four hours, if an inmate remains too agitated to be released, the inmate shall be moved to a municipal hospital prison ward.

Part VII - CONFIDENTIALITY

Section
7.1 Policy
7.2 Sharing of Information
7.3 Records

Section 7.1 *Policy*

The principle of confidentiality of information obtained in the course of treatment is to be upheld. The Departments of Correction and Health, with the approval of the Department of Mental Health, Mental Retardation and Alcoholism Services shall develop and implement a written policy governing the dissemination of information.

Section 7.2 *Sharing of Information*

(a) Mental health services shall promptly inform correction personnel when an inmate is identified as:

(i) suicidal;

(ii) homicidal;

(iii) posing a clear danger of injury to self or to others;

(iv) presenting a clear and immediate risk of escape or riot;

(v) receiving psychotropic medication; or
(vi) requiring transfer for mental health reasons.

(b) The Departments of Correction and Health shall develop and implement an explicit written procedure specifying which correction personnel are to be notified of information as described in Section 7.2(a) above, and the method of notification.

Section 7.3 *Records*

(a) Mental health records are to be maintained separately from the confinement record and kept in a secure file. Each significant inmate contact shall be reflected by a substantive progress note on the chart.

(b) Mental health records are to be transferred with an inmate when the inmate is transferred from one facility to another within the New York City Department of Correction. A record summary shall accompany each inmate transferred to a municipal hospital prison ward. When a request is received to transfer mental health records outside the jurisdiction of the Department of Correction, written authorization of the inmate is required unless otherwise provided by law.

Part VIII - COORDINATION

Section
8.1 Policy
8.2 Discipline
8.3 Meetings
8.4 Evaluation

Section 8.1 *Policy*

The Departments of Correction and Health shall consult and coordinate their activities on a regular basis in order to provide for the continued delivery of quality mental health care.

Section 8.2 *Discipline*

(a) The Departments of Health and Correction shall develop written procedures to provide for mental health services to be informed whenever an inmate in a special housing area for mental observation is charged with an infraction, and to be permitted to participate in the infraction hearing and to review any punitive measures to be taken.

(b) Any inmate to be placed in punitive segregation who has a history of mental or emotional disorders shall be seen by mental health services staff before being moved to punitive segregation. All inmates in punitive segregation shall be seen at least once each day by medical staff who shall make referrals to mental health services where appropriate.

Section 8.3 *Meetings*

Monthly meetings including the facility administrator, the chief representative of mental health services to that facility and representatives of the medical and nursing staff shall be held to discuss the delivery of mental health services. Meetings shall include a written agenda as well as the taking and distribution of minutes.

Section 8.4 *Evaluation*

The Department of Mental Health, Mental Retardation and Alcoholism Services shall annually conduct a formal evaluation of the quality, effectiveness and level of performance of mental health services provided to inmates in New York City correctional facilities.

Part IX - VARIANCES

Section
9.1 Policy
9.2 Variance Prior to Implementation Date
9.3 Variance Application
9.4 Variance Procedure
9.5 Granting of Variance
9.6 Renewal of Variance
9.7 Emergency Variance After Implementation Date
9.8 Emergency Variance Application
9.9 Granting of Emergency Variance

Section 9.1 *Policy*

Any Department affected by these minimum standards may apply for a variance from a specific Section or Part of these standards when compliance cannot be achieved or continued. A "variance" is an exemption granted by the Board from full compliance with a particular Section or Part for a specified period of time.

Section 9.2 *Variance Prior to Implementation Date*

A Department may apply to the Board for a variance prior to the implementation date of a particular Section or Part when:

(a) despite its best efforts and the best efforts of other New York City officials and agencies, full compliance with the Section or Part cannot be achieved by the implementation date; or

(b) compliance is to be achieved in a manner other than specified in the Section or Part.

Section 9.3 *Variance Application*

An application for a variance must be made in writing to the Board by the Commissioner of the Department at least forty-five days prior to the implementation date and shall state:

(a) the particular Section or Part at issue;

(b) the efforts undertaken by the Department to achieve compliance by the implementation date;
(c) the specific facts or reasons making full compliance by the implementation date impossible;
(d) the specific plans, projections and timetables for achieving full compliance;
(e) the specific plans for serving the purpose of the Section or Part for the period that strict compliance is not possible; and
(f) the time period for which the variance is requested, provided that this shall be no more than six months.

Section 9.4 *Variance Procedure*

(a) Prior to a decision on a variance application, the Board shall consider the positions of all interested parties.

(b) In order to receive this input the Board shall publicize the variance application in its entirety in a manner reasonably calculated to reach all interested parties, including direct mail. This shall occur at least thirty days prior to the implementation date of the Section or Part.

(c) The Board shall hold a public meeting or hearing on the variance application and hear testimony from all interested parties at least twenty-one days prior to the implementation date.

(d) The Board's decision on a variance application shall be in writing and shall include the specific facts and reasons underlying the decision.

(e) The Board's decision shall be publicized in the manner provided by Section 9.4(b) at least ten days prior to the implementation date.

Section 9.5 *Granting of Variance*

(a) The Board shall grant a variance only if it is convinced that the variance is necessary and justified.
(b) Upon granting a variance, the Board shall state:
(i) the time period of the variance; and
(ii) any requirements imposed as conditions on the variance.

Section 9.6 *Renewal of Variance*

An application for a renewal of a variance shall be treated in the same manner as an original application as provided in Sections 9.2, 9.3, 9.4 and 9.5. The Board shall not grant renewal of a variance unless it finds that, in addition to the requirements for approving an original application, a good faith effort has been made to comply with the Section or Part within the previously prescribed time limitation.

Section 9.7 *Emergency Variance After Implementation Date*

A Department may apply to the Board for a variance after the implementation date of a particular Section or Part when an emergency prevents continued compliance with the Section or Part.

Section 9.8 *Emergency Variance Application*

(a) A variance for a period of less than twenty-four hours may be declared by the Department or a designee when an emergency prevents continued compliance with a particular Section or Part. The Board or a designee shall be immediately notified of the emergency and the variance.

(b) An application for an emergency variance for a period of twenty-four hours or more, or for a renewal of an emergency variance, must be made by the Commissioner of the Department or a designee to the Board and shall state:
(i) the particular Section or Part at issue;
(ii) the specific facts or reasons making continued compliance impossible;
(iii) the specific plans, projections and timetables for achieving full compliance; and
(iv) the time period for which the variance is requested, provided that this shall be no more than five days.

Section 9.9 *Granting of Emergency Variance*

(a) The Board shall grant an emergency variance only if it is convinced that the variance is necessary and justified.

(b) A renewal of an emergency variance previously granted by the Board may be granted only if the requirements of Sections 9.7, 9.8(b) and 9.9(a) have been met.

(c) The Board shall not grant more than two consecutive renewals of an emergency variance.

Part X - EFFECTIVE DATE

Section 10.1
These standards (Parts I through IX) shall take effect February 1, 1985.

Part XI - IMPLEMENTATION DATES

The policies, procedures, criteria, plans, programs and forms required by the various sections of these standards shall be developed, approved and implemented within the time periods stated below. All time periods are computed from the effective date of these standards (see Part X).

Section	Development and Approval	Implementation
2.2 a-e	4 months	4 months
2.3 a	Not applicable (N/A)	8 "
2.3 b	9 months	9 "
2.3 c (i)	9 "	N/A
2.3 c (ii)	N/A	10 months
2.4 a, b and c	4 months	4 "

3.1	2 "	2 "
3.2 a	8 "	8 "
3.2 b (i) and (iii)	2 "	2 "
3.2 c	2 "	2 "
3.2 d	2 "	6 "
4.2 a	3 "	N/A
4.2 b	3 "	3 months
4.3 a (i)	2 "	2 "
4.3 a (ii)	2 "	N/A
4.3 a (iii)	8 "	8 months
4.3 a (iv)	5 "	5 "
4.3 a (v)	5 "	N/A
4.3 b (i) and (ii)	2 "	8 months
4.3 c (i), (ii) and (iii)	8 "	8 "
4.3 c (iv)	6 "	8 "
4.3 c (v), (vi) and (vii)	N/A	8 "
4.3 e	N/A	2 "
4.3 f	N/A	8 "
4.3 f (i) and (ii)	2 months	N/A
4.3 g	6 "	7 months
4.4	2 "	N/A
4.5 a-e	4 "	5 months
5.1	1 month	1 month
5.2 a (i) and (ii)	7 months	8 months
5.2 a (iii)	1 month	1 month
5.2 b (i)	1 "	1 "
5.2 b (ii)	7 months	8 months
5.2 b (iii)	1 month	1 month
5.3 a and b	1 "	1 "
5.4	1 "	1 "
6.1	3 months	4 months
6.2 b (i)	3 "	4 "
6.2 b (ii) and (iii)	1 month	1 month
6.3 a-h	1 "	1 "
7.1	3 months	3 months
7.2 a and b	2 "	2 "
7.3 a and b	2 "	2 "
8.2 a and b	1 month	1 month
8.3	1 "	1 "
8.4	1 "	1 "

Dated: December 21, 1984
New York, New York

Peter Tufo
Chair

Index